AF668672

Exam Preparatory Manual for Undergraduates

# Complete Dentures

## Exam Preparatory Manual for Undergraduates

# Complete Dentures

**Lovely M**
MDS (Prosth) DNB (Prosth) PhD
Professor
Department of Prosthodontics
Sree Mookambika Institute of Dental Sciences
Kulashekharam, Tamil Nadu, India

*Foreword*
**K Chandrasekharan Nair**

JAYPEE *The Health Sciences Publisher*
New Delhi | London | Philadelphia | Panama

**Jaypee Brothers Medical Publishers (P) Ltd**

**Headquarters**

Jaypee Brothers Medical Publishers (P) Ltd
4838/24, Ansari Road, Daryaganj
New Delhi 110 002, India
Phone: +91-11-43574357
Fax: +91-11-43574314
Email: jaypee@jaypeebrothers.com

**Overseas Offices**

J.P. Medical Ltd
83, Victoria Street, London
SW1H 0HW (UK)
Phone: +44 20 3170 8910
Fax: +44(0)20 3008 6180
Email: info@jpmedpub.com

Jaypee-Highlights Medical Publishers Inc.
City of Knowledge, Bld. 235, 2nd Floor, Clayton
Panama City, Panama
Phone: +1 507-301-0496
Fax: +1 507-301-0499
Email: cservice@jphmedical.com

Jaypee Medical Inc
325 Chestnut Street
Suite 412, Philadelphia, PA 19106, USA
Phone: +1 267-519-9789
Email: support@jpmedus.com

Jaypee Brothers Medical Publishers (P) Ltd
17/1-B Babar Road, Block-B, Shaymali
Mohammadpur, Dhaka-1207
Bangladesh
Mobile: +08801912003485
Email: jaypeedhaka@gmail.com

Jaypee Brothers Medical Publishers (P) Ltd
Bhotahity, Kathmandu, Nepal
Phone: +977-9741283608
Email: kathmandu@jaypeebrothers.com

Website: www.jaypeebrothers.com
Website: www.jaypeedigital.com

© 2016, Jaypee Brothers Medical Publishers

The views and opinions expressed in this book are solely those of the original contributor(s)/author(s) and do not necessarily represent those of editor(s) of the book.

All rights reserved. No part of this publication may be reproduced, stored or transmitted in any form or by any means, electronic, mechanical, photocopying, recording or otherwise, without the prior permission in writing of the publishers and the author.

All brand names and product names used in this book are trade names, service marks, trademarks or registered trademarks of their respective owners. The publisher and author are not associated with any product or vendor mentioned in this book.

Medical knowledge and practice change constantly. This book is designed to provide accurate, authoritative information about the subject matter in question. However, readers are advised to check the most current information available on procedures included and check information from the manufacturer of each product to be administered, to verify the recommended dose, formula, method and duration of administration, adverse effects and contraindications. It is the responsibility of the practitioner to take all appropriate safety precautions. Neither the publisher nor the author(s)/editor(s) assume any liability for any injury and/or damage to persons or property arising from or related to use of material in this book.

This book is sold on the understanding that the publisher is not engaged in providing professional medical services. If such advice or services are required, the services of a competent medical professional should be sought.

Every effort has been made where necessary to contact holders of copyright to obtain permission to reproduce copyright material. If any have been inadvertently overlooked, the publisher will be pleased to make the necessary arrangements at the first opportunity.

**Inquiries for bulk sales may be solicited at:** jaypee@jaypeebrothers.com

***Exam Preparatory Manual for Undergraduates: Complete Dentures***

*First Edition*: **2016,** Reprint: 2023

ISBN 978-93-86107-98-5

*Printed in India*

**Dedicated to**

*My dear husband Dr Biji Thomas George*
*&*
*My son Joshua*

# Contributors

**Anuroopa A** MDS
Reader
Sree Mookambika Institute of Dental Sciences
Kulashekharam, Tamil Nadu, India

**Kavitha Janardanan** MDS
Reader
Sree Mookambika Institute of Dental Sciences
Kulashekharam, Tamil Nadu, India

**Sangeeth K Cherian** MDS
Reader
Sree Mookambika Institute of Dental Sciences
Kulashekharam, Tamil Nadu, India

**Sudheer Arunachalam** MDS
Reader
Sree Mookambika Institute of Dental Sciences
Kulashekharam, Tamil Nadu, India

**Vini Varkey** MDS
Senior Lecturer
Sree Mookambika Institute of Dental Sciences
Kulashekharam, Tamil Nadu , India

# Foreword

*Exam Preparatory Manual for Undergraduates: Complete Dentures* by Dr Lovely M is an updated version of the *Review of Complete Dentures* that has emerged into a complete new title within a short span of seven years. Any branch of science will progress tremendously within this period. Dentistry has followed suit. But the science of complete dentures per se has not shown a voluminous change especially when we review the literature, but an intelligent integration with dental implantology has happened. In the clinical front, prosthodontists have started revalidating the unchallenged wisdom of many of the clinical practices. Advanced diagnostic tools like cone-beam CT has emboldened the intellectual and critical stand of the practitioners—may be the future of complete denture practice will have more factual foundations than logical assumptions!

Dr Lovely has recognized these facts and broadened the scope of her book. Usefulness of this title has merged the borders of undergraduate and postgraduate education. Question-answer format was not initially accepted by many teachers stating that students will refrain from reading textbooks. A brief market survey reveals the fact that this is the most successful model amongst the students. The review type books ensure that the students know the essentials of the subject. Ultimately, what do the teachers want? The student should learn the basics of the subject. In that respect, Dr Lovely has fulfilled her mission in making the students learn the subject.

**K Chandrasekharan Nair**
Professor
Department of Prosthodontics
AECS Maaruti College of Dental Sciences
Bengaluru, Karnataka, India

# Preface

*Exam Preparatory Manual for Undergraduates: Complete Denture* is primarily designed to be a quick revision tool just before the examinations for the Final Year BDS students as well as the postgraduates. Due to the good response from students and feedback received from the *Review of Complete Dentures* (the Mother Edition), it was decided to include viva, synopsis and recent advances in short to benefit the postgraduates also. However, I hope that this book will also be useful for practising dentists and a quick reference for anyone seeking to find answers for questions. I have put in great efforts to incorporate the best from all the standard textbooks in complete dentures in the writing of this book.

It is not, however, a replacement for textbooks, and students are expected to have gone through the textbooks during their study period. This will help them to grasp the concepts in this review better. The last ten years' question papers from all major universities in India have been collected and the solutions to almost all essay and short note questions have been included.

Such a venture could not have been possible without the help of many people. First of all I thank God, for enabling me to complete this book. I especially thank to Prof K Chandrasekharan Nair, for his invaluable help and time in going through and correcting the proofs of this review and also for writing a foreword and the section on tips for students on how to write the university examinations. Thanks are due to my many friends and colleagues all over India who sent me question papers from their universities. Special thanks to my department colleagues Dr James Rex, Dr Shibu A (Readers); Dr T Sreelal (Professor); Dr KS Arunachalam (Professor), for their encouragement and help. I must thank Ms Dhanya, for her help in drawing the diagrams which are included in this review. Last but not least, I thank my parents and in-laws, for their encouragement and support. I owe my gratitude to Mr Sudheer, for editing the contents of this book. I especially thank Dr Rema V Nair, Director, Sree Mookambika Institute of Dental Sciences, Kulasekharam, Tamil Nadu, for her support and encouragement.

I sincerely hope that students and dental practitioners will find this book useful.

Even though utmost care has been taken to ensure accuracy, mistakes could have inadvertently crept in and I do apologize in advance for the same. Any comments and suggestions are especially welcomed and I will try to implement them in future editions.

**Lovely M**

# Contents

## *Essays*

## *Short Notes*

# A Look into the Essay

A student of dentistry is trained to become knowledgeable, skilful in various clinical processes, laboratory procedures and communication and the student should develop an attitude to patients, colleagues and to the society at large, which is befitting to a professional. Essay question is an essential tool used to evaluate the knowledge of a student of dentistry. In a class examination or the final qualifying examination, essay is asked to evaluate the knowledge of the student. Very often it is used as a part of an assignment given to the student. Essay allows the student free expression and organization of thoughts. Essay gives an insight into the **depth of knowledge;** to be precise from a mere recall of facts to understanding and to application. The following examples will give an insight into "the depth of knowledge":

1. List five commonly used impression materials (**Recall**).
2. Classify impression materials into elastic and non-elastic based on the physical state of the set material (**Understanding**).
3. Select an appropriate impression material to be used in a partially edentulous situation (**Application**).

The first question can be answered if you learn by heart a list of impression materials. As such this will not be asked as an essay question but it can form part of an essay question. To answer the second question, the knowledge base must be broad and systematized. To answer the third question you should have the capability of reasoning and intelligence.

**The expression of the question** should be understood first. There will be a verb in the question which will decide precisely what the question is intended for. A few of such verbs are listed below:

| | |
|---|---|
| Analyze: | Various components of a concept is identified and the inter-relationship is described. |
| Compare: | Describe the similarities of two or more things. |
| Contrast: | Describe the differences of two or more things. |
| Define/Describe: | Give the definition and describe the components of the topic. |
| Discuss: | Different aspects of a problem are presented and a conclusion is drawn. |
| Enumerate: | Give a listing of the topics asked and briefly describe each. |
| Justify | Your point of view presented must be argued. |
| Outline: | Provide the main points of a topic. |
| Summarize: | Outline the main points briefly. |
| State: | Present the points clearly. |

**Outline of the essay:** Before answering the essay question, an outline of the essay must be made and it would indicate all the major points included in the essay. By doing this, the thoughts will be organized and no major point will be missed. The answering becomes fast and even if the answering is not complete, some credit will be given for the points given in the outline.

Between two answers sufficient space should be given so that at a later stage you can come back and more points can be added if necessary and if there is time. While starting the answer, immediately get to the point asked for. If the question asked is on vertical dimension, start with a statement on vertical dimension.

**Components of an essay:** There are three main components for an essay:
1. Introduction
2. Main body
3. Conclusion

**Introduction** is generally begun with a general issue on the topic asked and then narrowed down to the specifics that are discussed in the essay. Background information is given in the introduction which will make the subject content of the essay more relevant. A statement is also included on what you understand from the question. If possible a restatement of the question can be made with an outline of what is going to be discussed in the body of the essay.

The **body** should be arranged logically from a focal point and should contain a series of paragraphs which are packages of information. Each paragraph starts with a topic defining sentence which is expanded with details, examples and illustrations. There must be an uninterrupted flow of thought. Unnecessary statements which do not have relevance should be avoided because it is going to affect the time management.

Information in the **conclusion** moves from the specifics to the general and summarizes the content of the body. It provides a generalized answer to the question but new points cannot be made. Always devote some time to write the conclusion. Abrupt endings are never relished by the readers.

In the introduction you state what you are going to say, in the body state what you have to and in the conclusion state what you have already said.

**Time management:** Effective time management is essential in examinations or else you will find it difficult to complete the answering of all the required questions. Familiarize with the scheme of the examination and find out the marks for each question. Accordingly the time can be allocated for each question in a realistic fashion. Before answering, read the question carefully three times and this will give you clarity on what is asked. Make the outline and note down the key points and prioritize them. If the time allocated for one question is exhausted, leave it with some space to come back later if you get a chance to. Plan the time in such a way that at least five minutes are left at the end for correction of errors and to make a revisit to the questions which are not completed.

**Strategic approach:** Questions can be categorized as follows:
- Questions you *definitely know* and you can work out—these are the questions to be attempted first.
- Questions you think you know and you could guess—read these questions repeatedly and select logical answers without losing control over the time.
- Questions you are not sure of and have no clue about—read and reread the questions and think of the answers without making wild guesses and losing control over the time.

## On the Previous Night

- Confirm the time table and examination center
- Organize pen, pencils, rulers, etc.
- Refer the revision notes; not the texts
- Go to sleep early
- Practise yoga if you can
- Think of a time plan based on previous question papers.

## On the Examination Day

- Get up reasonably early
- To get energy for the examination have a good breakfast
- Briefly go through your notes

- Reach the examination center early; never rush
- To avoid distress do not talk too much on your preparation
- After reading the question do not look around to see other's reaction, every one will be stressed but that will be covered up by a smile and this smile might distress you
- Be positive; you can do it—remain as calm as possible.

## Helpful Tips

- Write clearly, concisely and legibly
- Answer the questions in the order of your preference unless specified but remember to put the number clearly—the first five marks are easier to get than the last five marks
- Draw relevant figures; it is equivalent to hundred words and more conspicuous
- Answer to the point. Writing more will not fetch more marks
- Do not get stuck to tough questions. Leave them and try later—if you run short of time and cannot come back, complete the sub-headings without describing the details—leave some space at the end of the answer
- If you get a point as a flash, immediately note it down somewhere or else you may forget it
- After the examination do not hang around and discuss.

## Examination Panic

- Once you read the question paper, you may suffer from examination panic, which is manifested by some or all of the following:
  - Nausea
  - Sweaty palms
  - Hot and cold feeling
  - Quick shallow breathing
  - Stomach churning
  - Lack of concentration
  - Rushing in of thoughts
  - Writer's block
  - Blank memory.

### *If you feel examination panic set aside 5 minutes to deal with it:*

- Concentrate on breathing
- Consciously relax the muscles
- Try tackling an easy question first
- If nothing works, switch off your mind for a while
- Think of something pleasant, pray to God
- Come back to the question.

## In Short

- Answer all the parts of the question—make an outline
- Define relevant terms in the question—cite examples, references
- Avoid incorrect observations
- Read the question paper thoroughly
- If the question is ambiguous, write your interpretation
- Prioritize the points
- Remember to put the question number
- Give space between answers
- Manage the time.

# ESSAYS

## 1. Classify mental attitude of a complete denture patient and how they can be managed?

Mental attitude of a patient was classified by Milus House and it has four classes.

### A. Philosophic

These patients accept the treatment plan without question. They accept their oral situation and have an ideal attitude for successful treatment, provided the biomechanical factors are reasonably favorable.

### B. Indifferent

Indifferent patients have little concern for their teeth or oral health. They often seek treatment because of family pressure and have no appreciation for the efforts of their dentist. They refuse to wear dentures if post insertion problems are encountered. Indifferent patients require more time to adjust with the use of dentures. Their attitude can discourage the dentist.

### C. Critical

They are quick to criticise the dentist at every stage of treatment planning. These patients will bring with them a collection of dentures pointing out faults in every denture made so far. These patients should be identified at the first appointment for a revision of their attitude. These patients generally have poor health which affects their overall personalities. Medical consultation is always advisable for critical patients before treatment is started.

The dentist should always direct all treatment and make decisions without patient involvement. These patients are a challenge to the dentist to complete treatment procedures which satisfy the patient, but their successful treatment can be most rewarding.

### D. Sceptical

These are patients who have had bad results with previous treatment and are therefore doubtful if anyone can help them. They also might be going through a recent series of personal tragedies not directly related to their denture problems. They have a negative outlook towards life and doubt the ability of anyone to help them with their problems. They are often in poor health, with severely resorbed residual ridges and other unfavorable conditions. They try to be good patients, but their problems seem countless. They need kind and sympathetic help as much as they need new dentures.

A careful and thorough examination can be the start of successful treatment. The dentist should take more time than usual in making examinations of sceptical patients, by which he can gain the confidence of these patients.

## IDENTIFYING THESE PATIENTS

From the initial appointment onwards the mental attitude of the patient can be analysed. Some patients keep on talking without listening to what the dentist has to say, others cry during talking, some criticize the previous dentist, or even suggest the treatment planning. Apart from the patient co-operation and trust in dentist, prosthodontic therapy for edentulous patients could be indicated as follows:

Clinical skill + Knowledge = Successful care

The prosthodontic experience demands technical and patient management skills, which helps in understanding the patient's mental attitude.

Attitude studies showed that many of these patients score highly on indices of neuroticism. Neurosis is regarded as a chronic anxiety state at the physiologic level and is known to affect the performance of tasks requiring neuromuscular coordination.

Whatever may be the type of patients,

A. A proper diagnosis and treatment planning.
B. Careful and thorough examination identifying the type of patient and gaining the confidence of the patient.
C. The duration of the time the patient has being edentulous to be noted, as longer the period greater the problem encountered in treatment procedure.
D. Other factors as residual ridge resorption, ridge form, accurate impression procedures, accuracy in each clinical steps all are factors which will aid in adequate retention of dentures thereby providing patient satisfaction.

## 2. Discuss the significance in diagnosis and treatment plan in complete denture patients.

Diagnosis is the examination of the physical state, evaluation of the mental or psychological makeup and understanding the needs of each patient to ensure a predictable result.

Treatment planning means developing a course of action that encompasses the ramifications and sequelae of treatment to serve the patient's needs.

## GENERAL DETAILS OF THE PATIENT

The patient's name, address, telephone number, age, occupation and other required general information such as how long the patient was edentulous is obtained.

## OBSERVATION OF THE PATIENT

### A. Motor Skills

Patient's gait, level of coordination and steadiness. Problems in motor skill can be due to Parkinsonism, Bell's palsy, nervous habits or possibly drug induced.

### B. Facial Features

Observe the philtrum, nasolabial fold and labiomental groove for hollowness or puffiness. Noting the profile view gives an indication of the patient's occlusal classification.

### C. Attitude and Adaptive Response

Previous experience with Dentist, a positive attitude, good general health, realistic expectation of the patient, good learning capacity, cooperative effort from patient.

## HEALTH HISTORY

1. The name of the patient's physician
2. A record of the status of all major body systems
3. A record of all medications the patient is currently taking
4. A record of any hospitalization
5. A record of any complication that was a result of previous dental treatment.

## CLINICAL EXAMINATION

1. Extraoral examination:
    a. *Head and neck region*: Examine for any existing facial lesions, nodules, nevi or ulcerations and the duration of the same are noted.
    b. *Lip Examination*: The lips are examined for cracking, fissuring at the corners and ulceration. The lips are then examined for support, fullness, thickness and length. This is needed for proper placement of anterior teeth.
    c. *Temporomandibular joint*: It is examined for pain, any joint sounds such as clicking, popping or crepitus upon opening and closing.
2. Intraoral examination of soft tissues:
    a. *The inside surface* of the cheeks, lips, residual ridge, floor of the mouth, hard and soft palate and the tongue are examined for abnormalities or pathological lesions. The anterior and posterior tonsillar pillars, oropharynx and nasopharynx should also be examined. Redundant tissue in maxilla and mandible should be examined. If present can cause shifting in denture bases leading to excessive ridge resorption.
    b. *Saliva*: The amount and consistency of saliva will affect the denture construction process Xerostomia will affect denture retention and can cause soreness.
    c. *Floor of the mouth*: If the floor of the mouth in the sublingual gland and mylohyoid areas are high and close to the ridge this crest can eliminate the alveololingual sulcus. The retromylohyoid space (lateral throat form) should be evaluated if this space can be filled, the mandibular denture will have good lingual seal and lateral stability.
    d. *Muscle and frenal attachments*: The attachments most often surgically corrected are the maxillary labial and mandibular lingual frena. If not relieved in denture can cause soreness in that region.
    e. *Tongue*: The tongue size should be noted. In patients with long period of edentulism without replacement of teeth or for patients who has worn a maxillary denture against the lower anterior teeth without replacement of lower posteriors, the tongue can become enlarged and powerful. Tongue movement and muscular coordination are important for border molding impressions and during normal physiological activity such as speech, mastication and deglutition.

    Wright classified tongue positions as follows:

    Class I—the tongue lies in the floor of the mouth with the tip forward and slightly below the incisal edges of the mandibular anterior teeth.

    Class II—the tongue is flattened and broadened but the tip is in a normal position and

    Class III—the tongue is retracted and depressed into the floor of the mouth with the tip curled upward, downward, or assimilated into the body of the tongue.

    Class I is favorable.
3. Intraoral examination of hard tissues:
    i. *Arch form*: Square, ovoid or tapered (opposing arches may not have the same form).
    ii. *Ridge contour*: The ideal ridge contour is a high ridge with a flat-crested parallel sides.
    iii. *Parallelism of ridges*: As the maxilla resorb the crest appears to move upward and inward. As the mandible resorbs, the crest of the ridge appears to move downward forward and laterally because it is wide at its inferior border than at its occlusal border.
    iv. *Hard palate*: The hard palate should be examined and its shape noticed. The U-shaped palatal vault is most favorable for retention.

v. *Soft palate*: There are three classifications of soft palate Fig. 1:
  - Class I: Large and normal with immovable band of resilient tissue, 5 to 12 mm distal to line drawn across the distal edge of tuberosities. Ideal for denture retention.
  - Class II soft palate turns downward at about a 45° angle to the hard palate and the amount of potential tissue coverage for the palatal seal is 3 to 5 mm.
  - Class III soft palate turns downward sharply at about a 70° angle just posteriorly to the hard palate. The available space for coverage by the posterior palatal seal is at a minimum. A 'V' shaped palatal vault is usually associated with a Class III soft palate.

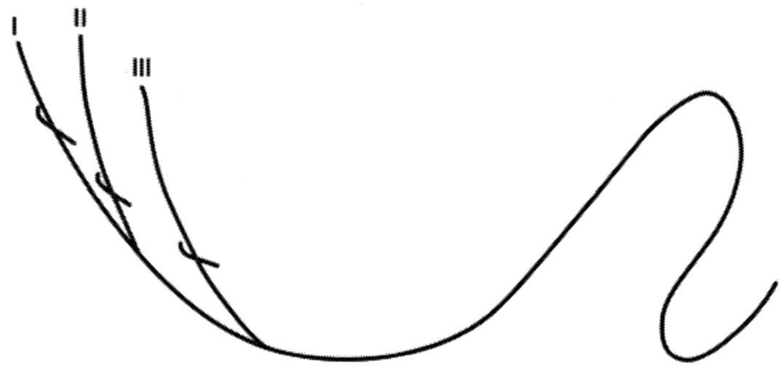


**Fig. 1:** Classification of soft palate

vi. *Bony undercuts*: Bony undercuts in maxillary are commonly seen on the anterior ridge and lateral to the tuberosities and in mandibular ridges is a prominent sharp mylohyoid ridge. Here surgical reduction and reattachment of the mylohyoid muscle can have beneficial results.

vii. *Torus palatinus* in maxilla is occasionally present on the midline to one that covers the entire hard palate. Generally surgical removal is contraindicated unless the torus is so large. Lingual tori are seen in the mandibular premolar region.

4 Gag reflex: The oral examination, medical history and conversation with the patient are important in identifying the existence of a problem and determining the treatment.

## RADIOGRAPHIC EXAMINATION

Panoramic examination of edentulous patients includes a five-step analysis as outlined by Chomenko.

a *Screen* jaws for defects, bone enlargement and displacement of jaw parts, any unerupted teeth or retained root fragments, foreign bodies, radiolucencies radio-opacities, rarefaction or sclerosis, expansion or bulging and any well-defined or ill-defined lesions. TMJ can be screened. In addition, the maxillary sinus can be checked for inflammation, cysts, polyps, tumors, infection or inflammation.

   Describe the appearance of the lesion and include location, size, shape, number and a description of the radiographic pattern.

b. *Correlate* the radiographic findings with the clinical, historical and laboratory findings.

c. *Perform a differential diagnosis* which includes all the diseases that could explain the findings.

d. *Estimate* the growth of the lesion.

e. *Document* the amount of ridge resorption which is classified as:
  - Class I (mild resorption) is a loss of up to one-third of the original vertical height,
  - Class II (moderate resorption) is a loss of from one-third to two-third of the vertical height,
  - Class III (severe resorption) is a loss of two-third or more of vertical height.

## EXAMINATION OF THE PRESENT PROSTHESES

If patient has an existing prosthesis then check for:

a. If the present prosthesis is acceptable or unacceptable.
b. Verify centric relation in which the first occlusal contact should be bilateral and distributed evenly anteroposteriorly to rate as acceptable.
c. Evaluate the occlusal vertical dimension in occlusion and speech.
d. Evaluate for proper basal seat coverage.
e. Examine the artificial teeth for wear or breakage.
f. Check for retention and stability of the complete dentures.
g. Evaluate the residual ridges and the patient's chief complaint.

## PRE-TREATMENT RECORDS

Diagnostic casts can detect the ridge relationships interridge distance or ridge shape and form.

Pre-extraction Records and Photographs showing natural teeth aids in determining tooth size, position and arrangement.

Old radiographs are also helpful in determining tooth size and bony changes.

## TREATMENT PLAN

After a thorough history taking, examination of the patient and verifying all diagnostic records, the treatment plan is decided. The treatment and expected level of achievement is explained to the patient. The fees for the procedure, the manner of payment, duration of treatment, any necessary tissue preparation, conditioning and corrective surgery are discussed. Limitations are pointed out if the complete denture patients present with different problems as in Hysterical or Critical patients, then medical consultation is always advisable before treatment is started. A trained professional is aware of all the patient's needs and educates the patient to overcome problems related to treatment procedures.

**3. Describe with diagrams the anatomical structures of**

**(i). Maxillary denture bearing area.**

**(ii). Mandibular denture bearing area.**

## (I) MAXILLARY DENTURE BEARING AREAS

### Stress-bearing Areas

The residual ridge and most of the hard palate are considered the primary stress-bearing area in the upper jaw. The crest of the residual alveolar ridge is covered with a layer of fibrous connective tissue and the bone in the region of the crest of the upper residual ridge may be compact in nature, being made up of haversian systems. The above features help to provide primary support for the upper denture.

### Anatomical Landmarks (Figs 2 and 3)

**A. Labial frenum:**

The maxillary labial frenum is a fold of mucous membrane at the median line with no muscle and has no action of its own. This band of tissue starts superiorly in a fan shape and converges

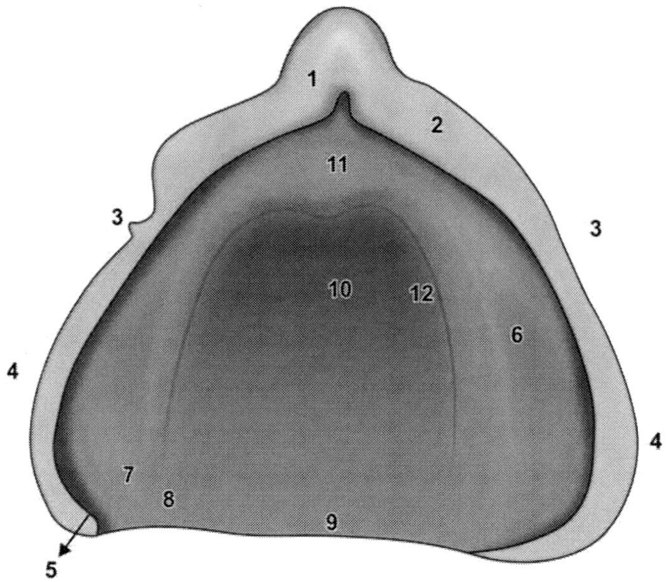


1. Labial notch
2. Labial flange
3. Buccal notch
4. Buccal flange
5. Coronoid contour
6. Alveolar groove
7. Maxillary tubercular fossa
8. Pterygomaxillary seal
9. Posterior palatal seal
10. Median palatine groove
11. Incisive fossa
12. Rugae

**Fig. 2:** Anatomical landmarks in the maxillary final impression

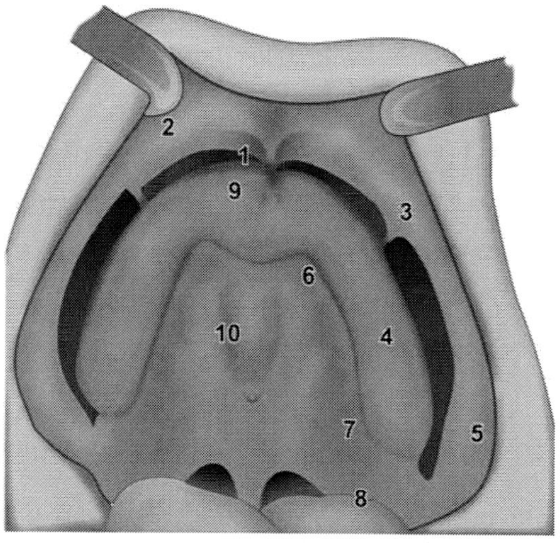


1. Labial frenum
2. Labial vestibule
3. Buccal frenum
4. Buccal vestibule
5. Coronoid bulge
6. Residual alveolar ridge
7. Maxillary tuberosity
8. Hamular notch
9. Incisive papilla
10. Median palatine raphe

**Fig. 3:** Anatomical landmarks of the maxillary area in the mouth

as it descends and attaches on the labial side of the ridge. The labial notch in the labial flange of the denture must allow the frenum to pass through it without manipulation of the lip.

**B. Labial flange**

The denture border between the labial and buccal frenum is known as the labial flange. The orbicularis oris is the main muscle resting on the labial flange and teeth of the denture. Its tone depends on the support it receives from the thickness of the labial flange and the position of teeth. The fibers of the orbicularis pass horizontally through the lips and anastomose with fibers of the buccinator muscle.

**C. Buccal frenum**

The buccal frenum can be a single or double fold of mucous membrane which is broad and fan shaped. The caninus (levator anguli oris) attaches beneath and affects the position of the buccal frenum. The orbicularis oris pulls the frenum forward and the buccinator pulls it backward. The buccal notch in the denture must be broad enough to allow this movement of the buccal frenum. The buccal frenum is a continuous band of tissue going from the maxilla through the modiolus to the buccal frenum on the mandible.

**D. Buccal vestibule**

The buccal vestibule is opposite the tuberosity and extends from the buccal frenum to the hamular notch. The size of the buccal vestibule varies with the contraction of the buccinator, the position of the mandible and the amount of bone loss from the maxilla. The thickness of the distal end of the buccal flange of the denture should accommodate the ramus and coronoid process and the masseter as they function. If too thick, the ramus will push the denture out of place during opening or lateral movements of the mandible.

**E. Incisive papilla**

The incisive papilla covers the incisive foramen and is located behind and between the central incisors. If adequate relief is not provided in this region it may cause interference with the blood and nerve supply.

**F. Rugae**

The rugae are irregularly shaped rolls of soft tissue in the anterior part of the hard palate which should not be distorted during impression procedures. The rugal area is set at an angle to the occlusal plane of the residual ridges and is thinly covered by soft tissues. It helps in secondary retention.

**G. Median palatine Raphe**

The submucosa in the region of the median palatal suture of the maxillary bones is extremely thin. Proper relief in the impression tray or the completed denture is essential for accommodation of the histologic nature of this tissue.

**H. Zygomatic process**

The zygomatic, or malar process, located opposite the first molar region, is a hard area found in mouths that have been edentulous for a long time. Some dentures require relief over this area to aid retention and prevent soreness of the underlying tissues.

**i. Palate**

Divided as anterior and posterior part. The posterior part consists of glandular tissue which aids in retention but does not provide significant support for the denture because of higher resiliency at this site. The mucus glands in this region are relatively thick and they cover the blood vessels and nerves coursing forward in the palate from the greater palatine foramen and they anastomose with vessels and nerves passing through the nasopalatine canal.

**J. Posterior palatal area**

As the posterior palatine foramina are thickly covered by soft tissue they do not need to be relieved except in extreme cases of resorption. Anterolaterally, the submucosa of the hard palate contains adipose tissue and posterolaterally it contains glandular tissue.

**K. Maxillary tuberosity**

The tuberosity region of the maxilla often hangs low if in cases where the maxillary posterior teeth are retained after the mandibular molars have been lost and not replaced, the maxillary teeth extrude, bringing the process with them. This excess soft tissue can prevent proper location of the occlusal plane if it is not removed.

**L. Pterygomaxillary (hamular) notch**

The hamular notch is situated between the tuberosity of the maxilla and the hamulus of the medial pterygoid plate. It is used as a boundary of the posterior border of the maxillary denture back of the tuberosity. The posterior palatal seal must be placed through the center of the deep part of the hamular notch, since no muscle or ligament is present at a level to prevent the placement of extra pressure.

**M. Palatine fovea region**

The foveae palatinae are indentations near the midline of the palate formed by a coalescence of several mucus gland ducts. They are close to the vibrating line and always in soft tissue, which makes them an ideal guide for the location of the posterior border of the denture.

**N. Vibrating line of the palate**

The vibrating line is an imaginary line drawn across the palate that marks the beginning of motion in the soft palate when the patient says "ah". It extends from one pterygomaxillary notch to the other and passes about 2 mm in front of the foveae palatinae. The vibrating line is always on the soft palate. The direction of the vibrating line varies according to the shape of the palate. In a mouth with a flat vault, the vibrating line is usually farther posterior and has a gradual curvature, with a broader posterior palatal seal area.

The distal end of the upper denture should end 1 or 2 mm posterior to the vibrating line and cover the tuberosities and extend into the hamular notches. The submucosa in the region of the vibrating line on the soft palate contains glandular tissue. The submucosa of the mucous membrane contained within the hamular notch is thick and made up of loose areolar tissue.

*The anterior vibrating line* is an imaginary line located at the junction of the attached tissues overlying the hard palate and the movable tissues of the immediately adjacent soft palate. One way to locate the anterior vibrating line is to have the patient perform the Valsalva maneuver, which requires that both nostrils be held firmly while the patient blows gently through the nose. Another method is to the patient to say "ah" with short vigorous bursts. Due to the projection of the posterior nasal spine, the anterior vibrating line is not a straight line between both hamular processes. The anterior vibrating line is always on soft palatal tissues.

*The posterior vibrating line* is an imaginary line at the junction of the aponeurosis of the tensor veli palatini muscle and the muscular portion of the soft palate. It represents the demarcation between that part of the soft palate that has limited or shallow movement during function and the remainder of the soft palate that is displaced during functional movements. The posterior vibrating line is visualized by instructing the patient to say "ah" in short bursts in a normal, unexaggerated fashion. The posterior vibrating line marks the most distal extension of the denture base. The posterior palatal seal area lies between anterior and posterior vibrating line and is cupids bow shaped.

## MANDIBULAR BASAL SEAT AREA (FIGS 4 AND 5)

**A. Crest of the residual ridge:**
Crest of the residual ridge is covered by fibrous connective tissue, if closely attached to the bone it can resist externally applied forces.

**B. Labial frenum**
The mandibular labial frenum contains a band of fibrous connective tissue that helps attach the orbicularis oris.

**C. Labial flange**
The part of the denture that extends between the labial frenum (labial notch) and the buccal frenum (buccal notch) is called the mandibular labial flange which is limited by the fibers of the orbicularis oris and the incisivus labii inferioris.

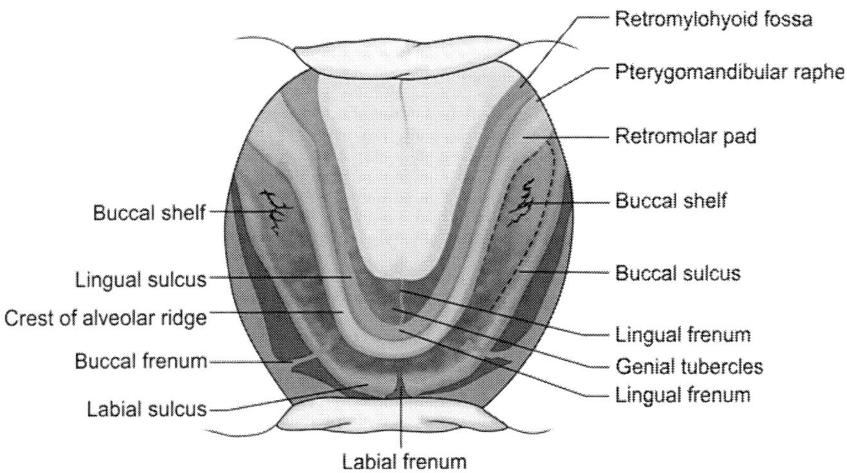


**Fig. 4:** Anatomical landmarks in the mandibular arch

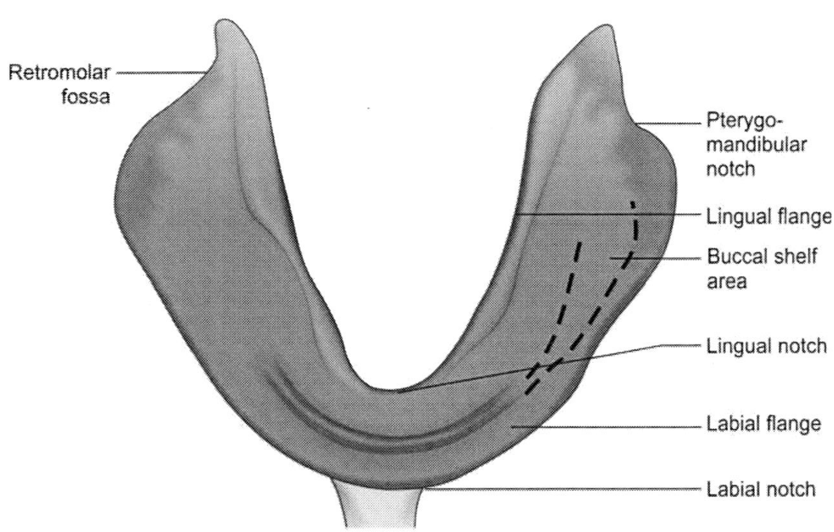


**Fig. 5:** Anatomical landmarks in the mandibular final impression

**d. Mental foramen area**

Severe resorption of bone near the mental foramina can result in a superficial location of mental foramen on the crest of the residual ridge. If relief is not provided in the denture base in this area this can lead to numbness of the lower lip due to pressure on the mental nerve.

**E. Buccal frenum**

The buccal frenum connects as a continuous band through the modiolus at the corner of the mouth to the buccal frenum in the maxilla.

**F. Buccal flange**

The buccal flange area starts immediately posterior to the buccal frenum and extends to the anterior portion of the masseter, swings wide into the cheek and is nearly at right angles to the biting force. Hence able to provide greatest surface for resistance to vertical occlusal forces. The buccal flange may extend to the external oblique ridge, or even over it, depending on the location of the mucobuccal fold.

**G. Buccal vestibule**

The buccal vestibule extends from the buccal frenum posteriorly to the outside back corner of the retromolar pad and from the crest of the residual alveolar ridge to the cheek. The buccinator, in the cheek, extends from the modiolus (anteriorly) to the pterygomandibular raphe (posteriorly). Its lower side attaches in the molar region in the buccal shelf of the mandible.

**H. Buccal shelf**

It is primary stress bearing area of the mandible denture base. Buccal shelf area extends from mandibular buccal frenum to the anterior edge of the masseter. It is bounded medially by the crest of the residual ridge, anteriorly by the buccal frenum, laterally by the external oblique line and distally by the retromolar pad. The inferior part of the buccinator is attached in the buccal shelf of the mandible and thus contraction of the muscle does not lift the lower denture. It is covered with good smooth cortical bone which is usually at right angles to the occlusal forces.

**I. Masseter muscle region**

The distobuccal borders of the mandibular denture converge rapidly to avoid displacement due to contracting pressure of the anterior fibers of masseter muscle, which passes outside the buccinator in this region. When the masseter contracts, it alters the shape and size of the distobuccal end by pushing inward against the buccinator muscle and suctorial pad of the cheek.

**J. Retromolar region and pad**

The retromolar pad is a triangular soft pad of tissue at the distal end of the lower ridge which must be covered by the denture to perfect the border seal. It contains glandular tissue, some fibers of the temporalis tendon, buccinator fibers enter it from the buccal side and fibers of the superior pharyngeal constrictor enter it from the lingual; the pterygomandibular raphe enters the pad at its superoposterior inside corner.

**K. Lingual frenum and lingual flange**

The anterior part of the lingual flange over the sublingual gland is usually shallow because of the mobility of the tissues controlled indirectly by the mylohyoid muscle hence only a short flange is usable.

**L. Mylohyoid ridge**

Soft tissue usually hides the sharpness of the mylohyoid ridge, which can be found by palpation. The lingual border of the mandibular impression extends into the undercut below the mylohyoid ridge. The mylohyoid muscle arises from the whole length of the mylohyoid line, extending from about 1 cm back of the distal end of the mylohyoid ridge to the lingual anterior portion of the mandible at the symphysis. Medially the fibers join those from the mylohyoid muscle of the opposite side and posteriorly they continue to the hyoid bone. The posterior part of the mylohyoid muscle in the molar region affects the lingual impression border in swallowing and moving the tongue. If the mylohyoid ridges are bulbous, irregular and severely undercut or extremely thin and sharp it is the cause aggravation and soreness for edentulous patients.

**M. Sublingual gland region**

It is in the premolar region on the lingual side of ridge. The sublingual gland rests above the mylohyoid muscle and when the floor of the mouth is raised, this gland comes close to the crest of the ridge reducing the vertical space available for flange extension.

**N. Alveololingual sulcus**

The alveololingual sulcus is the space between the residual ridge and the tongue extending posteriorly from the lingual frenum to the retromylohyoid curtain. The alveololingual sulcus is divided into three regions.

1. *The anterior region*

   Extends from the lingual frenum to where the mylohyoid ridge curves down below the level of the sulcus. The premylohyoid fossa can be palpated as a depression and a corresponding prominence, the premylohyoid eminence, can be seen on impressions. The premylohyoid fossa results from the concavity of the mandible joining the convexity of the mylohyoid ridge.

2. *The middle region*

   This part extends from the premylohyoid fossa to the distal end of the mylohyoid ridge curving medially from the body of the mandible. The curvature is caused by the prominence of the mylohyoid ridge.

3. *The posterior region*

   This part is the retromylohyoid space or fossa. It extends from the end of the mylohyoid ridge to the retromylohyoid curtain, being bounded on the lingual by the anterior tonsillar pillar and superior constrictor and on the buccal by the mylohyoid muscle, mandibular ramus and retromolar pad. The projection of the mylohyoid ridge toward the tongue and the existence of a retromylohyoid fossa at the distal end of the alveololingual sulcus causes the border of the lingual flange to assume an "S" shape when viewed from the impression surface.

## 4. What are the objectives of impression making? Explain various impression procedures in CD fabrication.

There are five main objectives in impression making. They are:

A. Preservation

   Preservation of the remaining residual ridges

   As the natural teeth are lost there is loss of stimulation resulting in alveolar ridge atrophy or resorption. Local factors such as occlusion, interocclusal distance, centric relation in harmony with centric occlusion, impression technique and the impression material all have its own effect on the continued health of both the soft and hard tissues. Pressure in the impression technique leads to pressure in the denture base and results in soft tissue damage and bone resorption.

B. Support

Support is defined as, "The resistance to vertical forces of mastication, occlusal forces and other forces applied in a direction towards the denture-bearing area."

Maximum coverage provides the "snowshoe" effect, which distributes applied forces over wide an area as possible. This helps in preservation, stability and retention.

C. Stability

Stability is defined as, "Resistance against horizontal movement and forces that tend to alter the relationship between the denture base and its supporting foundation in a horizontal or rotatory direction." The size and form of the basal seat, quality of the final impressions, the form of the polished surfaces and the proper location and arrangement of the artificial teeth help in maintaining the stability of the dentures.

Close adaptation to the undistorted mucosa increases stability.

D. Retention

Retention is defined as, "That quality inherent in the prosthesis which resists the force of gravity, adhesiveness of foods and the forces associated with the opening of the jaws"–GPT or it is the ability of the denture to withstand displacement against its path of insertion.

If the other objectives are achieved, retention will be adequate.

Atmospheric pressure, adhesion, cohesion, muscle control and patient tolerance affect retention.

*Atmospheric pressure*: Atmospheric pressure depends on peripheral seal. To ensure this seal, denture borders should extend into, but not to the extent to damage movable tissue.

*Adhesion*: Adhesion is defined as, "The physical attraction of unlike molecules to one another". Adhesion is the attraction of saliva to the denture.

*Cohesion*: Cohesion is defined as, "The physical attraction of like molecules for each other". The cohesive forces act within the thin film of saliva. Cohesion is the attraction of molecules of saliva to each other.

*Muscle control and patient tolerance*: Dentures are often retained in the mouth not because of the accuracy of conforming to the support but because of patient tolerance and the adaptability of the muscles of the lips, tongue and cheeks.

E. Aesthetics

Border thickness should be varied with the needs of each patient depending on the extent of residual ridge loss. The vestibular fornix should be correctly filled to restore facial contour.

F. Steps in complete denture impression making:

1. Ensure the health of tissues that comprise the denture-bearing surfaces:
   a. Leave denture out of the mouth.
   b. Adjust patient's present denture by tissue conditioning, occlusal adjustments.
   c. Prescribe pre-prosthetic surgery as in flabby tissues and prominent bony projections, etc.
2. Preliminary impression:
   a. Use rim locked stock tray and irreversible hydrocolloid impression material.
   b. Identify and mark the preferred peripheral outline of the custom tray. Make a laboratory stone cast.

3. Custom tray fabrication:
   a. Outline the stress-bearing surface for the denture and cover it with a wax spacer.
   b. Make an acrylic resin tray that extends just past the identified junction of the attached/ unattached mucosa.
4. Border Molding
   a. Try the tray in the mouth and correct for any overextensions.
5. Final Impression:
   a. Use the preferred final impression material.
6. Working cast preparation:
   a. Box and pour the final impression.
   b. Trim the cast.

## MANDIBULAR

G. Preliminary Impression
After assessing the space available in the mouth, the general form, size and health of the basal seat are evaluated. An edentulous metal stock tray is selected that will provide 6 mm bulk of impression material over the entire basal seat area and all supporting tissues including the retromolar pads.

H. Material of choice
   a. Alginate or
   b. Impression compound.
   (Depending on clinician's choice.)

I. Wax spacer design
Mandibular: A wax spacer about 1 mm thick is placed over the crest and slopes of the residual ridge. The buccal shelf on each side and the retromylohyoid spaces on the cast are left uncovered.

J. Tray
Autopolymerizing acrylic resin tray approximately 2 to 3 mm thick with an anterior resin handle centered over the approximate position of the anterior teeth without interfering with the position of the lip. Two posterior handles in the molar region are used as finger rests to complete the placement of the tray on the residual ridge and to stabilize the tray in the correct position. The flanges of the tray should be contoured like the flanges of the completed denture.
*Preparing the final impression tray*:
The acrylic resin tray is removed along with the spacer from the preliminary cast. The buccal and lingual flanges of the tray are marked in pencil and reduced until the borders are short of the limiting anatomic structures.

K. Border molding (Fig. 6)
   1. Modelling compound is added to the lingual borders in the molar regions on both sides of the tray (see steps 1 and 2 of the Figure 6) between the premylohyoid and postmylohyoid eminences. This area of compound is heated and tempered and the patient is asked to protrude the tongue. This develops the slope of the lingual flange in the molar region to allow for the action of the mylohyoid muscle. The distal end of the lingual flange should extend about 1 cm distal to the end of the mylohyoid ridge. The flange should be so

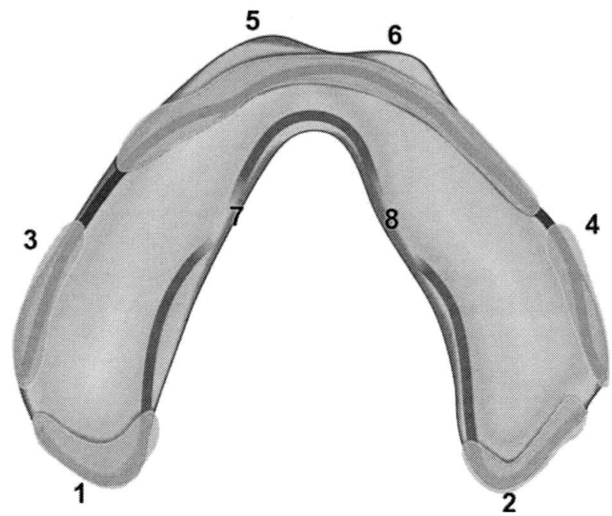


**Fig. 6:** Steps in border molding (mandibular arch) (see text for steps)

shaped that it turns laterally toward the ramus below the level of the retromolar pad and mylohyoid ridge. It assumes a typical "S" shape.

Compound on the distal end of the flange is heated and the tray placed in the mouth and patient is instructed to protrude his tongue to activate the superior constrictor, then he is asked to close as the dentist applies downward force on the impression tray. The resulting contraction of the medial pterygoid muscle, acting posteriorly on the retromylohyoid curtain, can limit the space available for the border of the impression in the retromylohyoid fossa. With the lower final impression tray is place in the mouth the patient should be able to wipe the tip of his tongue across the vermilion border of the upper lip without noticeable displacement of the lower tray.

2. *Buccal flange* is border molded on both sides (see steps 3 and 4 of the Figure 6) when the cheek is moved outward, upward and inward.

   *Buccal frenum:* The cheek is lifted outward, upward, inward, backward and forward to simulate movement of the lower buccal frenum.
3. *Labial flange* is border molded on both sides (see steps 5 and 6 of the Figure 6) when the lower lip is lifted outward, upward and inward.
4. The compound on the lingual surface from premolar to premolar of the flange, on both sides (see steps 7 and 8 of the Figure 6), is softened and the tray is placed in the mouth and the patient is asked to push the tongue forcefully against the front part of the palate. This functional activity molds the premylohyoid fossa in the canine-premolar region, the flange becomes longer and extends below the level of the mylohyoid line. After the tray is placed in the patient's mouth, the patient is instructed to protrude the tongue which raises the anterior part of the floor of the mouth. This functional activity molds the lingual frenum, both premylohyoid eminences and the lengths of the lingual flange on each side of the lingual notch will frequently be symmetric.

### Final Impression

The wax spacer is removed from the inside of the tray and several holes of about 12.5 mm apart are marked in the center of the alveolar groove and the retromolar fossae of the tray and are cut with a No. 6 round bur. The modelling compound borders are shortened approximately 0. 5 to 1 mm to make space for the final impression material.

Zinc oxide eugenol impression paste is used for final impression. The refined impression is removed from the mouth, washed with tap water, dried and boxed.
Sufficient stone is poured into the boxed impression with a base height of 9 to 15 mm from the deepest portion of the impression. It is separated after 30 minutes.
Another selective pressure technique in which Polyether is the material of choice. This is a single step border molding procedure.

## MAXILLARY

L. Maxillary preliminary impression
For the maxillary impression the tray should cover all the basal seat area including the hamular notches and maxillary tuberosities. The labial and buccal borders of the tray are observed in relation to the limiting anatomic structures.

M. Maxillary wax spacer design
The cast is made of artificial stone poured into the irreversible hydrocolloid impression or impression compound. The outline for a wax spacer is drawn in pencil on the cast. A wax spacer about 1 mm thick is placed over the incisive papillae and median palatine raphae or a full spacer short of posterior palatal seal area and 2 mm short of sulcus depth can be designed depending on the clinical situation.
Maxillary Impression Tray is fabricated in the same method as for mandibular.

N. Border molding procedure (Fig. 7)
1. Distal to the buccal frenum, including the hamular notch and across the posterior palatal seal area is molded first. After softening the stick compound ask the patient to open his mouth wide as in yawning, then protrude and move mandible to the right and left. This combined action develops the distal extent of the denture in the hamular notch and the space between the anterior border of the ramus and the tubercles. The impression compound across the posterior palatal seal area maintains contact with the tissues in this area. This is done bilaterally to ensure proper seating of the tray.
2. Add and soften stick compound at the buccal frenum attachment (unilaterally). Flame, temper, and seat to place. Gently massage the upper lip in a superior-inferior direction. Remove the tray and chill it.
3. Repeat for opposite side.
Soften impression compound in the buccal frenum area (unilaterally).
4. Add compound in the labial flange area and ask patient to suck gently on your finger to join the refined buccal border and seat. Repeat for opposite side
5. Soften impression compound in the labial frenum area, seat, grasp upper lip and extend directly, forward and to and fro.

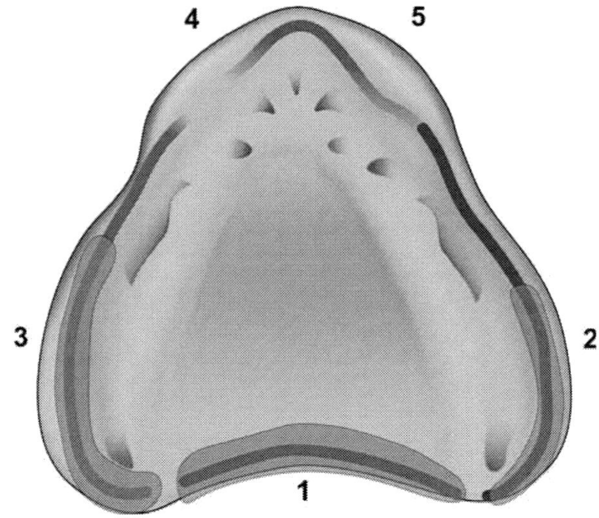


**Fig. 7:** Steps in border molding (Maxillary arch) (see text for steps)

## FINAL IMPRESSION

1 After the borders have been refined, the tissues are examined and palpated with a ball burnisher and the tray is relieved with a No. 8 round bur, three holes are placed in the tray. in the anterior section of the rugae area and two holes in the posterior area.
2. Apply petrolatum to the patient's face, as the impression material is sticky.
3. Mix the impression material according to manufacturer's instructions. Load the trays, including the borders, to a uniform thickness.
4. Place the loaded trays in the patient's mouth; seat them with positive pressure until the impression material is seen to flow from the borders and the posterior palatal seal area and the holes in the rugae area.
5. After which all pressure is released and the index and middle fingers are rested lightly, one on each side. The patient is instructed to flex his head forward and breathe through his nose.
6. When the zinc oxide-eugenol impression paste is thoroughly set, the refined impression is removed from the mouth, washed with tap water, dried with a gentle application of air and inspected. If needed, the impression can be reseated and checked for retention and stability.

### 5. Define impression. List the merits and demerits of various impression techniques.

## IMPRESSION

An impression is the negative form of the teeth and other tissues of the oral cavity, made in a plastic material which becomes relatively hard or set while in contact with these tissues. An impression is made in order to produce a positive form or cast of the recorded tissues.

A complete denture impression is a negative registration of the entire denture bearing, stabilizing and border seal areas present in the edentulous mouth.

## Types of Impression Techniques

1. Definite Pressure Impression or Mucocompressive Technique or Closed Mouth Technique.
2. Minimum Pressure Impression or Mucostatic Technique as open mouth or Passive Technique.
3. Selective Pressure Technique.
4. Controlled Subatmospheric Pressure.

**1. Definite-pressure Impressions or Mucocompressive Technique**

These are closed mouth techniques that record the tissues in their functional position. The patient applies pressure by closing against teeth or occlusion rims, that are attached to the impression trays which in turn exerts pressure and executes muscle actions such as swallowing, grinning, or pursing the lips while the impression material flows.

### Impression materials used for this technique

a. Impression compound.
b. Waxes that flowed at mouth temperature.
c. Soft liners.

Significance of closed mouth technique (Macmillan, 1947) is that this technique is capable of adequately trimming the lingual borders of the lower as the tongue movements are more forceful when the teeth are together than when the mouth is opened and the tongue is protruded.

### Disadvantages

1. Soft tissues that are displaced and recorded tend to return to their undisplaced position when the forces are released hence unseating the denture.
2. As the denture is constantly held in a displaced position, the pressure limits the normal blood flow.
3. Excessive bone resorption as due to lack of proper blood flow.
4. Inadequate retention.
5. Often the dentures made with closed-mouth impressions are overextended and must be arbitrarily trimmed.

Soft liners are good for refitting complete dentures and also possess the advantage retaining compliance for many weeks, good dimensional stability and excellent bonding to the resin denture base.

**2. Mucostatic, Open mouth, Passive or Minimal-Pressure Impressions**

This technique was proposed by Richardson and popularised by Harry Page hence also referred to as Page technique.

Open mouth techniques are those that record the tissues in their undisplaced position hence also referred to as a non-pressure or mucostatic technique. The main point of the mucostatic principle concerned Pascal's law which states that the mucosa, containing a percent of water, will react like liquid in a closed vessel and thus cannot be compressed. The impression is made in an oversized or spaced tray with no border seal or border refining. The completed denture borders are usually reduced to the stress-bearing mucosa depriving the denture of maximum coverage within tissue tolerance. Hence results in close adaptation of the denture base to the undistorted mucosa for stability but lacks in retention as no border seal is present.

The only advantage was that dentist can see whether muscle trimming is done properly or not.

## Disadvantages

1. The theory that mucosa is a closed vessel is not true as tissue fluids can easily escape under the border of a denture.
2. According to the principle of mucostatics, the impression material should record, every detail of the mucosa without distortion so that the completed denture would fit all minute elevations and depressions. Chrome alloy which were used did not copy all details as accurately as Gold alloys.
3. The mucosal topography is not static over a 24-hour period. There is a difference between the mucosal contours just after rising in the morning and that which exists after 12 hours in the upright position again losing all the infinite details achieved in the impression.
4. The adherents of the mucostatic principle considered interfacial surface tension as the only important retentive factor in complete dentures. They did not use conventional flanges because these did not resist vertical displacement, which was the only movement interrupting surface tension. The lack of flanges did not resist lateral displacement.
5. The mucostatic principle ignores the value of dissipating masticatory forces over the largest possible basal seat area.
6. Mucostatic denture minimized the retentive role of the musculature, as described by Fish.

**3. Selective Pressure Technique**

The selective pressure technique is a combination of extension for maximum coverage within tissue tolerance with light pressure or intimate contact with the movable, loosely attached tissues in the vestibules. The impression is refined with a minimum of pressure. This technique combines pressure over certain areas and little pressure over others. It utilizes a preliminary compound impression that is generously relieved over the midline and incisive papilla areas. The final impression is taken in plaster, which acts as a wash and also records the relieved areas with minimal pressure while the ridge areas are undergoing considerable pressure. Thus the midline and papilla sections of the denture will not make contact with the mucosa when the denture is not in function, but by the same token, they will not bear heavily when the patient is chewing.

This principle of impression making is based on the belief that the mucosa over the ridge is best able to withstand pressure, whereas that covering the midline is thin and contains very little submucosal tissue (Boucher, 1951).

## Disadvantage

This technique cannot be done on flabby ridges. This technique demands firm, healthy mucosal covering over the ridge.

**4. Controlled Subatmospheric Pressure**

Controlled subatmospheric pressure is a technique using individualized impression trays to which are attached small rubber hoses. Through these hoses a vacuum is created in the tissue side of the tray. The borders are refined, using an impression material such as Adaptol.

## Materials Used

Impression materials used in complete denture construction are elastic materials such as alginates, reversible hydrocolloids, rubber base and silicone compounds and inelastic materials such as plaster, compound, wax and metallic oxide pastes.

### 6. Enumerate and describe various physical factors of retention in complete denture prosthesis.

## FACTORS THAT ENHANCE THE RETENTION, STABILITY AND SUPPORT OF A DENTURE

1. Maximum coverage of the basal seat within the limits of the health and functions of the supporting and limiting tissues.
2. Borders that are in harmony with the anatomic and physiologic limitations of the oral structures.
3. A physiologic type of border-molding procedure.
4. Proper space ensured in tray for final impression material.
5. Selective pressure technique for final impression.
6. Ideal impression material to be used depending on clinical situation.
7. A guiding mechanism for correct positioning of the impression tray in the mouth.
8. The tray and final impression should be of dimensionally stable materials.
9. The completed final impression form is similar to the external form of the completed denture.
10. Accurately fitting final impression tray.

## FACTORS AFFECTING RETENTION OF DENTURES

Retention is defined as, "That quality inherent in the prosthesis which resists the force of gravity, adhesiveness of foods and the forces associated with the opening of the jaws"–GPT.
Retention is the ability of the denture to withstand displacement against its path of insertion.

*Factors that affect retention can be classified as:*

a. Anatomical factors.
b. Physiological factors.
c. Physical factors
d. Mechanical factors.
e. Surgical factors.
f. Psychologic factors.

## Anatomical Factors

1. Maximum coverage of the basal seat area.
2. Quality of denture bearing area, if the ridges are parallel and well formed better the retention.
3. Oral facial musculature.
4. Neuromuscular control.

*Oral and Facial Musculature*

a. The oral and facial musculature can supply supplementary retention provided

b. If the teeth are positioned in the neutral zone.
If the polished surfaces of the dentures are properly shaped.
The *buccal flanges* of the maxillary denture slope up and out from the occlusal surfaces of the teeth and the buccal flanges of the mandibular denture slope down and out from the occlusal plane.
The *lingual surfaces* of the lingual flanges should slope toward the center of the mouth so the tongue can fit against them. The "S" shaped area in impression copied on to denture also perfects seal in the posterior lingual aspect.
c. The denture bases must cover the maximum area without interfering with health and function.
d. The occlusal plane should be at proper level.

## Physiological Factors

***Saliva:*** The viscosity of saliva determines retention. Thick and ropy saliva leads to loss of retention. Thin and watery saliva also lead to compromised retention.
In ptyalism patient suffers from gagging sensation and in xerostomia dentures can produce soreness and irritation.

## Physical Factors

- Adhesion.
- Cohesion.
- Interfacial surface tension.
- Capillarity or capillary attraction.
- Atmospheric pressure and peripheral seal.
- Gravity.

### *Adhesion*

Adhesion is defined as, "The physical attraction of unlike molecules to one another." –GPT.
Saliva is very important for adhesion. A thin film of saliva aids in wetting the tissue surface of the denture and the mucosa. The amount of adhesion present is proportional to the denture base area.

Denture base materials that help in wetting have better retention by adhesion than materials that cause drops of water to form over their surfaces. Thick ropy saliva is formed by palatal glands tends to displace denture by hydraulic pressure.

### *Cohesion*

Cohesion is defined as, "The physical attraction of like molecules for each other".

The cohesive forces act within the thin film of saliva. The greater the denture bearing area, more effective is cohesion. Thin film of saliva is more cohesive than thick mucus saliva.

### *Interfacial Surface Tension*

Interfacial surface tension is defined as, " The tension or resistance to separation possessed by the film of liquid between two well-adapted surfaces." –GPT.

These forces are found within the thin film of saliva separating the denture base from the tissues which in turn resist the displacing forces. It plays a major role in the retention of a maxillary denture. This force is dependant on the presence of air at the margins of liquid and solid contact (liquid-air interface).

*Factors affecting interfacial surface tension:*

1. Consistency of Saliva. (Should be thin and even).
2. Perfect fit of the denture base.
3. Maximum coverage of basal seat area.
4. Good adhesive and cohesive forces, which aid to enhance interfacial surface tension.

### *Capillary Attraction*

Capillarity or capillary attraction is defined as, "That quality or state, because of surface tension causes elevation or depression of the surface of a liquid that is in contact with a solid."–GPT

Capillary attraction is a phenomenon in which a liquid tends to rise in a capillary tube by maximizing its contact along the walls of the tube at the interface between the liquid and glass. When there is close adaptation between the denture and the mucosa, thin film of saliva tends to flow and increase its surface contact thereby increasing the retention.

*Factors that aid to improve capillary attraction:*

- Good adaptation of denture base to soft tissue.
- Greater surface of the denture-bearing area.
- Thin film of saliva.

### *Atmospheric Pressure and Peripheral Seal*

Peripheral seal is the area of contact between the peripheral borders of the denture and the resilient-limiting structures which prevents air entry between the denture and the soft tissue. A good peripheral seal will have the denture borders resting on soft and resilient tissues. When displacing forces act on the denture, a partial vacuum (natural suction) is produced between the denture and the soft tissues, which aids in retention.

Hence, atmospheric pressure is referred to as emergency-retentive force or temporary-restraining force.

*Factors affecting atmospheric pressure*

- Good peripheral seal.
- Perfect fit of denture.
- Maximum coverage of basal seat.

## Mechanical Factors

- Undercuts
- Balanced occlusion
- Springs
- Magnets
- Denture adhesives
- Suction chambers and suction discs
- Gum Tragacanth.

***Undercuts:*** Unilateral undercuts aid in retention while bilateral undercuts will interfere with denture insertion and require surgical correction.

***Magnetic forces:*** Intramucosal magnets aid in increasing retention of highly resorbed ridges.

***Denture adhesives:*** They are available as creams or gels or powders. They should be coated on the tissue surface before wearing the denture.

***Suction chambers and suction discs:*** The suction chamber creates an area of negative pressure, which increases retention. But can also cause palatal hyperplasia.

***Surgical factors:*** Vestibuloplasty, Zygomaticoplasty, Tuberoplasty, Ridge augmentation procedures and implants.

***Psychologic factors:*** as Patient tolerance and patient education.

## 7. Define PPS. Describe various methods to record PPS and its advantages and disadvantages.

Posterior palatal seal (PPs) is defined as, "The soft tissues along the junction of the hard and soft palates on which pressure within the physiologic limits of the tissues can be applied by a denture to aid in the retention of the denture." (GPT) (Fig. 8)

### FACTORS IMPORTANT IN RECORDING PPS

- 1 to 2 mm distal to the expected denture border should be present in the impression tray
- Determine the type of soft palate classification.
- The "post-dam" should be located by the dentist.

### TECHNIQUES TO RECORD PPS

Marc Appelbaum (1979) reported the different techniques:
- Conventional Approach by Hardy and Kapur 1958
- Fluid Wax Technique Nelson 1970
- Arbitrary Scraping of Master Cast by Boucher

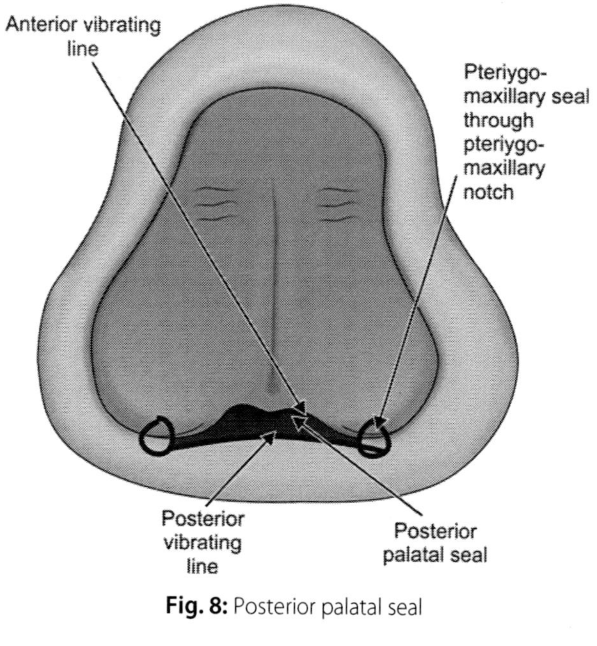


**Fig. 8:** Posterior palatal seal

- Adding a Posterior Palatal Seal to an Existing Denture by Moghadam and Scandrett 1974
- Extended palate technique by Silverman 1971
- Semi-physiologic method by Calamini.

## CONVENTIONAL APPROACH

- An accurate and fully extended final impression on which shellac or resin tray is made.
- Ask the patient to rinse with an astringent mouthwash and dry the PPS region.
- Locate the hamular processes with ("T" burnisher or mouth mirror) and mark with an indelible pencil.
- Locate pterygomaxillary notch and mark the notch and extend 3 to 4 mm anterolateral to the tuberosity, approximating the mucogingival junction. Repeat on opposite side and the outlining of the pterygomaxillary seal is complete.
- The patient is asked to say "ah" in short bursts meanwhile observe the movement of the soft palate between shallow displacement and marked muscular activity, the posterior vibrating line is marked with an indelible pencil.
- Connect the posterior vibrating line through the pterygomaxillary seal and ask the patient to keep the mouth open.
- The resin or shellac tray is then inserted and seated firmly in the mouth and the lines marked should have been transferred to the tray.
- The tray is then returned to the master cast to complete the transfer of the posterior border.
- Locating the anterior vibrating line with the "T" burnisher. It is the compressible tissue anterior to the Posterior vibrating line. The use of the Valsalva maneuver or visualizing the area while the patient says "ah" with short vigorous bursts may also be used. This line is marked with an indelible pencil and transferred to the master cast.
- The visual outline is in the shape of Cupid's bow. The area between the anterior and posterior vibrating lines is usually narrowest in the midpalatal region because of the projection of the posterior nasal spine.
- A Kingsley scraper is then used to score the cast. The deepest areas of the seal are located on either side of the midline, one-third the distance anteriorly from the posterior vibrating line and it is scraped to a depth of approximately 1 to 1. 5 mm.
- The median palatal raphe has little submucosa and hence, this area is scraped to a depth of approximately 0. 5 to 1. 0 mm only.
- As the seal approaches the anterior vibrating line there is just a slight scraping of the cast. Posterior to the deepest portion of the seal, is also tapered to the posterior vibrating line. If the seal is not tapered it may lead to tissue irritation.
- If a shellac tray is used, moisten the cast and readapt shellac to the scored cast, check the retention in the mouth by asking the patient to say "ah" in a short, unexaggerated manner. If no space is noted between the trial base and the soft palate then an adequate posterior seal has been created.
- If a resin tray is used, add small amounts of autopolymerizing resin until a good seal is achieved. Use separating medium.

### Advantages of Conventional Method

1. As the trial base has good retention, recording of jaw relation is accurate.
2. Patients will be ensured of good retentive complete denture prosthesis as they are able to experience the retentive qualities of the trial base.

3. The practitioner will be able to assess the retentive qualities of the finished denture.
4. The new denture wearer will be able to realize the posterior extent of the denture.

### Disadvantages of Conventional Approach

1. Not a physiologic technique and hence depends upon accurate transfer of the vibrating lines and careful scraping of the cast.
2. Potential for over compression of the tissues.

## FLUID WAX TECHNIQUE

After the transfer markings are copied on to the final impression as (Zinc oxide eugenol or plaster) same method as Conventional technique.

Any one of four types of wax can be used (Iowa wax, white, developed by Dr Earl S Smith; Korecta wax No. 4, orange, developed by Dr OC Applegate; H-L physiologic paste, yellow-white, developed by Dr CS Harkins; or Adaptol, green, developed by Nathan G. Kaye).

These waxes are designed to flow at mouth temperature and are painted onto the impression surface within the outline of the seal area after melting.

The impression is carried to the mouth and held in place under gentle pressure for four to six minutes to allow time for the material to flow.

A 30° flexion of the head and the tongue is firmly positioned against the mandibular anterior teeth (handle). The patient is asked to periodically rotate the head so that all functional positions of the soft palate are recorded.

If the tissue has been contacted, the wax will have a glossy appearance. Wherever it appears dull more wax should be added and procedure repeated.

The secondary impression is reinserted and held for three to five minutes under gentle pressure, followed by two to three minutes of firm pressure applied to the midpalatal area of the impression tray. During this time, the head and tongue positions must be maintained.

### Advantages

1. It is a physiologic technique displacing tissues within their physiologically acceptable limits.
2. Over compression of tissues is avoided.
3. Posterior palatal seal is incorporated into the trial denture base for added retention.
4. Mechanical scraping of the cast is avoided.

### Disadvantages

1. More time is necessary during the impression appointment.
2. Difficulty in handling the materials and added care during the boxing procedure.

## ARBITRARY SCRAPING OF MASTER CAST

This technique is the least accurate as it relies on the dentist's recollection of the palatal configuration and tissue compressibility to locate the anterior and posterior vibrating lines and the depth to which the cast should be scraped.

### Disadvantages

1. Underextension
   a. As a result of the practitioner's use of the fovea palatini as the landmark for terminating the denture base depriving 4 to 12 mm of tissue coverage, which can improve the retention of the denture.

b. If the hard and soft palates and the accurate marking of the vibrating lines are not carried out, the proper posterior border extension cannot be determined.
c. When the laboratory technician is asked to trim and polish the processed denture borders.

2. Underpostdamming
When the mouth is in the wide-open position, the pterygomandibular fold becomes taut. When the patient assumes any position other than a wide-open position, a space will be present between the denture base and the tissue, since the fold is no longer activated. The diagnosis of this condition consists of placing the wet denture base into the mouth and slowly pressing in the midpalate region until it is firmly seated, all the while observing the distal denture border. If air bubbles can be seen escaping from beneath the distal border, then at that point the denture base is underpostdammed.
3. Overpostdamming
If excessively overpostdammed upon denture insertion the posterior border will be displaced inferiorly. If it is moderately overpostdammed, tissue irritation will be seen across the posterior palatal region.
4. Overextension
If over extended the patient complaints that swallowing is painful and difficult. Small ulcerated areas in the region of the soft palate will be seen. Mark these lesions and transfer them to the denture base, the precise position of the overextension can be removed with a bur and then carefully repolished.
If the denture base covers the hamuli, the patient will experience sharp pain, especially during function.

## ADDING A POSTERIOR PALATAL SEAL TO AN EXISTING DENTURE

Only if the existing prosthesis has correct esthetic, phonetic requirements, proper vertical dimension and centric relation positions with proper denture border extensions then only correction of posterior seal area is done. If not a new prosthesis is the option.

### Techniques

1. Fluid wax technique.
2. Softened green stick modelling compound.
3. A combination of fluid wax and green stick compound.
4. Using Light cured resin.

### Fluid Wax Technique

Moghadam and Scandrett suggested this procedure. All of the steps outlined for locating, marking and placing the wax in the seal area are same except that the wax is placed on the processed denture base.

After the wax has flown adequately, the denture is removed from the mouth and the anterior extent of the seal is marked on the denture.

Utility wax is placed vertically across the palate, separating the posterior two-third from the anterior region and extended around the posterior portion of the denture.

Dental stone is vibrated into the denture-wax surface outlined by the utility wax.

After the stone has set, the wax is eliminated, the denture cleaned and the area distal to the anterior vibrating line is ground.

After applying lubricant to the unground areas, including the polished surface and a separating medium is applied to the stone cast, denture is replaced on the stone cast and held firmly with rubber bands.

Acrylic is added till the space between denture and cast is filled. After waiting till the initial set has taken place it is placed in a pressure pot with water (140°F) for 20 minutes under 30 psi pressure.

The cast and denture are separated, the excess acrylic is trimmed and the border polished lightly.

The above procedures can be done using green stick compound (by Carroll and Shaffer) and a combination of both (by Lauciello and Conte) and Light cured resin instead of Fluid wax alone.

Light cured resin allows for accurate placement of the seal by adding material selectively, similar to the fluid wax technique, curing it in stages. The curing procedure requires the use of a high-intensity white light.

### *Advantages*

1. No exothermic reaction to irritate the oral tissues
2. Minimal volumetric shrinkage during curing
3. More closely approximates a physiologic technique
4. Can be performed with relatively little chair time.

The only disadvantage is the cost of the curing unit.

## 8. Stability and support in complete denture.

Stability is defined as, "The quality of a denture to be firm, steady, or constant, to resist displacement by functional stresses and not to be subject to change of position when forces are applied." —GPT

### Factors Affecting Stability

1. Vertical height of the residual ridge:
   A parallel well rounded vertical ridge form offers better stability than resorbed ridges.
2. Quality of soft tissue covering the ridge:
   Firm resilient tissue is able to withstand masticatory forces better stability than thin or flabby tissues.
3. Quality of the impression:
   An impression should be accurate and should duplicate all the details without any voids.
   The impression should be made of dimensionally stable materials and should be poured immediately.
4. Occlusal plane:
   The occlusal plane should be oriented parallel to the ridge maintaining adequate interocclusal distance, this enhances stability.
5. Teeth arrangement:
   The teeth should be arranged in balanced occlusion and neutral zone.
   Balanced occlusion is the simultaneous contacting of the maxillary and mandibular teeth on the right and left and in the anterior and posterior occlusal areas when the jaws are in either centric or eccentric relation.
   Balanced occlusion facilitates the even distribution of forces across the denture. Absence of balanced occlusion lead to loss of stability.

The teeth in the denture should be arranged in the neutral zone. The neutral zone is defined as, "The potential space between the lips and cheeks on one side and the tongue on the other. Natural or artificial teeth in this zone are subject to equal and opposite forces from the surrounding musculature." –GPT

## Contour of the Polished Surface

From the cuspid to the posterior aspect the denture surface slopes slightly inward creating space for buccal corridor. The over all contour of the denture should be in terms with the Neutral zone concept.

**Support** is defined as, "The resistance to vertical forces of mastication, occlusal forces and other forces applied in a direction towards the denture-bearing area."

Maximum coverage provides the "snowshoe" effect, which distributes applied forces over wide an area as possible.

Confining the occlusal forces to stress-bearing areas and reliving the non-stress-bearing areas will aid to improve support.

## Factors affecting stability and support

1. Maximum coverage of the basal seat within the limits of the health and functions of the supporting and limiting tissues.
2. Borders that are in harmony with the anatomic and physiologic limitations of the oral structures.
3. A physiologic type of border-molding procedure.
4. Proper space ensured in tray for final impression material.
5. Selective pressure technique for final impression.
6. Ideal impression material to be used depending on clinical situation.
7. A guiding mechanism for correct positioning of the impression tray in the mouth.
8. The tray and final impression should be of dimensionally stable materials.
9. The completed final impression form is similar to the external form of the completed denture.
10. Accurately fitting final impression tray.

## 9. Explain the role of saliva in denture retention.

## Factors in Denture Retention

### *Extension of denture base:*

- Stensens duct—It is rare for a maxillary denture to cause obstruction to this duct.
- Whartons duct—Extension of the lingual flange in this region can lead to obstruction in which patient complains of swelling under the tongue while eating.
- Sublingual—It is rare for a denture to cause any significant obstruction.

### Amount of Saliva

- Excess saliva will affect the impression making procedure and in turn the final denture.
- Dry mouth will affect the retention of the denture and result in soreness of mucosa.
- When new dentures are worn for the first time increased salivation is seen in some patients and these patients need to be told that over a period of time salivary flow will come to normal.

### Consistency

Best to work with a serous type of saliva.

Thick saliva decreases complete denture retention, create hydrostatic pressure in the area anterior to the posterior palatal seal and results in a downward dislodging force.

Thick saliva also complicates impression making by forming voids in the impression surface.

Hence before impression making the palatal surface should be wiped free of saliva and the mucus glands massaged with a piece of gauze to eliminate as much as mucus as possible.

## Role of Saliva in Denture Retention

The physical forces in which saliva is involved are:
- Adhesion
- Cohesion
- Atmospheric pressure
- Capillary attraction
- Peripheral seal
- Viscosity of saliva and surface tension.

### Adhesion

- Adhesion is the physical attraction of unlike molecules for each other.
- It acts when saliva sticks and wets the basal surface of the dentures and at the same time to the mucous membrane. Watery saliva is quite effective, provided the denture base material can be wetted.
- Saliva that is thick and ropy adheres well to both the denture base and the mucosa; but the hydraulic pressure produced by the thick mucus secretion over power the adhesive forces of the denture and dislodge the denture.

#### Cohesion

- Cohesion is the retentive force that occurs in the layer of saliva between the denture base and the mucosa. To be effective the saliva should form a thin lager.

#### Interfacial surface tension

- Interfacial surface tension is the resistance to separation possessed by the film of liquid between two well adapted surfaces. It is found in the thin film of saliva which is similar in its action to cohesion and to capillary attraction.

#### Capillary attraction

- Capillary attraction is a force that causes the surface of a liquid to become elevated or depressed when it is in contact with a solid.

#### Peripheral seal

- Developed with the proper extension of the denture into the vestibule.
- Denture border merging against the mucosal border assembled by a thin film of saliva provides border seal as it prevents ingress of air, thus enabling the denture to be in their position.

#### Viscosity of saliva

The force required to displace a denture is proportional to the viscosity of saliva fluid film and the square of area of the denture and inversely proportional to the square of the distance separating denture from the supporting tissues and the time of force application.

Degree of retention possessed by the denture depends on the area of its fitting surface degree of closeness of fit and viscosity of the saliva.

The glycoproteins and the proteoglycans dissolved in the saliva increase the viscosity and provide it with pseudo plastic properties. When mastication is not taking place, saliva acts as a semisolid. In mouth the dentures are not immersed all the time, hence a meniscus can form at the periphery and surface tension can be included as a factor.

### 10. Describe the anatomy of TMJ in brief and add a note on the components of TMJ in detail.

#### Introduction

Temporomandibular joint (TMJ) or Craniomandibular joint found only in mammals is formed by the articulation of mandibular condyle at the base of the cranium with the squamous part of temporal bone.

#### SYNONYMS

Ginglymoid joint—As it provides hinging movement in forward and backward direction
Biarthrodial joint—As it provides gliding movement.
Ginglymo-arthroidal joint —As it provides both hinging and gliding movement
Modified ball and socket joint—As it allows movements in three planes (sagittal, transverse and coronal).
Compound joint—As the articular disc functionally serves as a non-ossified bone that permits the complex movements of the joints.

#### Functions of TMJ

Voluntary movements such as mastication, deglutition, phonation, and reflex actions such as grasping and yawning.

#### Development of TMJ

- The TMJ begins to develop by the 10th week of gestation from two separate blastemas -one for the temporal bone component and one for the condyle.
- Superior to the condylar blastema a band of mesenchymal cell develops that will eventually differentiate into the disc.
- Temporal condylar mesenchymal cell differentiate into osteoblasts which lay down membrane bone, from 12–32 weeks of gestation and there is a high degree of calcification of the condylar head.
- The developing TMJ shows all components of the mature joint by 14th week of gestation.

#### Histology of the articular surfaces composed of 4 distinct layers of zones:

1. Articular zone—Superficial layer adjacent to the joint cavity made of dense fibrous connective tissue
2. Proliferative zone—Undifferentiated mesenchymal tissue responsible for the proliferation of articular cartilage in response to functional demands placed in the articular surfaces during loading.
3. Fibrocartilaginous zone—Collagen fibers are arranged in bundles in a crossing pattern.
4. Calcified cartilage zone—Deepest zone composed of chondrocytes and chondroblasts

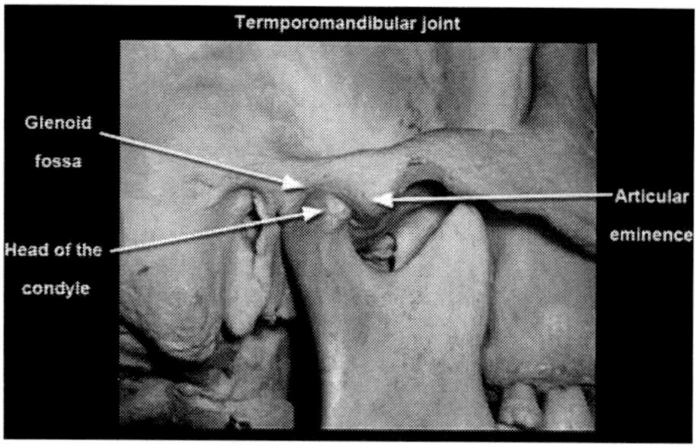


**Fig. 9:** Termporomandibular joint

**Articular eminence**—Is a small prominence on the zygomatic arch.
**Postglenoid tubercle**—Separates articular surface of fossa laterally from tympanic plate.
**Glenoid fossa**—Is the anterior articular area formed by the inferior aspect of squamous part of temporal bone. It acts as partition between middle cranial fossa and joint lined by dense avascular fibrocartilage. Posterior wall of glenoid fossa is formed by tympanic plate, separated by squamotympanic fissure.

## Components of TMJ (Figs 9 and 10)

- Cranial component
- Mandibular component.

*Cranial Component*

Are bounded anteriorly by Articular eminence and posteriorly by post-glenoid tubercle.

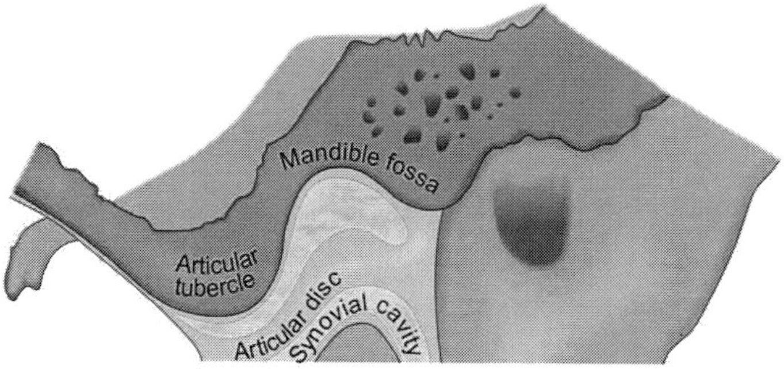


**Fig. 10:** Components of temporomandibular joint (TMJ)

### *Mandibular Component*

Condyle which is ovoid in shape with narrow neck forms the articular part of the mandible. It is broad laterally and narrows medially with a mediolateral width of 13–25 mm and anteroposterior width of 5.5–16 mm. It is convex in all direction and covered by fibrocartilaginous tissue.

## Clinical Anatomy of TMJ Components

A. Capsule
B. Ligaments of TMJ
C. Glenoid fossa
D. Condyle
E. Articular disc (meniscus)
F. Synovial membrane
G. Vascular supply and innervation
H. Musculature.

## A. Capsule

- Fibroelastic, highly vascular and highly innervated dense connective tissue
- Funnel shaped, blends with periosteum of mandibular neck and envelops meniscus
- Laterally—zygomatic tubercle, lateral rim of glenoid fossa, post glenoid tubercle
- Medially—medial rim of glenoid fossa (closely related to spine of sphenoid
- Sphenomandibular ligament, middle meningeal artery passing through foramen spinosum
- Anteriorly—anterior border of articular eminence
- Posteriorly—squamotympanic fissure and fuses with superior stratum of post-bilaminar zone (b/w post-capsule and post-glenoid tubercle-highly vascular tissue)
- Superiorly—circumference of cranial articulating surface
- Inferiorly—neck of condyle
- Inside lined by silky synovial membrane.

## B. Ligaments

These are composed of collagenous connective tissue and act predominantly as restraints to motion of the condyle and the disc.

The three functional ligaments are: Collateral ligaments, Capsular ligament and Temporomandibular ligament. The two accessory ligaments are Sphenomandibular ligament and Stylomandibular ligament.

## C. Articular Disc

- Dense, non-vascular, non-innervated fibrous connective tissue
- Biconcave in sagittal section
- Anatomically divided into three zones
  1. Anterior band.
  2. Central intermediate zone (Thinnest)
  3. Posterior band (Thicker)
- The intermediate zone is the area of function between mandibular condyle and temporal bone.
- Articular disc is attached to the capsular ligament anteriorly, posteriorly, medially and laterally. Anterior attachment of the meniscus is contiguous with the lateral pterygoid muscle
- Retrodiscal tissue - Posteriorly tissues are highly vascularized and innervated – bilaminar zone (involved in production of synovial fluid).

### D. Articular disc divides the joint into superior and inferior compartment

Superior compartment (temporodiscal complex)

- Permits translational movements
- Larger of the two compartments but less reinforced
- Extends further anteriorly than lower joint space
- Has a synovial fluid volume of 1.2 ml.

### E. Inferior compartment (condylodiscal complex)

- Permits rotatory movements
- Smaller, more tightly reinforced by disc attachments
- Has a synovial fluid volume of 0.9 ml.

### F. Synovial membrane

- Lines the joint spaces
- Responsible for secreting synovial fluid (nutrition and lubrication)
- Extremely thin, smooth connective tissue membrane
- Cells in the synovial membrane have the ability to differentiate into chondrocytes.

*Synovial fluid serves two purposes*

- Synovial fluid acts as a medium for providing metabolic requirements.
- Serves as a lubricant between articular surfaces by Boundary lubrication which is the primary mechanism of joint lubrication that prevents friction in the moving joint. The other mechanism is weeping lubrication by which metabolic exchange occurs and to eliminate friction in the compressed but not moving joint.

### G. Nerve supply

- The mandibular nerve innervates the joint.
- Three branches from the mandibular nerve send terminals to the joint capsule.
  - Auriculotemporal nerve (largest)—posterior, medial and lateral part of the joint
  - A branch from the posterior deep temporal nerve
  - Masseteric nerve—anterior part of the joint.

## 11. What are the different methods of registering vertical dimension? Differentiate vertical dimension at rest and vertical dimension at occlusion?

### VERTICAL RELATIONS

The vertical jaw relations are those established by the amount of separation of the maxillae and mandible under specified conditions.

**They are classified as:**

1. The vertical dimension of occlusion
2. Of rest and
3. Other positions.

The vertical dimension of occlusion is established by the natural teeth when they are present and in occlusion (In edentulous patients it is established by the vertical height of the two dentures when the teeth are in contact).

The vertical dimension of rest (or physiologic rest position of the mandible) is established by muscles and gravity. The mandible is in its physiologic rest position when all the muscles that close and open the jaws are in a state of minimal tonic contraction sufficient only to maintain posture.

## SIGNIFICANCE OF VERTICAL RELATIONS

The value of the vertical dimension of rest position in denture construction lies in its use as a guide to the lost vertical dimension of occlusion. The difference between the occlusal vertical dimension and the rest vertical dimension is the interocclusal distance. The interocclusal distance is the distance or gap existing between the upper and lower teeth when the mandible is in the physiologic rest position. It usually is 2 to 4 mm when observed at the position of the first premolars. The clinically recorded rest position is not the same as the electromyographically determined one. A range of reduced muscle tension up to an interocclusal distance of about 10 mm has been reported.

Failure to provide correct interocclusal distance will cause "clicking" of the dentures during speech, soreness of the tissues of the basal seat and rapid destruction of the residual alveolar ridges.

## RECORDING OF VERTICAL RELATIONS

### Two recordings are done

1. Rest position
2. Occlusion position.

### Methods for Recording Vertical Relations

1. Mechanical methods:
   a. Ridge relation—distance of incisive papilla from mandibular incisors and parallelism of ridges.
   b. Measurement of former dentures.
   c. Pre-extraction records—profile photographs, Lead wire adaptation, Face mask method by Swenson, Willis gauge, Dakometer and articulated models.
   d. Post-extraction methods—niswongers method, concept of equal thirds of the face, Boos biometer, Silvermans closest speaking space, electromyography.
2. Physiologic methods:
   a. Physiologic rest position
   b. Phonetics
   c. Esthetics
   d. Swallowing
   e. Tactile sense.

## 1. Recording Rest Position

Following are the few commonly used methods.

1. Facial Measurements:
   Instruct the patient to stand or sit comfortably upright with the eyes looking straight ahead. Insert the maxillary record base with the attached contoured occlusion rim. With either an indelible marker or a triangle of adhesive tape, place a point of reference on the end of the patient's nose and another on the point of the chin. Instruct the patient to wipe the lips with the tongue to swallow and to drop the shoulders. When mandible drops to rest position and then measure between the points with a millimeter ruler. Repeat the procedure until the measurements are consistent.
2. Tactile Sense:
   Then ask them to close slowly until the jaws reach a comfortable, relaxed position. The distance is measured between the points of reference and compared with the measurements made after swallowing.
3. Phonetics:
   Have patients repeat "M" until they are aware of the contacting of the lips as "M" is pronounced. Repeat this procedure and ask that they stop all jaw movement when the lips touch. At this time measure between two points of reference.

## 2. Occlusion Position Recording

### Pre-extraction Records

1. Profile Photographs:
   Measurements of anatomic landmarks on the photograph are compared with measurements using the same anatomic landmarks on the face.
2. Profile Silhouettes
3. Facial Measurements.

### Niswonger's Method

The distance is measured and these measurements are compared with measurements made between these points when the occlusal rims are tried in.

1. Closest speaking space
   The closest speaking space measures vertical dimension when the mandible and muscles involved are in physiologic function of speech. The 'F' or 'V' and 'S' syllables are used in locating closes speaking space.
2. Swallowing followed by Relaxing
   With denture in the mouth, instruct the patient to wipe the lips with the tip of the tongue, swallow and let the shoulders drop in a relaxed position. Watch the reference points and ask the patient to close the teeth together. If the teeth are together, it can indicate that no interocclusal distance exists.
   Another method is based on the theory that teeth make contact at or near centric occlusion. Two small cones of a soft wax are placed, one in each central sulcus of the mandibular first molars. Encourage the patient to swallow several times. If the vertical dimension of occlusion is correct, the wax will be penetrated and reduced to tooth contact.

3. Phonetics

Have the patient repeat these words:

"Three thirty-three"—there should be enough space for the tip of the tongue to protrude between the anterior teeth.

"Fifty-five"— incisal edges of the maxillary central incisors should contact the vermilion border of the lower lip at the junction of the moist and dry mucosa.

"Emma and Mississippi"—the teeth should not contact.

### Following are the some of the tests when the occlusion rims are placed in the mouth:

1. Judgment of the overall facial support.
2. When the patient closes jaw slowly until lips just touch, at this point mandible is at rest position. The lips are in constrained contact. Next ask the patient to close the jaw so that in closing through the interocclusal distance there is little or no movement of the lips. If patient has decreased vertical relation that is increased interocclusal distance, the lips close excessively, fold together and vermilion tend to disappear.
3. Visual observation of the amount of space between the rims when the jaws are at rest.
4. Measurements between dots on the face when the jaws are at rest and when occlusion rims in contact.
5. Observation made when sibilant - containing words are pronounced to ensure that occlusion rim come close together but do not contact.

## 12. Define face bow, its use and enumerate the steps in use of face-bow in complete denture fabrication.

Face-bow is a caliper-like device that is used to record the relationship of the jaws to the temporomandibular joints or the opening axis of the jaws and to orient the casts in this same relationship to the opening axis of the articulator.

### USES OF FACE-BOW

1. When cusp form teeth are used.
2. When balanced occlusion in the eccentric positions is desired.
3. When a definite cusp fossa or cusp tip to cusp incline relation is needed.
4. Interocclusal check records after face-bow transfer aid in verifying of jaw positions.
5. If the occlusal vertical dimension is changed and the alterations of tooth occlusal surfaces are necessary to accommodate the change.

### FACE-BOW TRANSFER PROCEDURE

### Preliminary Steps

1. The patient's head should be in an upright position and well supported.
2. Mark on skin or on adhesive tape the axis points by measuring 12 mm anterior to the middle of the tragus of the ear on a line drawn from the outer canthus of the eye to the middle of the tragus of the ear.

3. Contour the maxillary occlusion rim, establish the occlusal plane, mark the point of low lip line on the occlusal rims and a mounting index on the occlusal surface in the regions of the first molars.
4. Apply a thin layer of petrolatum to the occlusion rims to facilitate separating from the wax on the bite fork.
5. Reduce the mandibular occlusion rim to allow space for the fork and attached wax.
6. Adjust the condyle rods to the face for centering the bow by placing the ends over the marked points on the skin. Secure either the right or left condyle rod; lock and remove the bow from the face.

## Face-bow Record

1. A 6 mm thick horseshoe-shaped soften baseplate wax is rolled together and the prongs of the bite fork is embedded in it.
2. Fold the wax over at the margins to secure it to the fork.
3. Place the prongs of the bite fork with the attached soft wax between the occluding surfaces of the occlusion rims. Adjust the midline of the fork to coincide with the midline on the occlusion rim. Extend the stem of the fork forward and parallel to the sagittal plane.
4. Slide the stem of the fork through the opening in the clamp of the bow and adjust the width of the condyle rods equidistant bilaterally and secure the clamp of the bow to the stem of the bite fork.
5. Slide the condyle rods from the skin. Extend the condyle rods back to the axis points to countercheck.
6. If the infraorbital notch is used as the anterior point of reference, the infraorbital notch is located and marked. Place the point of the pointer over the mark and secure the clamp to the pointer. Remove the assembly from the face and allow the wax to set hard before removing the bite fork and face-bow record from the occlusion rims.

## Face-bow Mounting

1. Set the sliding condylar rods symmetrically on both sides over the articulator condyle shaft.
2. Raise or lower the face-bow to adjust until the low lip line, which was recorded on the labial surface of the occlusion rim, is on a level with the groove marked around the incisal pin.
3. Adjust infraorbital pointer to touch the pointer plate attached to the maxillary bow of the articulator.
4. Support the face-bow securely in position with the face-bow support.
5. Soak the maxillary cast in water for at least five minutes.
6. Secure the incisal guide pin with its top flush with the top of the maxillary bow of the articulator. Open the maxillary bow of the articulator and apply dental plaster to the top of the articulator until the incisal guide pin is stopped on the guide table and the mounting plate on the maxillary bow is embedded in the plaster.
7. Remove the excess plaster. After the plaster hardens remove the face-bow assembly. The maxillary cast is related to the opening axis in the articulator in the same anteroposterior and horizontal position as the maxillae in the skull are related to the arbitrarily located opening axis in the temporomandibular joints.
8. When the record bases, occlusion rims and interocclusal relations are satisfactory a tentative centric relation record with the jaws at the vertical dimension of occlusion is made and other records as right and left lateral records and protrusive records are made later.

## 13. Define face-bow. Classify face-bows. Mention the parts of facia type of face-bow. Discuss the use of face-bow.

### DEFINITION

Face-bow is a caliper-like device that is used to record the relationship of the jaws to the temporomandibular joints or the opening axis of the jaws and to orient the casts in this same relationship to the opening axis of the articulator.

### TYPES OF FACE-BOW

A. Arbitrary: Has two types : Ear piece face-bow and Facia type of face-bow
B. Kinematic or hinge-bow.

### 1. Arbitrary

1. The arbitrary face-bow is placed on the face with the condyle rods located approximately over the condyles.
2. Used in complete denture patients.
3. The condyle rods are positioned on a line extending from the outer canthus to the tip of the tragus and 13 mm in front of the external auditory meatus locating the rods within 5 mm of the true center of the opening axis of the jaws. (Facia type) Hanau Model C. Without clamping the condyle rods, the dentist center the device so equal readings are obtained on both sides and the wing nut of the clamp is tightened to hold the face bow in place on the occlusal fork.
4. The rods of another are designed to fit into the external auditory meatuses (Ear piece type)–WhipMix.

The fork of arbitrary face-bow is attached to the maxillary occlusion rim. Transverse axis of the articulator is 5/8 inch (15 mm anterior to the position of the ends of the face-bow).

This distance compensates for the distance between the external auditory meatus and the condyle.

### 2. Kinematic Face-bow

- The kinematic face-bow is so designed that the opening axis of the mandible can be located more accurately.
- The fork of kinematic face-bows is attached to the mandibular occlusion rim.
- As the patient retrudes the mandible and opens and closes the jaws, the movement of the points of the condyle rods are observed.
- As the condyle rods of kinematic face-bows have sharp points, their motion can be observed more accurately.
- When the points rotate only and do not translate, they are on the opening axis of the jaw.
- At this position the mandible is in centric relation for the occlusal vertical dimension that has been established. After the hinge axis center is located it is marked on the face with indelible pencil. The face-bow is now used in the regular manner by being fastened into place over the previously determined rotational points. This type of transfer will be exact in the positional relation of the cast and will permit a recording medium (as wax, zinc oxide-eugenol or plaster) for interocclusal records without usual inaccuracy being produced. This is important when the interarch distance is to be increased or decreased.

- Kinematic face-bow can aid in recording centric relation.

The difficulty of attaching the lower occlusion rim to an edentulous mandible and movement of the recording base on the jaw makes determining the exact center of the opening axis difficult hence, preventing its use for edentulous patients.

Aids in finding the appropriate vertical dimension clinically and does not change in the articulator.

## USES OF FACE-BOW

1. It supports the casts while they are being attached to the articulator.
2. When cusp form teeth are used.
3. When balanced occlusion in the eccentric positions is desired.
4. When a definite cusp fossa or cusp tip to cusp incline relation is needed.
5. Interocclusal check records after face-bow transfer aid in verifying of jaw positions.
6. If the occlusal vertical dimension is changed and the alterations of tooth occlusal surfaces are necessary to accommodate the change.

## PARTS OF FACE-BOW (FIG. 11)

It consists of a U-shaped frame or assembly that is large enough to extend from the region of the TMJs to a position 2 to 3 inches (5 to 7. 5 cm) in front of the face and wide enough to avoid contact with the sides of the face.

The parts that contact the skin over the TMJs are the condyle rods. The part that attaches to the occlusion rims is the fork. The fork attaches to the face-bow by means of a locking device, which serves also to support the face-bow, the occlusion rims and the casts while the casts are being attached to the articulator.

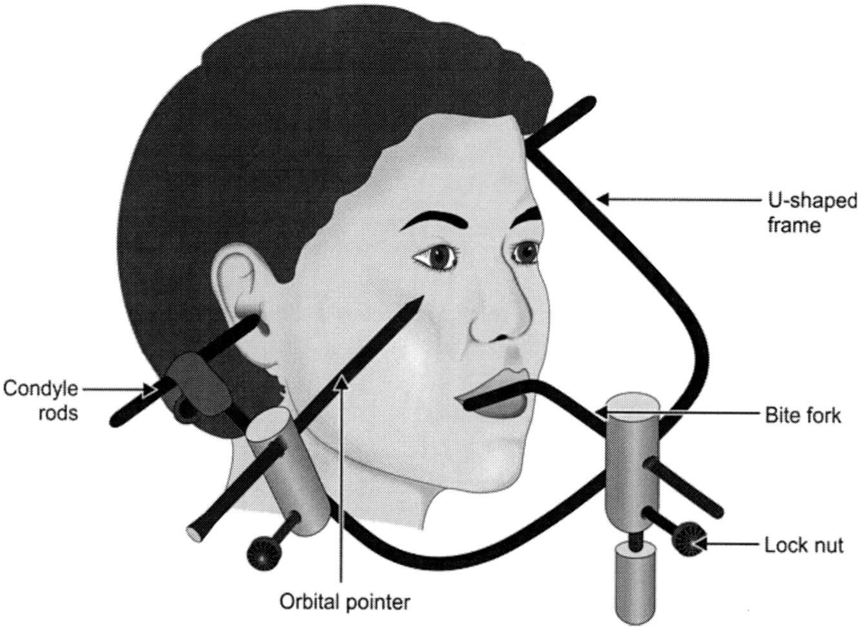


**Fig. 11:** Parts of a facia face bow

For the success of the complete denture, factors as evaluation of occlusion, denture stability, retention, and conditions of denture bearing tissues, together with patient satisfaction and adaptation, apart from an accurate Face-Bow transfer is important.

## 14. Define centric relation. Classify the methods of registering centric relation in completely edentulous mouth and describe any one method in detail.

### DEFINITION

The maxillomandibular relationship in which the condyles articulate with the thinnest avascular portion of their respective discs with the complex in the anterosuperior position against the shapes of the articular eminences.

### Methods of Recording

1. Minimal closing pressure:
   So tissue supporting the bases will not be displaced while the recording is made.
   Opposing teeth to touch uniformly and simultaneously at their first contact.
2. Heavy closing pressure:
   So the tissues under the recording bases will be displaced while the record is being made.
   Same displacement of soft tissues as could exist when heavy closing pressures are applied on the denture.
   Clinical experience and empirical data seem to endorse use of minimal closing pressure.

**The above concepts are otherwise classified as:**

1. Static
   a. Extraoral
   b. Intraoral
2. Functional
   a. Extraoral
   b. Intraoral

Centric relation record is made at the correct occlusal vertical dimension. At the correct occlusal vertical dimension, the patient is asked to relax as much as possible and the dentist guides mandible into a retruded position. This method is passive method. The second method is active method in which the patient responds to instructions by actively retruding the mandible.

**Methods for assisting the patient to retrude the mandible:**

1. Instruct the patient by saying "let your jaw relax, pull it back, close slowly and easily on your back teeth."
2. Instruct the patient by saying "get the feeling of pushing your upper jaw out and closing your back teeth together".
3. Instruct the patient to protrude and retrude the mandible repeatedly while he holds his fingers lightly against his chin.
4. Instruct the patient to turn the tongue backward towards the posterior border of the upper denture.
5. Instruct the patient to tap the occlusal rims of back teeth together repeatedly.
6. Tilt the patient's head back while the various exercises just listed are carried out.
7. Palpate the temporal and masseter muscles to relax them.

## Methods

1. Extraoral tracing devices:
   A needlepoint tracing made on a tracing table coated with carbon or wax can be used to indicate the relative position of upper and lower jaws in the horizontal plane. These tracings are shaped like a gothic arch and therefore are referred to as "gothic arch tracings". Also known as "arrow point tracings".
2. Intraoral tracing devices:
   A hole may be drilled in the plate at the apex of the intraoral tracing or a plastic disc with a hole in it may be placed over the apex of the tracing. The hole or the depression is used to ensure that the patient's jaw is in the retruded position while the registration is being done with plaster or some such material.
3. Other methods:
   Heat the surface of one of the rims and have the patient close into this softened surface to make a new maxillomandibular relation impression.
   Soften the wax rims by deep heating posterior portion of the mandibular wax rim and leaving the anterior portion cool to maintain the predetermined vertical dimension of occlusion. Deep heating is referred to as Pooling. The heated portion will readily collapse under closing pressure. Swallowing method: when swallowing the jaws go back to centric and cones of wax are compressed against maxillary occlusal rims.
   Chewing records.

## Intraocclusal Centric Relation Records in Detail

After establishing the vertical dimension record, 3 mm of wax from the mandibular rim is removed from the first premolar area both on right and left sides.

Cut 2 or 3 notches on the corresponding maxillary rim.

After lubricating this surface with petrolatum place both the upper and lower rim in the patient's mouth.

Check for any interferences and train the patient to close in centric relation by assisting the patient in retruding the mandible by placing the index fingers on the buccal flanges of the mandibular occlusal rim in both premolar regions with the thumbs under the patient's chin.

Instruct the patient to close slowly and gently on the back teeth, if centric relation position satisfactory, soft Alu wax or bite registration paste is placed from where 3 mm of wax was removed.

The registration material should be placed 1 ½ mm above the original height of the rim.

If Alu wax is used then place the mandibular base in warm water as to soften the wax evenly.

After the registration material is placed, the patient is guided in retruding the jaw and closing it slowly with minimum force until the anterior occlusal rims are within ½ mm of the original accepted occlusal vertical dimension.

Trim the excess material from the buccal and lingual sides and recheck to see if the bases contact simultaneously and in the proper position.

## 15. Define centric relation and explain graphic methods in detail.

## DEFINITION

The maxillomandibular relationship in which the condyles articulate with the thinnest avascular portion of their respective discs with the complex in the anterosuperior position against the shapes of the articular eminences.

## GRAPHIC METHODS

These methods use graphs or tracings to record the centric jaw relation. Graphic methods are of two types:

a. Arrow point tracing
b. Pantograph.

The arrow point tracing is a graphic record measured in a single plane whereas the pantograph is measured three-dimensionally.

### Factors affecting accuracy of graphic tracing

1. Stability of the denture base.
2. Resistance by the occlusal rims against occlusal forces.
3. Difficulty in placing the central-bearing device in certain clinical situations.
4. Presence of flabby tissue.
5. Height of the residual alveolar ridge.
6. Interference from the tongue.
7. Efficiency of the recording devices.
8. Obtaining a pointed apex in the tracing pattern.
9. Lack of coordinated movement can cause double tracing.
10. The graphic tracing should harmonize with the centric relation and centric occlusion.

### Arrow Point Tracing

It is a single plane graphic tracing using an arrow-point tracer. The characteristic pattern created is called a central arrow-point tracing.

It is defined as, "The pattern obtained on the horizontal plate used with a central-bearing tracing device."–GPT

The apex of the arrow point tracing gives the centric relation.

### Parts of the tracer

A pen-like pointer is attached to one occlusal rim and a recording plate is placed on the other rim. When the mandible moves the pointer draws characteristic patterns on the recording plate.

The pointer is known as the central-bearing point and the recording plate is known as the central bearing plate. The pointer and the plate together are called as the central-bearing device.

Central-bearing device is defined as, "A device that provides a central point of bearing or support between the maxillary and mandibular dental arches. First attributed to Alfred Gysi, Swiss Prosthodontist, in 1910."

It is a triangular plate of metal with a central metal pointer and with extensions to attach itself to the occlusal rim. The pointer in the center can be adjusted in height. It is usually attached to the mandibular occlusal rim, also can be attached to the maxillary rim.

Central bearing plate is a triangular piece of metal with extensions at the three corners provided to attach the plate to the maxillary occlusal rim. A mixture of denatured spirit and precipitated chalk is coated on this plate and when the spirit dries, a fine layer of precipitated chalk is left behind. The tracing is marked on this layer of precipitated chalk.

### Types of arrow point tracers (Based on the location of the tracer)

- Intraoral tracers
- Extraoral tracers.

## Intraoral Arrow Point Tracers

The central bearing device is located intraorally and hence the name.

### *Procedure*

1. The central bearing point and the central-bearing plate (coated with chalk) attached to record bases are inserted into the patient's mouth.
2. The central bearing point is adjusted to a predetermined vertical dimension such that it contacts the central-bearing plate when the patient closes his mouth.
3. When the patient is asked to make anteroposterior and lateral movements, the central-bearing point will draw the tracing pattern on the central-bearing plate.
4. After completing the movements, the tracing should resemble an arrow point with a sharp apex. If the apex is blunt, the record is repeated.

### *Disadvantages*

1. The tracer is not visible during the procedure.
2. The size of the tracing is very small, hence to determine the apex of the tracing is difficult.
3. It cannot be used in patients who cannot retract the tongue and in cases of macroglossia.

## Extraoral Arrow Point Tracers

The concept is same as for intraoral tracer.

### *Parts of Extraoral Tracers* (Fig. 12)

Central-bearing device attached to the occlusal rims (central bearing point and central bearing plate).

Extraoral tracing pointer attached to maxillary rim.

Recording plates are attached to mandibular rim.

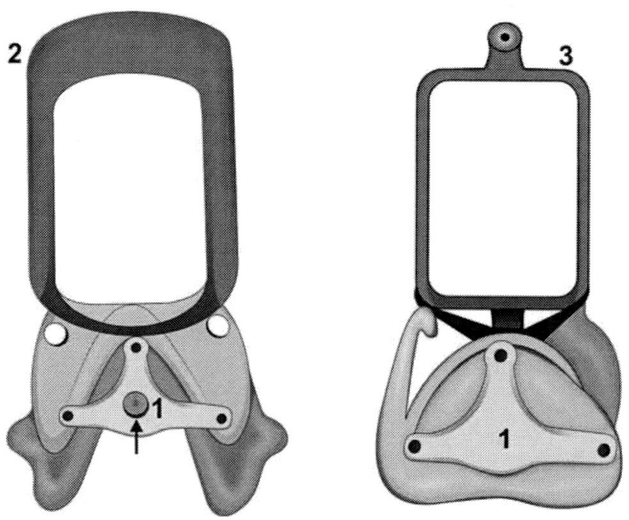


1. Central bearing plate
2. Tracing plate (Mandibular Rim)
3. Needle point tracer (Attached to maxillary rim)

**Fig. 12:** Extraoral tracer

### *Procedure*

1. A tentative vertical dimension is established.
2. The maxillary cast is mounted in the articulator using face-bow transfer and mandibular cast is positioned against the maxillary in a tentative centric relation and articulated.
3. The mandibular occlusal rim is reduced to obtain interocclusal distance.
4. The recording plate is attached to the mandibular occlusal rim coinciding with the midline of the rim.
5. The stylus or the central bearing point is attached to the maxillary occlusal rim.
6. The record bases attached to the recording devices are inserted in the patient's mouth.
7. The Ney excursion guide can be used to train the patient for proper jaw movements.
8. The recording plate projecting extraorally (attached to the mandibular rim), is coated with precipitated chalk and denatured alcohol.
9. Intraorally, the central-bearing point should touch central-bearing plate at the predetermined vertical dimension.
10. The patient is asked to perform protrusive, lateral and anteroposterior movements.
11. It is an extraoral tracing on the recording plate by the tracing pointer. The tracing should have a sharp apex.
12. After finalising the records, quick setting plaster is injected between the occlusal rims.
13. The assembly is removed and articulated and should be checked using an interocclusal check record.

### *Advantages*

1. Extraoral tracing can be examined as it is made.
2. The size of the tracing pattern is easily seen.
3. The apex can be identified easily.

## Pantographic Tracing

It is defined as, "A graphic record of mandibular movement in three planes as registered by the styli on the recording tables of a pantograph; tracings of mandibular movement recorded on plates in the horizontal and sagittal planes."–GPT

The instrument used to do a pantographic tracing is called a pantographic tracer. A pantographic tracer is defined as, "An instrument used to graphically record one or more planes paths of the mandibular movement and to provide information for the programming of the articulator."–GPT

### *Parts of a pantograph*

A pantographic tracer has six flags (The surface over which the tracing is done is called a flag). A stylus (tracing pointer) is present for each flag (It draws tracing patterns on the flags).

### Location of the flags

Two flags located perpendicular to one another near the condyles. Two for the right and two for the left condylar guidances. They locate the actual (true) hinge axis.

Two flags are placed in the anterior region. They record the anteroposterior movements.

### Advantages

1. Most accurate method available to record centric jaw relation.
2. Eccentric jaw relation can be recorded using these instruments.
3. Used for full-mouth rehabilitation of dentulous patients.

### Disadvantages

1. Are very sophisticated
2. Cannot be used in the fabrication of complete dentures as the complete dentures have a relief factor that aids to compensate for minor fabrication errors.

## 16. Define articulator. Classify articulators and add a note on the advantages of an articulator.

### ARTICULATOR

An articulator may be defined as "a mechanical device that represents the temporomandibular joints and jaw members to which maxillary and mandibular casts may be attached to simulate jaw movement".

### ADVANTAGES OF ARTICULATOR

1. Properly mounted casts gives a better view of the patient's lingual occlusion
2. For a proper occlusal scheme to be developed adequate lingual view is needed.
3. Patient cooperation is not a factor after interocclusal records are obtained.
4. After obtaining interocclusal records complete denture occlusion can be refined on an articulator, as it is difficult to do it in the mouth due to shifting of denture bases and resiliency of the supporting tissues.
5. Less chair time and patient appointment time.
6. More procedures can be delegated to auxiliary personnel.
7. The patient's saliva, tongue and cheeks are not factors when using an articulator.

### CLASSIFICATION OF ARTICULATORS

Articulator classification was based on the instrument's function, instrument capability, intent, registration procedure and registration acceptance.

### A. University of Michigan in 1972

#### Class I

Simple holding instruments capable of accepting a single static registration with possible vertical motion.

#### Class II

Instruments that permit horizontal and vertical motion but do not orient the motion to the temporomandibular joint via a face-bow transfer as:

1. Eccentric motion permitted is based on average or arbitrary values.
2. Eccentric motion permitted is based on theories of arbitrary motion.
3. Eccentric motion permitted is determined by the patient using engraving methods.

#### Class III

Instruments that simulate condylar pathways by average or mechanical equivalents for all or part of the motion, Face-bow transfer is possible.

A. Instruments that accept a static protrusive registration and use equivalents for the rest of the motion.
B. Instruments that accept static lateral protrusive registrations and use equivalents for the rest of the motion.

### Class IV

Instruments that will accept three-dimensional dynamic registrations with face-bow transfer. The cams representing the condylar paths are formed by registrations engraved by the patient. Instruments that have condylar paths that can be angled and customized.

## B. Articulator of Different Classes with Examples

### Class I (Gariot's articulator 1805, Barn Door Hinge)

Instruments in this Class accept a single interocclusal record with vertical motion. The hinge-joint articulator is representative of this Class. J. B. Gariot articulator consisted of a simple hinge with a set screw in the posterior against a metal plate to serve as a vertical stop.

### Class II-A (Grittman, Simplex, by Alfred Gysi)

Instruments in this Class permit eccentric motion based on averages and will not accept a facebow transfer.

Grittman's articulator had the condyles on the lower member and their paths were inclined at 15°. According to Bonwill's triangle, the casts are mounted. (four-inch equilateral triangle from condyle to condyle and to the lower central incisor).

Simplex, designed by Alfred Gysi of Zurich in 1914. The condyles are on the lower member and the condylar paths are inclined at 30°; the incisal guidance is fixed at 60°.

### Class II-B (Maxillomandibular Instrument by Monson)

Instruments in this class permit eccentric motion based on arbitrary theories of motion and will not accept a face-bow transfer. Monson's instrument is based on spherical theory of occlusion, in which each cusp and incisal edge conforms to a segment of the surface of a sphere eight inches in diameter with its center at the glabella. The upper member of the instrument moves anteroposteriorly and mediolaterally.

### Class II-C (House Articulator)

Instruments in this class permit eccentric motion based on engraved records obtained from the patient and will not accept a face-bow transfer. The instrument is adjusted by means of a Needles-House "chew-in", which employs four metal studs in the upper occlusion rim against a lower compound occlusion rim.

### Class III (Hanau-Mate)

It is an arcon instrument and will accept a face-bow transfer. It has an average horizontal condylar guidance of 30° and a Bennett angle of 15°. The incisal guide table has average values of 10° for both protrusive and lateral movements. As this will not accept static protrusive or lateral interocclusal records, it cannot be Classified as III-A or III-B.

### Class III-A (Hanau Model H, by Rudolph Hanau and Dentatus)

Instruments in this Class accept a face-bow transfer and a protrusive interocclusal record. The horizontal condylar inclinations are set by means of a protrusive interocclusal record. The condyles are on the upper member. The Bennett angle (L) was calculated from the horizontal condylar inclination (H) by means of Hanau's equation, $L = (H/8) + 12$. If the horizontal condylar inclination = 30°, then the Bennett angle would be approximately 16.

Another articulator similar to the Hanau Model H is the Dentatus, designed in 1944 in Sweden. In this articulator the upper and lower members can be standardized with a "gauge block", so that casts can be transferred from one articulator to another in the same relationship.

### Class III-B (Trubyte articulator by Gysi and Panadent, designed by Robert Lee)

It is a non-arcon instrument with a fixed intercondylar distance. The horizontal condylar inclinations are individually adjustable and individual Bennett adjustments are located near the center of the intercondylar axis. The incisal guide table is adjusted to the patient's Gothic arch angle. This instrument can accept only some lateral interocclusal records.

Panadent, designed by Robert Lee, utilizes interchangeable preformed curved analog fossae for condylar pathways. It is an arcon instrument with a fixed intercondylar distance. Fossa analogs are available with average lateral pathways and immediate side shifts from 0.5 to 2.5 mm. Lateral interocclusal records or the Axi-Path recorder is used to determine the amount of side shift and the steepness of the horizontal condylar inclination. Then the corresponding side shift analog is selected and set to the recorded steepness of the horizontal condylar inclination.

### Class IV-A (TMJ instrument by Kenneth Swanson)

It will accept three-dimensional dynamic registrations and utilize a face-bow transfer. The condylar pathways or cams are formed by registrations engraved by the patient.

An intraoral registration is generated by studs in autopolymerizing called as "stereographic" recording. The stereographic recording is then placed on the articulator and used to mold fossae in autopolymerizing resin supposed to be an accurate analog of the patient's temporomandibular joint function.

### Class IV-B (D5A, Simulator)

Instruments in this Class will accept three-dimensional dynamic registrations and utilize a face-bow transfer. The condylar pathways can be selectively angled and customized. The tracings are produced by the pantograph which consist of six styli and tracing tables attached to the mandible and maxilla. Two tracing tables are located adjacent to each condylar area in the horizontal and vertical planes. Two additional tracing tables are located in the anterior and in the horizontal plane. Mandibular movements such as the right and left lateral border pathways of the mandible and the protrusive pathway of the mandible are traced. All are repeatable except for the protrusive pathway.

These tracings are then transferred to the articulator using Pantronic. It is an electronic pantograph which provides a computer printout of numerical condylar measurements in the same relationship in which they exist in the patient. All articulators in this Class are arcon instruments with adjustable intercondylar distances. The condylar housings can be adjusted in the horizontal, sagittal and frontal planes. Each has a Bennett guide adjustment. They are called as gnathologic instruments.

**17. List various uses and requirements of articulators and describe in detail semi-adjustable articulators.**

## USES OF ARTICULATOR

A. Is to act as the patient in the absence of the patient.

B. It is used to simulate the patient's temporomandibular joints, muscles of mastication and the complex neuromuscular mechanism that programs mandibular movements.
C. Mounting of dental casts for diagnosis, treatment planning and patient presentation.
D. Fabrication of occlusal surfaces for dental restorations.
E. Arrangement of artificial teeth for complete and removable partial dentures.

### Requirements of an Articulator

1. To maintain the correct horizontal and vertical relationship of the patient's casts.
2. The cast should be easily removed and attached to the articulator without losing their correct horizontal and vertical relationship.
3. It should have an incisal guide pin with a positive stop that is adjustable and calibrated.
4. The articulator should be able to open and close in a hinge-like fashion.
5. The articulator should accept a face-bow transfer utilizing an anterior reference point.
6. The articulator should be accurate, rigid and of a noncorrosive material able to resist wear. The adjustments should be freely movable and secure.
7. There should be adequate distance between the upper and lower members with good rear vision.
8. The articulator should be not be too bulky and heavy.

### Additional Articulator Requirements

If dentures are to be fabricated with balanced occlusion.

1. The condylar guides should allow right lateral, left lateral and protrusive movements.
2. The condylar guides should be adjustable horizontally.
3. Provisions for adjustment of Bennett movement.
4. The incisal guide table should be a mechanical table that can be adjusted in the sagittal and frontal planes or customized table.
   Optional articulator capabilities are adjustable intercondylar distance and an immediate Bennett adjustment. The articulator may either be arcon or non-arcon.

## HANAU ARTICULATORS (FIG. 13)

### Hanau H2

The Hanau H2 articulator is non-arcon type with the condylar guidance controls attached to the lower member of the articulator. "

It has a fixed intercondylar distance of 110 mm and does accept a face-bow transfer. The lateral horizontal condylar inclinations are set by protrusive interocclusal record.

The amount of Bennett movement is calculated from the lateral horizontal condylar inclinations and the vertical condylar posts are rotated accordingly.

The mechanical incisal guide table is adjustable both in sagittal and frontal planes.

### Procedure

The maxillary cast is mounted on the Hanau H2 articulator by means of a face-bow transfer. The facia face-bow or earpiece face-bow can be used.

Hinge axis is located (the axis around which the mandible may rotate without translation).

The facia face-bow has adjustable condylar rods that are placed lightly against the face over the center of rotation of the condyles.

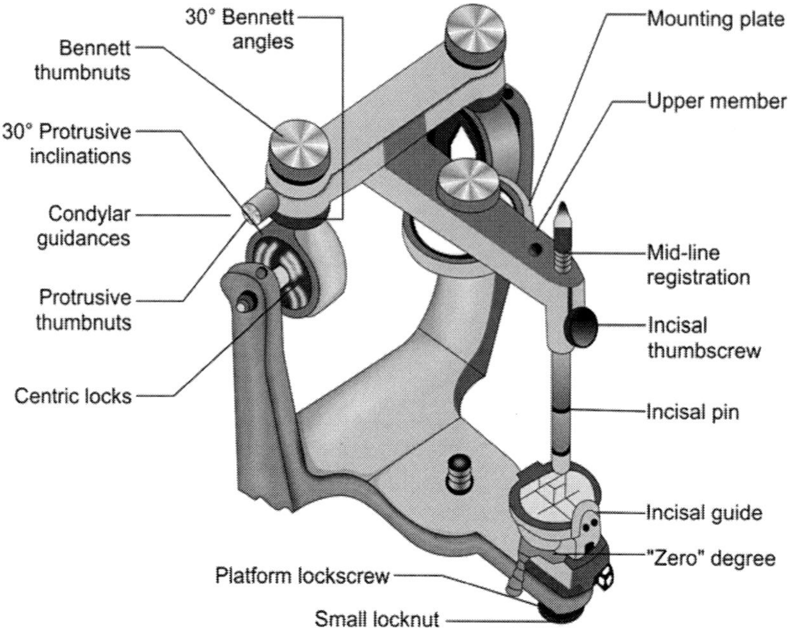


**Fig. 13:** Parts of the hanau articulator

The earpiece face-bow are placed in the external auditory canals and while transferring to the articulator, the earpieces are seated on the auditory pins of the centric locks which relates to the patient's horizontal axis.

The anterior reference point of the facia and earpiece face-bows can either be the orbitale or the incisal plane.

The anterior reference point along with the two posterior reference points form the axis-orbital plane, which has the same occlusal plane has that is in the patient's skull. The incisal plane is adjusted so that it is level with the upper notch on the incisal pin when making the face-bow transfer.

If orbitale is the anterior reference point then the orbitale pointer in the face-bow assembly should touch the orbitale indicator on the upper member of the articulator when making the transfer.

The Hanau Twirl-Bow relates the maxillary arch to the Frankfort horizontal plane and this can be transferred to the articulator without physically attaching the face-bow to the articulator. This face–bow allows the operator to open and close the earpieces simultaneously and equidistantly.

A horizontal orbitale pointer is attached to the right temple arm. The relationship is recorded by a transfer rod, which is attached to the bite fork perpendicular to the Frankfort horizontal plane.

A mounting guide is utilized to mount the transfer rod and attached bite fork to the articulator.

## ADVANTAGES

### Ease of Manipulation

Maxillary cast can be mounted on the articulator without the face-bow.

## RECORDS

Horizontal condylar inclinations is determined by means of a protrusive interocclusal record. The patient should protrude approximately 6 mm. The horizontal condylar guidances are adjusted until the maxillary cast seats into the protrusive interocclusal record.

The amount of Bennett movement is calculated from the horizontal condylar settings by Hanau's equation,

Bennett angle (L) = (H/8) + 12

Where H is the horizontal condylar inclination determined by the protrusive interocclusal record. If the horizontal condylar inclination is 30°, then the Bennett angle would be approximately 16°. The vertical condylar posts are then rotated to the calculated Bennett angulation.

## INCISAL GUIDE PIN AND INCISAL TABLE

Mechanical incisal guide table is adjustable in sagittal and frontal planes.

There is a single sagittal adjustment and right and left frontal adjustments.

These adjustments are made to compensate for the amount of horizontal and vertical overlap incorporated in the anterior teeth arrangement.

The setting of the incisal guide table protects the anterior teeth from dislodgment when arranging the posterior teeth.

The sagittal inclination is determined by bringing the central incisors into an end-to-end relationship and the frontal adjustments are determined by bringing the cuspids into an end-to-end relationship.

The incisal guide pin is straight or angled.

The angled incisal guide pin always maintains an exact center of the table position even with a change in vertical dimension of 5 mm. In case of the straight incisal pin any change in vertical dimension will alter the position of the incisal guide pin in relation to the incisal guide table and a readjustment of the incisal guide table is needed.

### 18. Given condylar and incisal guidance in articulator, what are other factors in considering balanced occlusion? Give a note on each factor.

## BALANCED OCCLUSION

Balanced occlusion is the simultaneous contacting of the maxillary and mandibular teeth on the right and left and in the anterior and posterior occlusal areas when the jaws are in either centric or eccentric relation.

Balanced sliding occlusion is the even contacting of teeth as the mandible moves to and from eccentric and centric maxillomandibular relations.

Balanced occlusion is associated with cusp form posterior teeth and nonbalanced occlusion with noncusp form posterior teeth.

### Advantages of Bilateral Balanced Occlusion

Enables the denture to be seated during activities such as swallowing saliva, closing to reseat the dentures. If teeth are not arranged in balanced occlusion, the constant unseating of the denture bases create soreness and inflammation, which may lead to accelerated bone resorption. The denture is compromised in stability, retention and comfort.

## Factors Affecting Occlusal Balance (Hanau's Quint)

- Condylar guidance
- Incisal guidance
- Plane of occlusion
- Compensating curve
- Angulation of the teeth / Cuspal height.

### *Condylar Guidance*

Condylar guidance can be defined as, "Mandibular guidance generated by the condyle and articular disc traversing the contour of the glenoid fossa." —GPT

The condylar path should be determined on the patient and set on the instrument so that the patient's temporomandibular joint is in harmony with the occlusion as programmed on the articulator. A steep condylar path needs a steep compensating curve for occlusal balance. If a lesser compensating curve is substituted for a steep condylar guidance it would result in a steep incisal guidance resulting in loss of molar balancing contacts.

### *Incisal Guidance*

It is defined as, "The influence of the contacting surfaces of the mandibular and maxillary anterior teeth during mandibular movements." —GPT

Incisal guidance is the effect of contact of the upper and lower anterior teeth on the movement of the mandible. It is usually expressed in degrees of angulation from the horizontal by a line drawn in the sagittal plane between the incisal edges of the upper and lower incisor teeth when closed in centric occlusion.

If the incisal guidance is steep, it requires steep cusps, a steep occlusal plane, or a steep compensating curve to effect an occlusal balance. A steep inclined plane is detrimental to the stability and equilibrium of the denture base hence for complete dentures the incisal guidance should be as flat as esthetics and phonetics will permit. When the arrangement of the anterior teeth necessitates a vertical overlap, a compensating horizontal overlap should be set to prevent dominant incisal guidance (anterior interference) from upsetting the occlusal balance on the posterior teeth.

### *Plane of Occlusion*

It is defined as, "An imaginary surface which is related anatomically to the cranium and which theoretically touches the incisal edges of the incisors and the tips of the occluding surfaces of the posterior teeth. It is not a plane in the true sense of the word but represents the mean curvature of the surface." —GPT

It is established in the anterior by the height of the lower cuspid and in the posterior by the height of the retromolar pad. It is also related to the ala-tragus line, or Camper's line. Its position can be altered only slightly without creating serious functional problems.

### *Compensating Curve*

Compensating curve is defined as, "The anteroposterior and lateral curvatures in the alignment of the occluding surfaces and incisal edges of artificial teeth which are used to develop balanced occlusion." –GPT

**Types of compensating curves**

- Anteroposterior curves
- Lateral curves.

**Curve of Spee** is defined as, "Anatomic curvature of the occlusal alignment of teeth beginning at the tip of the lower canine and following the buccal cusps of the natural premolars and molars, continuing to the anterior border of the ramus as described by Graf Von Spee." —GPT. It is an imaginary curve joining the buccal cusps of the mandibular posterior teeth starting from the canine passing through the head of the condyle.

**Significance:** In protrusion the posterior teeth arranged incorporating this curve will remain in contact without disocclusion.

## Lateral Compensatory Curves

This curve runs across the palatal and buccal cusps of the maxillary molars. During lateral movement the mandibular lingual cusps on the working side should slide along the inner inclines of the maxillary buccal cusp. In the balancing side the mandibular buccal cusps should contact the inner inclines of the maxillary palatal cusp. This relationship forms a lateral balance

It is determined by the inclination of the posterior teeth and their vertical relationship to the occlusal plane so that the occlusal surface results in a curve that is in harmony with the movement of the mandible as guided posteriorly by the condylar path.

A steep condylar path requires a steep compensating curve for occlusal balance.

A lesser compensating curve for the same condylar guidance would result in a steeper incisal guidance (anterior interference), which would cause loss of molar balancing contacts.

## Cusps on Teeth or the Inclination of Cuspless Teeth

Cusp angle is defined as, "The angle made by the average slope of a cusp with the cusp plane measured mesiodistally or buccolingually." —GPT

The mesiodistal cusp heights that inter-digitate lock the occlusion so that reposition of the teeth due to settling of the base cannot take place. To prevent this problem, it is advocated that all mesiodistal cusp heights be eliminated, hence only the buccolingual inclines are considered as determinants of balanced occlusion in anatomic-type teeth.

Once the vertical and horizontal overlaps of the anterior teeth have been established incisal guidance, the plane of occlusion, the compensating curve and the tooth form must harmonize with the three guiding elements, if balanced occlusion is to be achieved on the articulator. The incisal guidance and the plane of occlusion can be altered only a slight amount because of esthetic and physiologic factors. The compensating curve and the cuspal inclinations can be adjusted by the dentist.

### *Factors affecting Protrusive Balance*

1. Condylar inclination represents the path of the condyle in protrusion modified by the combined action of all of the tissues of the temporomandibular joint and the ridges covered by the recording bases.
2. The inclination of the incisal guidance is chosen for the patient.
3. The inclination of the plane of occlusion set to physiologic factors.
4. The compensating curve set to harmonize with 1 and 2.
5. Cusp heights and tooth inclination of the posterior teeth can be adjusted depending on other factors.

### *Factors affecting Lateral Balance*

1. The inclination of the condylar path on the balancing side.
2. The inclination of the incisal guidance and cuspid end-to-end contact.

3. The inclination of the plane of occlusion on the balancing side and working side.
4. The compensating curve on the balancing side and working side.
5. The buccal cusp heights or inclination of the teeth on the balancing side.
6. The lingual cusp heights or inclination on the working side.
7. The Bennett side shift on the working side.

The forces of occlusion should be balanced from right to left and anterior to posterior in complete dentures.

### 19. Describe types of occlusion, factors affecting types of occlusion and add a note on balanced occlusion.

Balanced occlusion is the simultaneous contacting of the maxillary and mandibular teeth on the right and left and in the anterior and posterior occlusal areas when the jaws are in either centric or eccentric relation.

Balanced sliding occlusion is the even contacting of teeth as the mandible moves to and from eccentric and centric maxillomandibular relations.

Balanced occlusion is associated with cusp form posterior teeth and nonbalanced occlusion with noncusp form posterior teeth.

Organic occlusion employs cusp form posterior teeth that are not arranged in protrusive and bilateral balance.

## TYPES OF OCCLUSION

1. Balanced occlusion.
2. Nonbalanced occlusion.

When forces act on a body in such a way that no motion results, there is balance or equilibrium.

### Factors in Balance

1. The wider and larger the ridge in which teeth are close to the ridge, the greater the lever balance.
2. Wider the ridge and the narrower the teeth buccolingually, the greater the balance.
3. The more lingual (inside) the teeth are placed in relation to the ridge crest, the greater the balance.
4. Maximum denture base coverage greater the balance.
5. The more centerd the force of occlusion anteroposteriorly, the greater the stability of the base.
6. Occlusal balance with stable contacts at the centric and in long centric.
7. Right and left eccentric occlusal balance by simultaneous contacts at the limit of functional and parafunctional activity.
8. A minimum of three contacts for establishing a teeth in centric and eccentric occlusion
9. Intermediate occlusal balance for all positions between centric occlusion and all other functional or parafunctional excursions to the right, left and protrusive.
10. It is important that balance, due to tooth position and tooth contact, complement.

### Types of Balance

- Unilateral
- Bilateral
- Protrusive.

### *Unilateral Lever Balance*

This is present when there is equilibrium of the base on its supporting structures when a bolus of food is interposed between the teeth on one side and a space exists between the teeth on the opposite side.

### *For Good Unilateral Lever Balance*

1. Teeth are arranged so that direction of force on the functioning side is over the ridge or slightly lingual to it.
2. Maximum coverage of denture base.
3. Teeth arranged close to the ridge.
4. Occlusal food table with narrow buccolingual width.

### *Unilateral Occlusal Balance*

This is present when the occlusal surfaces of teeth on one side articulate simultaneously, as a group, with a smooth uninterrupted glide.

### *Bilateral Occlusal Balance*

This is present when there is equilibrium on both sides of the denture due to simultaneous contact of the plane of equilibrium.

This type of balance depends on the interaction of the incisal guidance, the plane of occlusion, the angulation of the teeth, the cuspal height, the compensating curve and condylar inclination.

### *Protrusive Occlusal Balance*

This is present when the mandible moves essentially forward and the occlusal contacts are smooth and simultaneous in the posterior both on right and left sides and on the anterior teeth.

Protrusive occlusal balance requires a minimum of three contacts, one on each side posteriorly and one anteriorly and is dependent on the interaction of the same factors as bilateral occlusal balance.

**20. Explain the various concepts proposed to attain balanced occlusion in complete denture.**

## CONCEPTS

1. Gysi's concept
2. French's concept
3. Sear's concept
4. Pleasure's concept
5. Hanau's concept
6. Trapozzano's concept
7. Boucher's concept
8. Lott's concept
9. Levin's concept.

## 1. Gysi's Concept

Gysi proposed the concept in 1914. For complete denture arrangement 33° anatomic teeth were used to enhance the stability of the denture.

### 2. French's Concept

The mandibular cuspal plane was lowered to increase the stability of the dentures along with balanced occlusion. Individual tooth was designated a particular inclination such as:

- Maxillary 1st Premolar - 5° inclination
- Maxillary 2nd Premolar - 10° inclination
- Maxillary 1st Molar - 15° inclination.

### 3. Sear's Concept

He proposed balanced occlusion for non-anatomical teeth using posterior balancing ramps or an occlusal plane which curves anteroposteriorly and laterally. The use of the second molar ramp, provided the tooth contacts for the balanced occlusion.

### 4. Pleasure's Concept

This concept was proposed by Max Pleasure in 1937 in which a pleasure curve or the posterior reverse lateral curve was used to align and arrange the posterior teeth in order to increase the stability of the denture. This was achieved by modifying lower posterior teeth to a reverse curve by tilting teeth buccally. This curve runs from the palatal cusp of the 1st PM to the distobuccal cusp of the 2nd molar which provides occlusal balance and second premolar provides lever balance.

#### The reverse curve was set as:

- 2nd PM (Premolar)—buccally tilted
- 1st M (Molar)—horizontally
- 2nd M—lingually tilted.

### 5. Hanau's Concept

The nine factors involved in balanced articulation are:

1. Horizontal condylar inclination
2. Compensating curve
3. Protrusive incisal guidance
4. Plane of orientation
5. Buccolingual inclination tooth axes
6. Sagittal condylar guidance
7. Sagittal incisal guidance
8. Tooth alignment
9. Relative cusp height.

He combined the 9 factors into 5, such as:

1. Condylar guidance
2. Compensating curve
3. Relative cusp height
4. Incisal guidance
5. Plane of orientation.
   He showed how they affected one another by a diagram called "The articulation quint".

## 6. Trapozzano's Concept

## The 3 factors were:

1. Condylar guidance
2. Relative cusp height
3. Incisal guidance.

### *Reasons for eliminating the other two factors*

Plane of orientation was eliminated as its location is highly variable within the available inter-ridge space. The length of the cusp inclines is sufficient to permit the teeth to maintain contact within the limits of the eccentric functional movements.

Compensating curve was eliminated as the cuspal angulations which produce the balanced occlusion is determined, a compensating curve of varying concavity or convexity is created.

### 7. Boucher's Concept

1. Factors in balanced occlusion
   - Orientation of occlusal plane
   - The incisal guidance
   - The condylar guidance
2. The angulations of cusp is more important than the cusp height
3. The compensating curve enables one to increase the effective cusp height without changing the form of the teeth

## 8. Lott's Concept

The laws of occlusion were related to the posterior separation that is the resultant of guiding factors. The greater the separation of posterior teeth, the greater or higher must be the compensating curve.

## 9. Levin's Concept

The plane of orientation was eliminated as it was considered that the patients have an adaptive capacity for a slight change in the plane of occlusion (1–2 mm at most).

### *Levin's Quad*

1. The condylar guidance is fixed and recorded from the patient. The balancing condylar guidance includes the Bennett movement, which may or may not affect lateral balance.
2. The incisal guidance is obtained from patient's esthetic and phonetic requirements.
3. The compensating curve is the most important factor for obtaining balance. Monoplane or low cusp teeth must employ the use of a compensating curve.
4. Cusp teeth have the inclines necessary for obtaining balanced occlusion but nearly always are used with a compensating curve.

## 21. Describe the methods of selecting anterior teeth for an edentulous patient.

The selection of anterior teeth is done to satisfy esthetic requirements. The anterior and posterior teeth must function in harmony and be anatomically and physiologically compatible with the surrounding oral environment.

## ANTERIOR TEETH SELECTION

### Size of Anterior Teeth

Seven anatomic factors are used as guides to selection of anterior teeth for size:

1. *Size of the face:* The average width of the maxillary central incisor will be approximately one sixteenth of the width of the face measured between the zygoma.
   The Trubyte Tooth Indicator is useful in determining the size of the maxillary central incisors. The combined width of the six maxillary anterior is slightly less than one-third of the bizygomatic breadth of the face. The face-bow can be used as a caliper to record the bizygomatic breadth of the face.
2. *Size of the maxillary arch:* The mold selector can be used to make measurements of the maxillary cast. Measurements are made from the crest of the incisal papilla to the hamular notches and from one hamular notch to the opposite hamular notch. The combined length of the three legs of the triangle in millimetres is used on the selector. When there is a discrepancy between face size and arch size the selection of anterior teeth should be done by face size.
3. *Incisal papilla and the cuspid eminences or the buccal frenum:* Measure the distance from the distal of one cuspid eminence to the distal of the other and in the midline, the maxillary central incisors are situated labially to the papilla. The combined width of the six maxillary anterior teeth is determined in millimeters.
   Another method is to mark in the occlusion rim at each corner of the lips. The marker is passed on a line parallel to the pupils of the eyes. The distance between the marks following the contour of the arch measured in millimeters is the combined width of the six maxillary anterior teeth.
4. *Maxillomandibular relations:* Any disproportion in size between the maxillary and the mandibular arches influence the length, width and position of the teeth.
5. *The contour of the residual ridges:* The artificial teeth should be placed to follow the contour of the residual ridges that existed when the natural teeth were present.
6. *The vertical distance between the ridges:* The length of the teeth is determined by the available space between the existing ridges.
7. *The lips:* The labial surfaces of the maxillary anterior teeth support the upper lip. The labial incisal third of the maxillary anterior teeth supports the superior border of the lower lip and the incisal edges contact the lower lip at the junction of the vermilion border when the letter F is pronounced.

### Form of Anterior Teeth

Three factors are used as guides in the selection of anterior teeth for form.

1. *The form and contour of the face:*
   The general outline of the tooth should conform to the general outline of the face in frontal view and the mesial or distal outline conform to the contour of the profile.
   The square, tapering, ovoid and combinations of face forms helps in selecting the tooth form. By using a tooth indicator on the patient's face, face form as square, square tapering or ovoid can be assessed from the relationship of the face form with the vertical lines of the indicator. Profile is observed by checking forehead, the base of the nose and the point of the chin. If in line, the profile is straight.

2. Sex:
   Curved facial features are associated with femininity and square features are associated with masculinity.
3. Age:
   As age progress the lips lose their curves and the teeth wear at the incisal edges and interproximal surfaces. The labial surfaces seem flatter and the outline form appears squarer.

### Color or Shade of Anterior Teeth

Shade is the degree of darkness of a color with reference to its mixture with black. The yellow is more prominent in the gingival third and the gray is more prominent in the incisal third. To check the shade, the patient's mouth should not be opened too wide. White light after 10 o'clock in the morning and before two in the afternoon is preferred. The tooth and the shade guide should be viewed from a distance of six or eight feet and in different angles.

Harmony should exist between the color of the teeth and the color of the skin, hair and eyes.

To check the size, form and shades, the anterior and posterior teeth of both arches should be arranged in their anatomic positions on accurately adapted record or trial bases.

### Composition of Material of Anterior Teeth

Artificial teeth for complete dentures are made either of porcelain, or processed acrylic resins. The porcelain teeth are either air fired or vacuum fired. The vacuum fired are denser than the air fired. Porcelain teeth are hard to abrade and will retain their finish. Gold pins must attach the porcelain teeth to the supporting base mechanically. Although porcelain is brittle, its hardness and resistance to abrasion from foods and brushing make it the material of choice for esthetic purposes when space is available. Acrylic resin teeth are not as hard as porcelain and can be abraded more readily. The acrylic resin teeth can be bonded to the denture base without mechanical means.

The commonly used one is a reinforced cross-linked acrylic tooth, which has better abrasion strength.

## 22. Explain selection of posterior teeth in complete denture fabrication.

The selection of posterior teeth involves shade, size, number and form.

### Shade of Posterior Teeth

The shade of the posterior teeth should harmonize with the shade of the anterior teeth.
The maxillary bicuspids used more for esthetic than for functional purposes and the shade will be same as canine tooth.

### Size and Number of Posterior Teeth

This depends on the anatomy of the surrounding oral environment and the physiologic acceptance by the supporting tissues. The posterior teeth must support the cheeks and tongue and function in harmony with the musculature in swallowing and speaking as well as in mastication.

### Form of Posterior Teeth

The occlusal form will be decided by the type of occlusion to be developed. If the teeth are to be balanced in the centric and eccentric positions, a cusp form tooth is indicated. If the posterior teeth are to disocclude when an eccentric jaw movement occurs, either cusp or monoplane teeth can be used. If the posterior teeth are to be arranged on a plane and balanced in centric position only, monoplane teeth are used.

### Buccolingual Width of Posterior Teeth

The buccolingual widths of artificial teeth should be less from the widths of the natural teeth they replace. Artificial posterior teeth that are narrow in a buccolingual direction are better to develop the correct form of the polished surfaces of the denture allowing the buccal and lingual denture flanges to slope away from the occlusal surfaces.

### Mesiodistal Length of Posterior Teeth

The length of the mandibular residual ridge from the distal of the canine to the beginning of the retromolar pad is usually available for artificial posterior teeth.
After the six anterior mandibular teeth have been placed in their final position, a point is marked on the crest of the mandibular ridge at the anterior border of the retromolar pad. A ruler can be used to measure from the distal surface of the mandibular canine to the point that has been marked at the end of the available space. The total mesiodistal width in millimetres of the four posterior teeth is often used as a mold number. For example, mold 32L of the Dentists' Supply Company signifies that the four posterior teeth have a total mesiodistal dimension of 32 mm and a long occlusocervical length.

### Vertical length of the Bucco Posterior Teeth

It is best to select posterior teeth corresponding to the interarch space and to the length of the anterior teeth. The length of the maxillary first premolars should be comparable to that of the maxillary canines or, the denture base material will appear unnatural distal to the canines. The ridge laps that are thin and long can be easily positioned in full ridges posteriorly.

### Commonly used Materials

Vacuum-fired porcelain teeth are more resistant to abrasion and therefore, maintain their lustre longer than acrylic resin teeth. Acrylic resin teeth can be altered and will bond with the denture base for retention in instances of limited interarch space. Acrylic resin teeth are preferred when the teeth in the opposing arch have been restored with gold; as the porcelain has a higher coefficient of wear than gold.

## 23. Define denture esthetics. Discuss in detail esthetic requirements of complete denture.

A denture is esthetic when the teeth and bases are in harmony with the facial musculature and to the size and shape of head.

To arrange esthetically, the composition, size, shape and color of the six anterior teeth are important.

### Factors influencing the size and form of the anterior teeth are

1. The size of the face.
2 The amount of available interarch space.
3. The measured distance between the distal of the right and left maxillary cuspids, using the arch and incisal papilla as measuring guides.
4. The length of the lips.
5. The size and relation of the arches.

### The color of teeth is influenced by:

1. Age
2. Habits
3. Complexion
4. Color of the eyes.

### The arrangement is influenced by:

1. Age
2. Sex
3. Personality
4. Cosmetic factor
5. Artistic reflection.

### AGE

Age changes take place throughout the entire body and also on the teeth. These include:

1. *Loss of lip support:* The denture borders are contoured to fill the vestibules and the teeth are arranged to support the lips and the cheeks.
2. As *cheeks sag,* the horizontal overlap of the posterior teeth is increased to prevent cheek biting.
3. The *interincisal distance* increases with age; therefore, the mandibular teeth become more visible.
4. Teeth *abrade* with age. The central and lateral incisors abrade in a straight line, this flattens the arch. The cuspids abrade in a curve. This is in harmony with the flattening of the lips as the Cupid's bow of the upper lip disappears and the fullness of the lower lip diminishes with the aging processes.
5. As the *gingival tissues recede* with age, selecting a long tooth, contouring the wax and positioning the tooth properly can reproduce this recession.
6. The *smile line is sharp* in young people and less sharp in older people and care should be taken not to alter occlusal plane.

If natural restorations were present in the dentition it can be duplicated in the artificial teeth arrangement.

### SEX

As the contours of the bodies of males and females are different, the individual contours and the arrangement of the teeth differ. Depending on the male or female features the positions of the incisal edges, the prominence of the gingival portions of the necks of the teeth and the positions of the body of the teeth are arranged accordingly.

### The differences in male and female arrangement

1. Roundness of the arch form denotes femininity and squareness denotes masculinity.
2. In the male, the central incisors are on a horizontal plane parallel with the lip, the lateral incisors are above the plane and the cuspids are on the plane, the mesial surface of the lateral incisor is often hidden behind the distal surface of the central incisor. The distal surface of the lateral incisor is rotated very slightly in a posterior direction. The cuspid is made more prominent as a result of this arrangement.
3. The incisal edges of the maxillary anterior teeth of females follow the curve of the lower lip viewed from front, the distal surfaces of the central incisors of females are usually rotated

in a posterior direction, the mesial surface of the lateral incisor is often seen in an anterior relation to the distolabial surface of the central incisor. The distal surface of the lateral incisor is rotated in a posterior direction. The smile is softened as a result of this arrangement.

## PERSONALITY

Self-consciousness is possible with either natural or artificial teeth. An unselfconscious person may have had natural teeth pleasant in appearance or dentures with natural appearing artificial teeth. It is the obligation of the dentist to arrange the artificial teeth in a manner to encourage the development of an attractive personality.

## COSMETIC FACTOR

The cosmetic factor involves personal grooming. When a person dresses neatly and keeps generally well groomed, the dentist needs to observe and arrange teeth accordingly.

## ARTISTIC REFLECTION

Artistic reflection is the arrangement of the teeth to reflect the dentist's concept of what he thinks appears natural for the patient. The arranged teeth should harmonizes with the surrounding features and should be acceptable to the patient. The dentist should advice and discuss with the patient the advantages of placing teeth in particular positions, after the physiologic requirements are satisfied.

**Few changes that will harmonize with patient features**

1. Varying the slant of the long axis placing the teeth so that the tips of the lateral incisors show when the patient speaks.
2. Create asymmetry in the divergences of the proximal surfaces of the teeth from the contact points.
3. Use an eccentric midline.
4. Place one central and lateral incisor parallel to the midline and rotate the other central and lateral incisors slightly in a posterior direction.
5. Place one maxillary central incisor slightly in an anterior direction to the other central incisor.
6. Place the neck of one maxillary central incisor in a posterior direction and the neck of the other central incisor in an anterior direction.
7. Create asymmetry for the maxillary right and left cuspids. Rotate one in a more posterior direction than the other. Place the neck of one in a more labial direction than the other.
8. Create a good smile line by the proper placing of the maxillary posterior teeth mediolaterally in relation to the cheek.

The similarity in shape and size of the mandibular anterior teeth presents a problem in positioning for esthetics. The esthetic acceptance can be enhanced by:

1. Grinding the incisal edges rotating and overlapping the teeth to give an irregular appearance creating asymmetry in the divergences of the proximal surfaces of the teeth from the contact points.
2. Creating a slight diastema between the lateral incisor and the cuspid on the one side.
3. Physiologically they must be in a position compatible with the lips, tongue and cheeks whether the mandible is in a relaxed position or in motion.
4. The teeth must function in harmony with the surrounding oral environment in masticating, swallowing, speaking, yawning and all parafunctional mandibular movements.

*Frush and Fisher concept:* Convex, rounded and shortened papilla, exposure of more cervical root to simulate recession, stippling of denture and tinting of dentures were proposed by them.

Kayon denture base stains as Basic pink for attached gingiva, Light red for papilla and muscle attachments enhance denture esthetics.

## 24. Define golden proportion with its significance in dental esthetics and add a note on the applications of various proportions in dental esthetics.

### According to GPT

Golden proportion is the ratio between succeeding terms in a mathematical progression called the Fibonacci series (Leonardo Pisano: nickname Fibonacci) in which each number is the sum of the two immediately preceding it (i.e., 1, 1, 2, 3, 5, 8, 13, 21, 34, 55, 89, 144, and so on). The ratio converges on approximately 1.618 to 1. Claims have been made that the Golden Proportion exists in natural dentitions in the ratio of the widths of incisors and canines as seen from the facial surfaces.

### Golden Proportion in Dentistry

Lombardi (1973) was the first to suggest the application of the golden proportion in dentistry. Levin (1978) suggested the golden proportion to relate the successive width of the anterior teeth as viewed from the labial aspect.

### Application of Golden Proportion in Dental Esthetics (Fig. 14)

- To develop ideal size and shape relationships for maxillary teeth and to determine the width of the teeth.
- Golden proportion can be applied only after determining the incisal edge position, incisal plane, gingival plane, and central incisor length.
- As applied to the maxillary teeth, the Golden Proportion requires a 62% reduction in the viewing width of each tooth, beginning with the central incisor, and proceeding posteriorly.
- To apply the concept of the Golden Proportion, a lateral incisor can be arbitrarily assigned a viewing width of 1, in which the central incisor width should be 1.6, the cuspid 0.62, the first premolar 0.38, and the second premolar 0.23. This allows for a smile dominated by the central incisors, with the other teeth becoming progressively smaller.

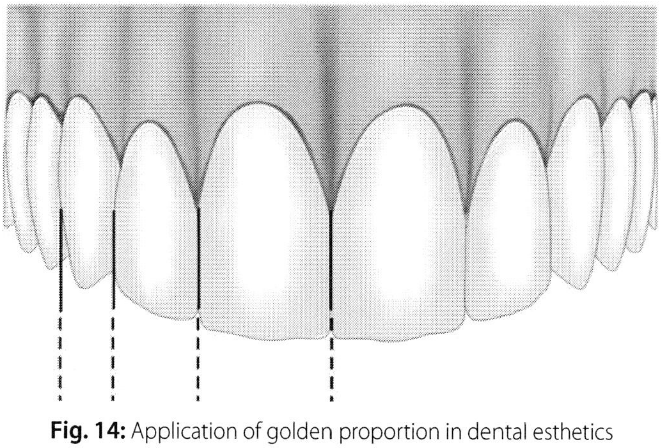

**Fig. 14:** Application of golden proportion in dental esthetics

## Modifications of Golden Proportion

**Snow** proposed that the Golden Proportion could be used to develop symmetry, dominance, and proportion for esthetically pleasing smiles.

The assigned values for the six anterior teeth were added (assigning 1.6 to the central, 1 to the lateral, and 0.62 to the cuspid) (Fig. 15). Then the assigned width of each tooth was divided by the total to determine the relative percentage. The resulting percentages were: central incisor 25%, lateral incisor 16%, and cuspid 9%.

These percentages illustrate the dominance of the central incisors, which are 50% of the cuspid-to-cuspid width.

**Dr Stephen Marquardt**, an eminent Oral Surgeon in California, discovered that," The Height of the central incisor is in the Golden Proportion to the Width of the Two central incisors".

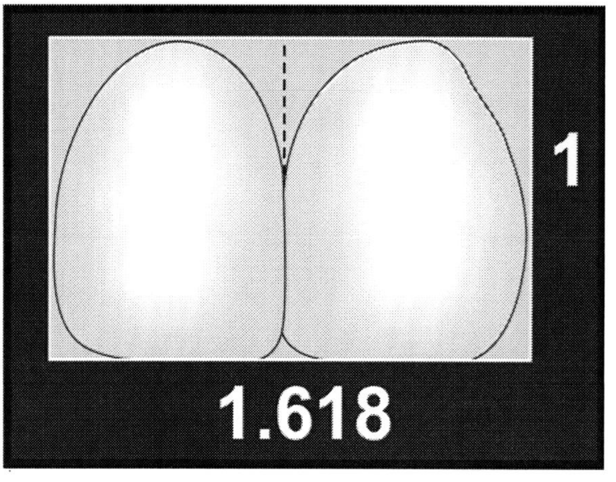


**Fig. 15:** Central incisor to lateral incisor ratio

**Daniel H Ward** proposed the recurring esthetic dental proportion (red) (Fig. 16.)
When golden proportion is used, lateral incisors seem to be too narrow and canine is not prevalent enough and hence proposed a RED proportion or Recurring Esthetic Dental Proportion.

According to this, the dentist can establish his own proportion and remain consistent while moving distally. 70% seems to be more pleasing but should be modified to fit face skeletal structure and general body type.

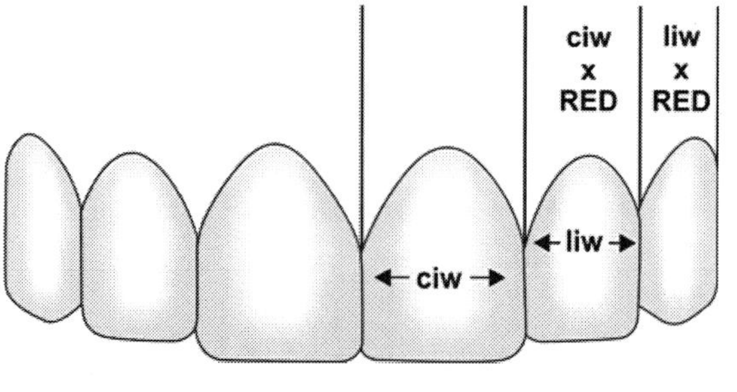


**Fig. 16:** RED proportion

***Red Smile Design (Recurring esthetic dental proportion)***

The equation used to determine the ideal width of a central incisor from a predetermined RED proportion is:

(Frontal Intercanine View width of the anterior 6 teeth)/2(1+RED + RED2) = width of central incisor

Using this formula, if the frontal intercanine view width of the maxillary anterior 6 teeth is 37.2 mm and the desired RED is 70%, the calculated width of the central incisor would be 8.5 mm.

## Preston and RED Proportion (Fig. 17)

The central incisors are identical in size in both the Preston and 70% RED proportions. The lateral incisors are slightly wider in the 70% RED proportion, while the canines are slightly wider in the Preston proportion.

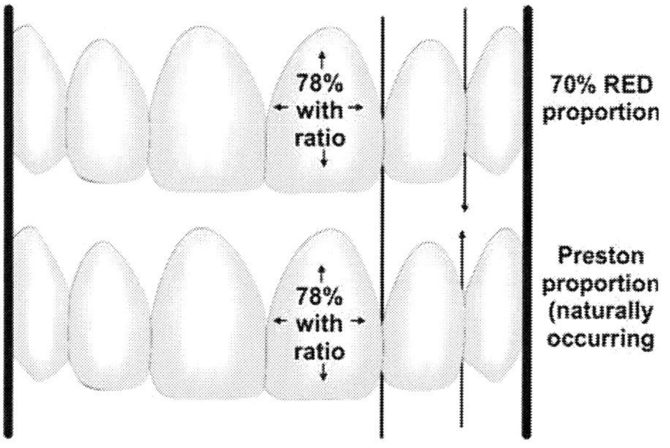


**Fig. 17:** Preston and RED proportion

Once the width of the central incisor has been established, the height can be determined by using the formula:

(Width of central incisor / Width-to-height ratio) = height of central incisor
(The width-to-height ratio should be expressed as a decimal <1)

- If the teeth are relatively short and the patient will not allow a change in length, a larger RED should be used.
- When there are no possible changes to the widths of the central incisors, the heights may be altered either by lengthening the incisal edges or performing elective periodontal crown lengthening surgery.
- The final length of the teeth and RED proportion used should ideally coincide with the patient's facial and body structure.
- The RED Proportion is an objective method of evaluating and designing smiles.

## 25. Explain the dynesthetic interpretation of the dentogenic concept proposed by John P Frush and Roland D Fisher.

The dentogenic concept of denture esthetic has been explained as sex, personality and age to construct a dentogenic restoration effectively.

The secondary factors of a dentogenic restoration is called as Dynesthetics (DYN = Power).

### Consideration in Dynesthetics

Artificial tooth shades should be classified according to the physiologic color changes seen in progressively aging, undiseased natural teeth.

Color texture always appears with age but it may not darken the tooth.

Creating illusion of natural dentition for an older person, we would select a shade of artificial tooth which represents this aging process.

### Dynesthetic Considerations for a Dentogenic Restoration

1. Mold
2. Lip support
3. Midline
4. Labioversion
5. Speaking line
6. Smiling line
7. Central incisor position
8. Lateral incisor position
9. The cuspid
10. Spaces
11. Embrasures
12. Buccal corridor
13. Long axes
14. Gum line
15. Interdental papilla
16. Lingual cutaway
17. Labial and buccal denture base contour.

#### *Mold*

Selection of mold involves its subsequent treatment for abrasion, erosion, depth grinding, masculinity or feminity, shaping and polishing.

#### *Lip Support*

This is the bodily anteroposterior position of teeth supporting the upper lip in a natural and pleasing manner. The placement of upper anterior teeth for proper lip support is an independent procedure not controlled by any other consideration of cranial relation or opposing tooth position.

#### *Midline*

The mid-axis is important to general composition and should be vertical to the incisal and occlusal plane.

### *Labioversion*

This effect is obtained when the long axes of the central incisors are either vertical or with a slight labial inclination. This determination is made by observing the teeth in profile when the patient is standing in normal posture.

### *Speaking Line*

The speaking line is the incisal length or vertical composition of anterior teeth. It is spoken of as the speaking line because the final evaluation of the incisal length is made when the patient is speaking. A guide to vertical composition using the incisal edges of the central incisors in their relationship to the lip line, at rest, as a measure is as follows:

- *Young woman*—3 mm below lip line at rest
- *Young man*—2 mm below lip line at rest
- *Middle age*—1½ mm below lip line at rest
- *Old age,* senility—0 mm below lip line at rest to 2 mm above lip line at rest.

### *Smiling Line*

The smiling line is a curve whose path follows the incisal edges of the central incisors up and back to the incisal edges of the lateral incisors and, then to tips of cuspids. Its arc is determined by the age of the patient and decreases as the patient gets older. The smiling line is a secondary vertical composition of the individual six anterior teeth and is subject to the interincisal distance.

### *Central Incisor Position*

Their shape is controlled by the physical personality of the patient, and their position determines the strength and action of dentogenic composition.

The central incisors must be depth ground. The central incisors must dominate the lateral incisors in their positions within general curve of anterior dental arch.

### *Lateral incisor position*

The position of lateral incisor is subordinated in importance to that of the central incisor. Its rotation however will either harden or soften the dental composition.

The right and left lateral incisors should have asymmetric long axes.

The lateral incisors should be positioned so that at least a portion is seen when patient speaks seriously.

The sex determination comes from either rounding the incisal edge for feminine effect or from squaring the incisal edge for masculine effect.

### *Cuspid*

The position of the cuspid supports the anterior arch form in its widest part and controls the size of buccal corridor.

The cuspid should be positioned to dominate the lateral incisor and to complete the desired upward curve of smiling line.

Cuspid should be abraded to convey the physiologic age of the patient in the dental composition.

The three basic requirements of the cuspid tooth position are:

- Tooth should be rotated to show its mesial surface
- Cervical end should be out
- Observed from side, long axis of cuspid should be vertical.

### *Spaces*

All spaces must be V-shaped to shed food.
Diastema between the central incisors is unsightly and should be avoided.
Diastemas should be asymmetrically placed on either side of arch.
Width of diastema should be controlled.

### *Embrasures*

An embrasure gives freedom to dental composition and represents a divergence of the proximal surface of the anterior teeth from the contact point. There is no separation of proximal surface since the contact areas are touching.

### *Buccal Corridor*

It is a space created between the buccal surface of the posterior teeth and the corner of lips when the patient smiles.

The buccal corridor begins at the cuspid, and its size and shape are controlled by the position and slant of cuspid even though the actual corridor exists posterior to the cuspid tooth.

The use of buccal corridor prevents the "sixty tooth smile" or the "molar to molar smile" which is often characteristic of a denture.

### *Long Axes*

Long axes of each tooth vary in minute degrees and it should be exaggerated in the dentogenic restoration as an artistic device.

### *Gum Line*

The gum line at the cervical ends of the teeth should vary in height.
Slightly below high lip line at central incisors.
Lower than the central incisor gum line at the lateral incisor
Higher than the central or lateral incisor gum line at the cuspid.
Slightly lower than the cuspid for the bicuspid and variable for the molars.

### *Interdental Papilla*

It forms the main part of the tooth matrix and occupies one-third of total importance of the dental composition. The other two-third are occupied by the tooth and tooth position.

The correctly formed interdental papilla accomplishes four definite purposes.

- It creates a hygienic, self-cleansing interdental area.
- It is a complimentary factor in age interpretation.
- It determines the outline form of a tooth and makes the two-dimensional outline form of a tooth incidental to other esthetic requirements.
- It brings a degree of color reflection to the interdental area which creates the illusion of a natural dental composition.

### *Lingual Cutaway*

The lingual cutaway is a groove in the lingual interdental surface which begins at the contact points of the teeth if they are together or at the tip of the interdental papilla if there is a diastema.

It widens and deepens according to the natural divergence of the lingual proximal tooth surfaces. It fades away into the palatal surface of the denture.

***Labial and Buccal Denture Base Contour***

The denture base contour beyond the matrix (visible denture base) should provide a self-cleansing surface and therefore, should not be over accentuated with depressions, grooves, wrinkles, folds or any shape which would defeat the smooth cleansing action of the cheek or lips.

## 26. Discuss in brief the post-insertion management of complete denture prosthodontics.

Educating patients to the limitations of dentures must be a continuing process from the initial patient contact until adjustments are completed. Forewarning about the problems makes the patient more tolerant and doesn't relate them incorrectly to the fit of the dentures.

### Instructions to patient:

1. Individuality of patients:
   They should be educated not to make comparison with the experience of other denture wearers.
   Chewing and speech patterns experience with new dentures are different for each patients.
2. Adaptability to new dentures:
   Younger the patient, the more adaptable to dentures.
   Some patients tend to mislead the new denture wearer by stating that, they never had to adjust to any problem with their new dentures, even though they had problems which they tend to forget over the years.
3. Appearance with new dentures:
   Appearance with new dentures will become more natural with time as initially the dentures will feel strange and bulky in the mouth.
   The lips will not adapt immediately to the fullness of the denture borders and may initially present a distorted appearance.
   Muscle tension may cause an awkward appearance
   Patients should be instructed to refrain from exhibiting their dentures until they are more confident or they may become unfairly critical of the dentures.
   During the period of edentulism a gradual reduction of the interarch distance and collapsing of the lips will have occurred which could change the patients appearance even if proper dentures are replaced. This new change in appearance can be overcome only with the passage of time and patients are advised to persevere during the period.
4. Mastication with new dentures:
   As learning to chew with new dentures requires at least 6 to 8 weeks patients are made aware that this learning period is to be expected.
   The muscles of the tongue, cheeks and lips must be trained to maintain the dentures in position on the residual ridges during mastication
   Excess flow of saliva for the first few days after placement of new dentures also affects mastication which the patient should be made aware of.
   Patients are instructed to chew soft food cut into small pieces and the chewing is best done on both sides of the mouth at the same time.

Also, during the learning period, patients are advised to avoid observation by friends or members of the family, since the patients will feel awkward in the beginning phases of chewing as this may lead to negative attitude in the patient.

When biting with dentures, patients should be instructed to place the food between their teeth toward the corners of the mouth, rather than between the anterior teeth. Then the food should be pushed inward and upward to break it apart.

5. Position of the tongue:

   Ideal position is to position the tongue on the lingual surfaces of the lower anterior teeth. This will help develop stability for the lower denture.

6. Speaking with new dentures:

   The adaptability of the tongue to compensate for changes is so great that most patients master speech with new dentures within a few weeks.

   Initially the additional bulk over the palate and the linguogingival border of the anterior teeth would cause a speech defect, especially in the production of "S" sounds. But as the tongue is very adaptable it doesn't cause phonetic changes that are too great to be readily compensated.

   Speaking normally with dentures requires practice. Patients are advised to read aloud and repeat words or phrases that are difficult to pronounce.

7. Oral hygiene with dentures

   Patients must be convinced of the importance of maintaining good oral hygiene. Plaque, stain and calculus accumulate on dentures and oral mucosa of edentulous patients.

   Dental plaque can cause denture stomatitis, inflammatory papillary hyperplasia, chronic candidiasis and offensive odours.

   Patients should be instructed to rinse their dentures and their mouths after meals. Leaving the dentures in the cleanser (Kleenite) overnight is needed for effective killing of microorganisms and removal of all stain. An alternative soaking cleanser is one that can be made up using 1 teaspoon of Clorox and 2 teaspoons of Calgon in 8 ounces of water.

   After the dentures are removed from the soaking cleanser, they should be brushed gently with a soft brush and rinsed thoroughly.

   Patients should be discouraged from using toothpastes, as most contain an abrasive material that will wear away the surface of acrylic resin.

   The mucosal surfaces of the residual ridges and the dorsal surface of the tongue should also be brushed daily with a soft brush which will increase the circulation and remove plaque.

8. Preserving the residual ridges

   The residual ridges were not intended to bear the stresses of mastication created by complete dentures. Hence, the patient should be told of factors as some irritation, discomfort of the oral tissues and in the long run residual ridge resorption. Patients must be made aware of these varying and unpredictable conditions.

   If some irritation of the tissues is experienced, patients are advised to remove their dentures and rest the mouth for a time.

   Patients must be cautioned not to do any adjustments to the dentures.

   Patients should be told that dentures must be left out of the mouth at night to provide needed rest from the stresses they create on the residual ridges. When dentures are left out of the mouth, they should be placed in a container filled with water to prevent drying and possible dimensional changes.

Adhesives and home-reliners, should not be encouraged as they can cause invariably a change of both vertical and centric relations; the residual ridges can be irreparably damaged in a short time.

9. *Periodic recall of patients* is a must the tissues supporting dentures change with time, depending on local and general factors. All edentulous patients should be examined by a dentist at least once a year and should be placed on a recall list.
10. Educational material for patients
    Written instructions or other formal educational material is helpful to educate the patient and follow instructions without doubt.
    In studying the material, patients become aware that dentures are not permanent and maintaining good oral hygiene is an essential deciding factor in the success with dentures.

## 27. Explain the various relining techniques and add a note on the advantages and disadvantages of each technique.

There are two major relining techniques:
- Open-mouth
- Closed-mouth.

## Indications for Relining or Rebasing

- Immediate dentures at three to six months after their original construction.
- When the residual alveolar ridges have resorbed and the adaptation of the denture bases to the ridges are poor.
- When the construction of new dentures with the accompanying series of appointments can cause physical or mental stress, such as for geriatric or chronically ill patients.
- When the patient cannot afford the cost of having new dentures constructed.

*General considerations*
- The occlusal vertical dimension should be satisfactory.
- The centric relation should coincide with centric occlusioln.
- Oral tissue should be in optimum health.
- Denture base extension should be adequate.
- Inter-occlusal distance should be correct,

*Contraindications*
- When excessive amount of resorption has taken place.
- When abused soft tissues are present.
- When the patient complains of TMJ problems.
- If the dentures have poor esthetics.
- If the dentures create major speech problems.

## Steps in Relining Technique

### *Tissue Preparation*

- Excessive hypertrophic tissue should be surgically removed. The dentures can be used as a surgical splint.
- The oral mucosa should be free of areas of irritation.
- Removal of the dentures from the mouth during sleep is a must for several weeks before treatment commence.

- The dentures should be left out of the mouth at least two or three days before making the final impression.
- Daily massage of the soft tissues is helpful to stimulate their blood supply.

### *Denture Preparation*

- Pressure areas on the tissue surface of the dentures should be relieved.
- Minor occlusal disharmony is corrected by selective grinding.
- Small border inadequacies are corrected.
- A correct posterior palatal seal area should be established before the final impression. Stick compound and autopolymerizing acrylic resin can be used for this purpose.

### *Factors to take Care During Relining*

- Do not increase the occlusal vertical dimension.
- Multiple even contacts (maximum intercuspation) should be present in centric relation.
- Do not permit the maxillary denture to move forward during impression making.
- Ensure that centric relation and centric occlusion are identical.
- Ensure that an accurate posterior palatal seal has been established.
- An equal thickness of final impression material should be used.

## CLOSED-MOUTH RELINING TECHNIQUES – MAXILLARY DENTURE

Done using the existing centric occlusion and intercuspation of the dentures. The various techniques in closed mouth are

### Technique A

**Centric relation** is recorded before the impression is made, using the medium of choice (modeling compound or wax).

**Denture preparation**—Denture is relieved of all large undercuts and a space of 1.5–2 mm made on tissue surface for impression material. The borders are reduced 1–2 mm except the posterior border of maxillary dentures. Large part of the middle of the palatal portion of the maxillary denture is removed for visibility in positioning the maxillary denture during the impression making.

**Border molding**—Borders of the dentures are reformed to their functional contours by using low-fusing modeling compound.

**Impression**—Zinc oxide-eugenol impression paste is used. During the border molding and impression making, the patient closes lightly into the premade interocclusal record. The impression of the exposed part of the palatal section is made with quick-setting plaster.

### *Advantages*

- The opening of the palatal portion will allow better seating of the maxillary denture and alleviate the increase in vertical dimension.
- The premade interocclusal record helps to position the dentures during the impression making and to orient the dentures on the articulator.
- The two-step impression technique will reduce the possibility of moving the maxillary denture forward during the final impression making.

### *Disadvantages*

- The possibility of moving the maxillary denture forward is still a major problem.
- The wax interocclusal record is not an accurate and safe record This technique does not suggest any solution for difficulties of relining both dentures at the same time.

## Technique B

**Centric relation**—Existing centric occlusion and intercuspation are used as a means to seat the dentures.

**Denture preparation**—The same as for technique A. For easy removal of palatal portion the outline of the area is drawn and deepened on the polished surface up to half the thickness of the base. Holes are drilled at 5- to 6mm intervals inside this groove.

**Border molding**—Low-fusing modeling compound (green stick) is suggested for border molding.

**Impression**—Kerr's impression wax (Iowa wax) is the material of choice in this technique. The impression is made in two steps. The impression of the labial flange and the crest of the alveolar ridge between the canines is made as a second step.

### *Advantage*

The two-step impression technique will reduce the possibility of extreme forward movement of the maxillary denture.

### *Disadvantages*

- Wax impression material is difficult to work with and the possibility of distortion exists.
- Errors of existing centric occlusion can produce an inaccurate impression.

## Technique C

**Centric relation**—Same as in technique B.

**Denture preparation**—Same as in techniques A and B.The labial and palatal flanges of the denture are perforated. The perforations will decrease the pressure inside the denture during the impression-making procedure, thereby preventing displacement of maxillary denture.

**Border molding**—The same as techniques A and B.

**Impression**—No specific impression material recommended.

### *Disadvantages*

The same as in techniques A and B.

## Technique D

**Centric relation**—The existing centric occlusion is used to seat the maxillary denture.

**Denture preparation**—The same as in the other technique.

- Denture periphery should be shortened to create a flat border.
- A large opening should be prepared in the palatal portion of the maxillary denture.
- Adhesive tape is attached over the buccal and labial surfaces of both dentures 2 mm away from the denture borders.

- With a knife-edge stone, a fairly deep groove should be cut into the buccal and labial surfaces of the dentures at the junction of the impression material and filled with molten base-plate wax.

**Border molding**—During the impression making it has been emphasized that a slight amount of impression material should be left on the flattened borders.

**Impression—**Plaster of Paris or zinc oxide-eugenol is suggested for the first step of impression making, and plaster of Paris for the second step (the palatal portions).

### *Advantages*

The same as in technique A.

### *Disadvantage*

Even though it has been suggested that the patient should not seat the denture by closing on it, the existing errors of centric occlusion may produce some pressure points and a faulty impression can result.

## CLOSED-MOUTH RELINING TECHNIQUE–MANDIBULAR DENTURE

### Technique E

**Centric relation**—Existing centric occlusion is used as a means to seat the mandibular denture during the secondary impression. The occlusion is corrected during the establishment of a new occlusal vertical dimension.

**Denture preparation**—Loss of vertical dimension is corrected by luting softened modelling compound to the occlusal surfaces of the mandibular posterior teeth. The patient is directed to repeatedly pronounce the letter "m". The record is chilled, trimmed and slightly heated before returning it to the patient's mouth. The procedure is repeated until the occlusal vertical dimension is established to the operator's satisfaction. The denture is luted to the maxillary denture in maximum intercuspation. Softened modeling compound is placed inside the mandibular denture and the articulator closed against the lower cast to contact the incisal guide pin. With this procedure, the amount of vertical dimension indicated by the thickness of the compound on the surface of the mandibular teeth is transferred to the base of the mandibular denture. The mandibular denture at this stage is used as a tray for making the final impression.

**Impression**—Modeling compound at the early stage and zinc oxide-eugenol for making the secondary impression are suggested.

### *Advantages*

- The loss of vertical dimension can be compensated for during the relining procedures.
- The error in centric occlusion can be reduced during the laboratory stages.

### *Disadvantages*

- This technique is very time consuming from the standpoint of clinical and laboratory procedures.
- The procedure for establishment of occlusal vertical dimension is highly questionable.

## OPEN-MOUTH IMPRESSION TECHNIQUE

Boucher's technique (technique F) is the only one that explains a method for relining the mandibular and maxillary dentures at the same time.

## Technique F

**Centric relation**—Utilizing both dentures as recording bases, the jaw relation is recorded after making the secondary mandibular and maxillary impressions.

**Denture preparation—**A posterior palatal seal is formed in modeling compound on the maxillary denture. One millimeter of space is provided inside the denture for the new impression material. The borders are shortened 1 mm to allow space for the impression material to form a new border.

In lower denture the buccal surfaces of the lingual flanges are ground to minimize the pressure against the mylohyoid ridges and between the tissues of the floor of the mouth and buccal sides of the lingual flanges. The lingual flange between the premylohyoid eminences is shortened by 1 mm. The labial flange between the buccal notches is shortened by 1 mm. Two grooves are cut on the buccal sides of the lingual flanges to facilitate removal of the retromylohyoid eminences after the cast is poured. A modeling compound handle formed over the lower anterior teeth facilitates handling the denture when it is carried to the mouth. Adhesive or masking tape is adapted over the polished surfaces of both dentures and over the teeth.

**Border molding**—If the flanges are inadequate, the borders should be corrected with modeling compound.

**Impression**—Zinc oxide-eugenol impression material in which the patient is asked to pull his upper lip down and to open his mouth wide. These actions mold the impression material over the border of the denture. The upper denture is laid aside until the lower impression has been made.

### *Advantages*

- The special trimming of the denture and making room for the impression material will facilitate the making of a reasonable impression during the selective pressure impression technique without any occlusal interference.
- A separate interocclusal record using already made impressions as the recording bases will allow the operator to concentrate on recording the jaw relation.
- It is possible to verify the centric relation record, if necessary.
- The interocclusal record, which is made with quick-setting plaster, is a reliable one.

### *Disadvantage*

- The technique requires more clinical and laboratory time.

## Suggested Technique

Functional impression with fluid resin (tissue conditioning material).

## Clinical Procedures

- Dentures not to be worn overnight before impression making.
- Examination of old dentures for errors of occlusion and centric occlusion (maximum intercuspation).
- The basal surface of the denture is reduced to allow room for the tissue conditioning material.
- This surface is dried before the material is placed into the denture.
- A minimum thickness of tissue conditioning material is placed over the tissue surface of the denture.
- After removal from the mouth, the tissue conditioner is trimmed to remove all excess material.

**Instructions given to patient on care of resilient liners**

- When the patient returns to the dentist after three to five days, the denture should be examined for denuded areas. Mark the denuded areas with an indelible pencil and relieve the pressure areas on the denture before the next application of tissue conditioner.
- Underextended borders should be corrected with impression compound before the next application of material.
- The material is never allowed to remain in a denture for more than a week, as the material itself may become a source of irritation.
- When the tissue has returned to a clinically discernible healthy state, the patient is scheduled for making impressions.
- All of the tissue conditioning material on the tissue surface of the dentures should be replaced with new impression material.
- The patient is instructed to wear the dentures for 3 minutes while in the waiting room and he or she may eat a light meal if desired.
- If there are no pressure areas, this impression could be considered as a master impression for relining the dentures.

## Laboratory Procedure

- After the final impression is made, a cast must be poured immediately.
- Mount the maxillary cast on a semi-adjustable articulator using the face-bow transfer record.
- Relate the mandibular denture to the maxillary denture, which is already mounted on the articulator, using an interocclusal record.
- If an occlusal discrepancy exists, it should be corrected before separating the impressions from the casts, by using a selective grinding procedure.
- The procedures of relining and rebasing are the same until this stage. During the laboratory phase of a rebasing procedure, the entire old denture base is replaced by new material without changing the arrangement of the teeth. The presence of all porcelain teeth greatly facilitates a rebasing procedure. If resin teeth are present, relining is usually indicated, as it is difficult to rebase a denture with resin teeth.
- When the dentures are finished, plaster remount casts are made and the maxillary cast mounted on the articulator.

## Insertion Procedure

- Use a pressure-indicating paste to locate pressure areas. They are carefully relieved by grinding with mounted stones.
- A new interocclusal record is used to mount the lower denture in centric relation.
- It is necessary to verify the mounting before adjusting the occlusion.
- With a selective grinding procedure, the occlusion can be preferred at the correct occlusal vertical dimension.
- Before dismissing the patient at the initial placement visit, check the occlusion once again.

## 28. Classify denture lining materials and elaborate on permanent and temporary denture liners.

The material may be classified as follows:

- Permanent lining materials
  1. Heat-cured acrylics
  2. Cold-cured acrylics

3. Light-cured acrylics
4. Plasticized acrylics
5. Silicones
6. Polyolefins
7. Phosphazines
8. Silastics

- Temporary relining materials
    1. Tissue conditioners
    2. Functional impression materials.

## Permanent Lining Materials

Long-term soft lining materials distribute stress more evenly and absorb impacts that can arise from masticatory function. They can therefore be said to have a shock-absorbing or cushioning effect. Long-term soft lining to a complete lower denture improves the ability to bite and chew and provides general improvement in comfort when compared with hard relines.

### *Indications for use*

1. Persistent pain under a denture.
2. Thin atrophic mucosa.
3. Para function.
4. Replacing an existing denture, having a soft liner.
5. Sharp bony ridges or spicules on which the denture-bearing mucosa, in essence, becomes impaled.
6. Superficially placed mental nerve.

## Types of Permanent Lining Materials

Silicone rubber or soft acrylic. The silicone materials may be cold-curing or heat-curing. The soft acrylics are heat-curing; cold-curing soft acrylics are only used as temporary soft liners.

## Acrylic Resin Materials

### *Composition*

**Polymer**: Can be either poly (ethyl methacrylate) or poly (methyl methacrylate)/poly butyl methacrylate

**Monomer**: Can be methyl methacrylate, nbutyl methacrylate or a combination of ethyl acetate and methyl methacrylate.

**Plasticizers**: Butyl phthalyl butyl glycolate, di-n-butyl glycolate or 2 ethylhexyl-diphenyl phosphate.

Most of the materials use polyethylmethacrylate or polybutylmethacrylate as the basic polymer. The materials are heavily plasticized to create softness.

## Manipulation

Available as powder and liquid. 2:1 or 1.5:1 polymer/monomer ratio is taken normally.

### *Disadvantages*

1. Water solubility is high.
2. Bacterial growth and fungal growth is prevalent.
3. Color changes are marked with these materials.

## Plasticized Vinyl Acrylics

Composition of vinyl acrylics is similar to acrylics except that the vinyl major function groups are present. They have a higher concentration of plasticizer that is in the range of butyl phthalyl butyl glycollate in the concentration of about 58.8%.

### *Properties*

Tensile strength : 20-37 kg/cm$^2$
Percent elongation: 250-280
Hardness shore A number : 35-55
Tear resistance : 5-11 kg/ cm.

### *Visible Light Cure Resins (VLC)*

- Polymerization shrinkage for each of the three materials is nearly equal in value.
- Tensile strength for VLC resin was slightly higher than the values for HC and AP acrylic resin.
- The transverse deflection values at 3500 and 5000 g showed that deflection of the VLC resin was less than that of the HC and AP acrylic resins materials, indicating that VLC resin is comparatively stiffer.
- The elastic modulus (bending) was slightly higher than in HC and AP acrylic resin.
- Dimensional changes were evaluated by fabricating VLC, HC and AP bases on identical casts with metal markers in five locations. After 10 days in water, the AP resin shows a +0.05% expansion from ridge crest to ridge crest but no expansion was seen with HC or VLC.

## Phosphazines

These materials have higher bond strengths than other materials.

## Manipulation

Available as tubes base and catalyst. Two equal lengths of catalyst and base are taken in glass slab and mixed so that uniform color is obtained.

### *Properties*

Tensile strength : 37 kg/cm$^2$
Percent elongation: 240
Hardness shore A number : 50
Tear resistance : 9 kg/ cm.

## Cold-curing Silicone Rubber Materials

### *Composition*

Polymer—Alpha dihydroxy end blocked poly (dimethyl siloxane) whereas the catalyst may be triethoxy silanol, ethyl polysilicate, Tetraethoxy silane, methyltriacetoxy silane, Acryloxyalkyl silane.

Catalyst—Dibutyl tin dilaurate, stannous octoate, moisture or heat with benzoyl oxide. commonly used catalyst, dibutyl tin dilaurate, has been found to be a mucosal irritant.

## Manipulation

Available as tubes base and catalyst. Two equal lengths of catalyst and base are taken in glass slab and mixed so that uniform color is obtained.

### *Properties*

Tensile strength : 25–44 kg/cm$^2$
Percent elongation: 325–340
Hardness shore a number : 25–45
Tear resistance : 5–7 kg/cm.
The abrasion resistance of these materials is poor.

## Heat-cure Silicone Rubber Materials

### *Composition*

Polymer—Alpha dihydroxy end blocked poly (dimethyl siloxane)
Catalyst—Acryloxyalkyl silane.

The adhesive used with this is gamma methacryloxypropyl trimethoxysilane.

## Manipulation

Available as tubes base and catalyst. Two equal lengths of catalyst and base are taken in glass slab and mixed so that uniform color is obtained.

## Properties

Tensile strength : 25–48 kg/cm$^2$
Percent elongation: 325–400
Hardness shore a number : 25–50
Tear resistance : 11–14 kg/cm.
Water absorption of these materials is low.
Dimensional stability is improved and accuracy of fit is good.

# RECENT ADVANCES

A soft denture liner is made from an envelope covered with a polyethylene film which is filled with a viscous silicone liquid allowing continuous adaptation of the denture base.

## Temporary Lining Materials

### Tissue conditioners—Plasticized acrylics

Tissue conditioners are soft elastomers used to treat an irritated mucosa supporting a denture. These materials will conform to the anatomy of the residual ridge, gel in that position and continue to flow slowly after application. They are used only for short term applications and should be replaced every 3 days.
Supplied as powder/liquid or ready sheet forms.

## Composition

Powder—Polyethylmethacrylate or copolymers of polyethyl/methylmethacrylate.
Liquid—A mixture of an aromatic ester, such as dibutyl phthalate which acts as a plasticizer and Ethyl alcohol.

## Properties

- Hardness—13 to 49 shore A hardness units 24 hours after mixing.
- They show a loss in weight due to loss of alcohol and become harder over a period of time.

- Easily deformed—When a stress of 200 gm/cm$^2$ applied 15 minutes after the set of the material, the compression will range from 60 to 83% of the original length. Those materials with a low alcohol content exhibit good dimensional stability for the first few hours after mixing.
- Viscoelastic and elastic behavior, cushions the cyclic forces of mastication and bruxism. Viscoelastic behavior can be modified by altering the powder/liquid ratio.

### 29. What is an immediate complete denture? Mention the advantages and disadvantages of immediate complete dentures. Describe briefly the clinical procedure of managing a patient with immediate complete dentures.

## INTRODUCTION

A patient who is not esthetically conscious of the loss of anterior teeth generally prefers a complete denture treatment after the extraction of all natural teeth. This patient remains without teeth not only during the healing phase, but also during the time required for the fabrication of the complete denture. For patients who find it difficult to go around without anterior teeth two options remain, one is to convert an existing removable partial denture into an interim complete denture another is to make a conventional immediate complete denture.

The "Glossary of Prosthodontic Terms" defines an immediate denture as "the complete or removable partial denture constructed for insertion immediately following the removal of natural teeth".

**There are usually two surgical appointments for the removal of the natural teeth**

The posterior teeth are removed except for the first premolars. Six to eight weeks later, after the ridges are healed impression procedures are performed. The immediate denture is fabricated during several appointments prior to the extraction of the remaining anterior teeth and inserted at the second surgery appointment.

## ADVANTAGES

1. There is no time that the patient will be without teeth; hence they are able to continue their social and business activities without embarrassment.
2. The digestive function is uninterrupted but for a short period following insertion of the prosthesis.
3. The general appearance of the patient is less affected as there is only a minimal change in muscle tone and the occlusal vertical dimension is maintained.
4. There is no change in the masticatory and facial muscles, for unfavorable speech and chewing habits and centric relation is easier to record.
5. As early functional loading is done chances of ridge resorption is less and support for a complete denture is better.
6. The immediate denture acts as a matrix or bandage with negative pressure over the surgery site, hence this controls hemorrhage, prevents contamination and provides a protective covering over the wound. It can be used to maintain medications in place, also the patient usually experiences less pain.

7. The artificial teeth can be set in the identical positions occupied by the natural teeth. The size, shape and shade of the natural teeth as well as their individual positions can be copied exactly.

## DISADVANTAGES

1. After insertion, the alveolar bone and soft tissue around the extraction sites will remodel and resorption occurs. Hence, the denture will not fit well and relining is needed.
2. Treatment with an immediate complete denture is expensive as there is more of postoperative adjustments and needs to be often relined following healing.
3. The esthetics of the immediate denture cannot be evaluated until the insertion appointment as there is no anterior trial done.

## DIAGNOSIS AND TREATMENT PLANNING

A diagnosis and treatment plan is carried out. A clinical examination of hard and soft tissues is performed. The patient's radiographs are evaluated to detect the extent of bone loss due to periodontal disease. A panoramic radiograph can be used to determine the presence of impacted teeth, retained roots, foreign bodies, exostoses, osteoporosises, cysts and other pathology.

Mounted diagnostic casts are used to evaluate tooth position, jaw relationships and occlusal plane discrepancies. It also helps to reveal and analyze undercuts.

An immediate denture for one arch is initially done and only after the healing and stabilization of this arch is the opposite arch treated for immediate denture.

## TREATMENT PROCEDURES

### Initial Impressions

Initial impressions are made with alginate in a stock tray, this is poured with dental stone. A custom tray is fabricated with autopolymerizing acrylic resin on the preliminary cast and the remaining teeth are covered with a double thickness of baseplate wax to provide space for the impression material around the teeth. Any undercut areas are blocked out with wax. The tray borders are ensured to have sufficient thickness to support border-molding material and refined for sharp borders.

### Secondary Impressions

After the custom tray is adjusted for proper extension. The posterior palatal seal area is determined and transferred to the tray. The tray is trimmed back to the line and heated stick compound is added sequentially to the borders of the tray and border molded in the mouth. Perforations are placed in the tray to enhance the flow of the impression material and increase its retention within the custom tray. A final impression material as light bodied polysulfide rubber is used.

If excessive undercut or tooth mobility is present, those areas should be blocked out with soft wax and lightly coat the mobile teeth with petrolatum. In severe cases a vacuum formed resin stent can be used as a protective sheath while making the impression.

The impression is made with the tray being seated in the mouth and allowed to remain there for curing. The tray is removed on a line parallel to the long axes of the remaining teeth. After the impression is inspected for detail, voids and thickness of the impression material it is poured with vacuum-mixed dental stone.

## Alternative Impression Procedure

In this technique the edentulous areas and periphery are recorded in zinc oxide-eugenol paste and the teeth are recorded with irreversible hydrocolloid (alginate). A custom tray is fabricated that covers only the edentulous area. The tray is border molded with stick compound and a zinc oxide-eugenol impression is made. After applying alginate adhesive to the outer surface of the tray, the impression is reseated. A stock tray is loaded with irreversible hydrocolloid and another impression is taken over the initial impression. After the irreversible hydrocolloid sets, the stock tray is removed along with the custom tray which is embedded in the impression. The impression is poured with vacuum mixed dental stone.

## Jaw Relation Records

A recording base of autopolymerizing acrylic resin and an occlusal rim of baseplate wax is made. A face bow record is made to orient the maxillary cast on the articulator. If posterior tooth are present evaluate the existing vertical dimension including supra eruption, drifting of natural teeth and occlusal wear by phonetics and other methods. If the patient has no posterior occlusion, the tentative occlusal vertical dimension should be determined as in totally edentulous patient.
The centric relation record is made at a slightly increased vertical dimension with impression plaster or zinc oxide-eugenol impression paste. This record is removed from the mouth trimmed and verified and the mandibular cast is mounted using the centric relation record. A protrusive interocclusal record is made to set the condylar guidance on the articulator.

## Tooth Selection and Arrangement of Posterior Teeth

If natural teeth are present the same shade is selected, and if opposing natural tooth is present anatomic tooth form is used. Acrylic denture teeth is the choice of artificial teeth as porcelain denture teeth cannot be ground and adjusted. The posterior teeth are arranged as to provide multiple bilateral posterior contacts in centric relation and there should be no anterior contact in centric relation. Bilateral balancing contacts are provided in lateral and protrusive excursions unless it opposes a natural dentition.

## Posterior Try-in

If the trial base is not retentive, denture adhesive may be used. Centric relation and occlusal vertical dimension are verified. The position of the posterior palatal seal is verified and scribed in the maxillary master cast.

## Arrangement of Anterior Teeth

The anterior denture teeth are arranged after the posterior try-in appointment. The anterior teeth are removed one at a time at the level of the gingival margin with a rotary instrument or sharp knife and the remaining ridge is smoothed with a hand instrument. Denture teeth are placed alternatively and selectively ground to the ridge lap portion of the tooth. Modifications in anterior arrangement is done as to the patients liking. The wax up of the denture is completed to provide proper contour and thickness of the denture base. After boil out the cast can be modified as needed and the denture is processed using conventional techniques. The denture is disinfected prior to insertion.

## Insertion Procedures

Under local anesthesia the remaining teeth are removed with a minimum of trauma and bony spicules, sharp edges of bone are removed. A clear surgical stent is made to evaluate the prepared surgical site. After the surgical procedures the denture is inserted and if the denture base will not seat completely, relining or tissue conditioner is used and occlusal, interferences are also eliminated.

### *Instructions*

1. Cold packs are suggested.
2. The patient must not remove the denture during the first 48 hours as tissue inflammation and edema from the surgery may prevent the reinsertion of the denture for several days.
3. A soft diet (E.g. milk shakes, jelly, ice cream) is advised to minimize trauma.
4. Appropriate pain control medication should be prescribed if necessary.

## Post-insertion Care

1. The patient is seen 24 hours following insertion during this appointment.
2. The occlusion is checked with articulating paper before the removal of the denture.
3. The denture is evaluated for any ulceration from denture pressure or overextension of the base on the tissue side.
4. The tissue surface of the denture is cleaned and patient is instructed to rinse mouth gently with a mouthwash.
5. During the check up denture insertion and removal are done sparingly.
6. After 48 hours the patient is recalled and all the above procedures are repeated.
7. The patient is instructed to keep denture clean and use warm saline rinses and also instructed to keep the denture in at night for three days following insertion. Once adequate healing takes place patient can remove denture in the night time and can shift from soft diet regimen.
8. The next appointment is after a week during which, occlusion, tissue surface of denture, soft tissues are evaluated for any changes. If a tissue conditioner was placed at insertion, it should be replaced at this time and every succeeding week until replaced with a resilient liner.
9. After three to four weeks of healing the patient is seen again, subjective complaints are addressed. A clinical remount is performed and the occlusion is refined on the articulator.
10. After the patient has worn the immediate denture for about four to five weeks and after the extraction sockets have filled, treatment linings with a resilient self-curing chairside liner is given, which will be comfortable for the patient and maintain the denture in its normal relationship by preventing it from settling.

These resilient linings are repeated four- to six-week intervals until the sockets are completely filled in with bone which usually takes about six months. After six months the denture can either be relined, if the patient is satisfied with the esthetics and function of the denture or remade if the patient has complaints about the esthetics of the immediate denture.

## SUMMARY

An immediate denture provides restoration of esthetics, phonetics and masticatory function with immediate replacement of artificial teeth. The immediate denture also facilitates the transition to the edentulous state. A proper follow-up care is essential for the success of an immediate denture.

**30. Define overdenture. Mention the biomechanical rationale of over-denture prosthesis. Discuss the advantages and disadvantages of over-denture.**

## DEFINITION

A tooth-supported complete denture is a dental prosthesis that replaces the lost or missing natural dentition and associated structures of the maxillae or mandible and receives partial support and stability from one or more modified natural teeth.

## CLASSIFICATION

Based on the method of abutment preparation.
1. Noncoping
2. Coping
3. Attachments.

### Noncoping Abutments

In noncoping, selected root abutments are reduced to a coronal height of 2 to 3 mm and then contoured to a convex or dome-shaped surface. These abutments commonly require endodontic therapy and are prepared conservatively to receive an amalgam or composite type restoration.

#### *Abutments with Copings*

Cast metal copings with a dome-shaped surface and a chamfer finish line at the gingival margin are fabricated and cemented.

Two types of copings are prepared
1. Short coping
2. Long coping.

Short cast copings are 2 to 3 mm long and as coronal root reduction would expose the pulp, endodontic therapy is done. As the cast coping is small a post is fitted to the canal hence soft gutta percha-like material is used.

As long cast copings are normally 5 to 8 mm long endodontic therapy is not done. The long cast coping is ellipsoidal-shaped coronal coping and has a larger crown-root ratio hence require good bone support.

#### *Abutments with Attachments*

Attachments are used to improve retention of the denture base and generally are secured to the abutment by a cast coping. As long as the tooth-supported complete dentures remain functional, the resorption rate of the remaining residual ridge is significantly reduced.

#### *Goals*

1. Over denture maintains teeth as part of the residual ridge and can withstand a greater occlusal load without movement.
2. Overdenture decreases the rate of resorption as the remaning teeth supports the alveolar bone.

### Indications

For young patients who face the loss of the remaining natural teeth.

### Requirements of an Overdenture

1. Teeth used as over denture abutments should be free of any periodontal dieases.
2. Good plaque control measures is to be taken to preserve the existing abutment tooth.
3. The abutment tooth should be nonmobile, some mobile tooth can be salvaged after periodontal therapy but need good attached gingiva to act as a vertical stop.
4. A well-fitting base is needed to distribute the load over a wide area and also prevent food and plaque accumulation under the base.
5. The appliance should be simple to construct and maintain.

## ADVANTAGES

1. The retained natural tooth in over denture aids in providing tensile stimulation to the residual alveolar ridge preserving it.
2. Preservation of proprioceptive response.
3. The modified teeth provide a definite vertical stop for the denture base.
4. Horizontal and torquing forces are minimized.
5. Stability and support are increased.
6. The retention of only one tooth frequently makes for a more favorable prognosis.
7. Less post insertion problems.
8. Convertibility: Can be easily relined or rebased into a conventional complete denture.

## DISADVANTAGES

1. Caries susceptibility of the abutment teeth.
2. Periodontal disease can cause failure in overdenture functioning
3. Encroachment of the interocclusal distance when internal attachment is used.
4. Bony undercuts adjacent to the overlaid teeth (usually buccally), prevent close adaptation of the denture flange to the underlying tissue.
5. If undercuts are blocked it causes spacing between denture and tissue creating a food trap.
6. Esthetics, bony under cuts cause overcontouring of denture resulting in improper lip fullness.
7. Under contouring leads to improper retention and stability.

### 31. Define overdenture and discuss in detail the clinical procedures in overdenture.

## DEFINITION

A tooth-supported complete denture is a dental prosthesis that replaces the lost or missing natural dentition and associated structures of the maxillae or mandible and receives partial support and stability from one or more modified natural teeth.

## OTHER TECHNIQUES

Other techniques for the preparation of teeth to serve as abutments for overdenture include simple tooth modification and reduction, tooth reduction and cast coping, endodontic therapy with amalgam plug, endodontic therapy and cast coping and endodontic therapy and cast coping utilizing some form of attachment.

## Clinical Procedure

1. Remove the hopeless teeth and insert the removable prosthesis.
2. During the healing period, the periodontic and endodontic treatment is carried out and the clinical crowns of the retained teeth may be reduced at this time.
3. Preparation of the retained teeth.

**Tooth preparation is of two types**

1. For minimal retention utilizing only the clinical crowns.
2. For positive retention using endodontically treated root.

## Tooth Preparation for Minimal Retention

1. Sufficient tooth structure is removed to provide favorable crown-root ratio, acceptable esthetic position for prosthesis and a favorable occlusal relation with the opposing arch.
2. The prepared tooth is tapered in an occlusogingival direction with a chamfer margin extending beneath the free gingival margin.
3. The finished tooth with attached coping is the male member of the denture. The female member is a part of the denture base
4. The occlusal and/or incisal surface is prepared as to accommodate a cobalt chromium bearing.
5. Coping fabrication: Carve the wax pattern on the die made from an accurate impression placing the concavity in the occlusal surface of the pattern, using a wax tool. Cast the coping, using a hard type of Class III gold. Cement the polished coping to the tooth.

***Steps in Clinical Procedure***

1. *Preliminary impression* with alginate, cast is poured in dental stone and a custom-made impression tray is made by applying one thickness of baseplate wax (1 to 2 mm) over the abutment teeth.
2. *Final impression* is made using Elastomeric impression material. A master cast is obtained on which record Bases and Occlusion Rims are made with the incorporation of the metal bearing in the record base. This is done by adapting one thickness of baseplate wax to the abutments, leaving the occlusal surface exposed. The bearing is seated in the concavity and sealed in place with wax over which a stable record base is made.
3. *Jaw relation* is made in the same manner as for conventional complete dentures.
4. Teeth arrangement
   Acrylic resin artificial teeth are used commonly, but if the opposing arch tooth is gold or porcelain then the same material is preferred for replacement. The metal bearing is retrieved after removing record base and repositioned in the concavity. The acrylic resin tooth is made hollow with an acrylic bur until metal bearing is properly positioned. Occlusion is adjusted, after the bearing is positioned to the acrylic resin tooth with sticky wax and rest of teeth are arranged in maximum occlusion.
5. At trying-in:
   1. Verify the centric and eccentric jaw relation records.
   2. Assure esthetic and phonetic acceptability by the patient.
6. Laboratory Procedures
   1. Contour the wax.
   2. Flask the denture.
   3. Eliminate the wax.

The metal bearings are retrieved from the acrylic resin tooth, cleaned with boiling water, dried and the metal bearing is seated in the concavity and a coping of activated acrylic resin is made, using the "shake on" technique. This allows trial packing of the heat-cured acrylic resin denture base.

Remount procedures for processing errors are completed.

7. Denture insertion

   Using pressure-disclosing paste, the contacts between the female member in the denture base and the male abutments are assessed. There should be no contact except between the convex surface of the metal bearing and the concave bearing surface of the coping. After evaluating the tissue side and the borders for pressure areas and overextension, remount procedures are completed to perfect the occlusion. The patient is recalled once a month for the first six months and once every three months thereafter.

8. Tooth preparation to provide retention

   In positive retention, the attachment used is the endodontically treated root of the tooth and not the clinical crown.

   A. The clinical crown is prepared to the level of the gingiva.
   B. A root cap preparation is made after opening the root canal to the desired diameter and depth for retention and rigidity.
   C. An individual impression of the root preparation and canal is made, stone poured and die is prepared.
   D. A dowel is fitted with an acrylic knob attached into the canal in the die. Hence, the knob is securely imbedded in the irreversible hydrocolloid impression and also used to position the die accurately for cast pouring.
   E. A full arch impression is made of Alginate.
   F. The dies are fitted to the transfer dowels and the impression is poured in dental stone.
   G. Remount indices are placed in the base of the cast.
   H. The die is covered with one thickness of baseplate wax before making a record base.
   I. Jaw relation records are made and the casts mounted on to the articulator.
   J. The male member is placed as close to the center of the root as possible sometimes in a slight lingual position if more favorable for the esthetic positioning of the artificial tooth.
   K. The cap, post and male member are waxed and invested in a flask and cast in a hard gold alloy.
   L. Teeth are arranged, try in done, Waxed up and denture is processed.
   M. Cast is retrieved and remounted to correct processing errors.

## Endodontic Therapy with Cast Coping Utilizing Some Form of Attachments

Endodontic therapy is used in situation in which stability and retention are desired. This requires sufficient interridge distance.

### Attachments used are

1. Stud attachments
2. Gerber attachment
3. Dalbo attachments: rigid, resilient and stress broken
4. Ceka attachment
5. Ancrofix system
6. Magnets as cobalt-samarium

7. Bar attachments of two types: Bar units and bar joints. Examples: Hader bar, Dolder bar and the Dolder bar joint. Clips as Baker clip, Ackermann clip and CM clip (Fig. 18).
8. Quinlivan attachment (Fig. 18).

Photoelastic tests concluded that the best design for uniform distribution of occlusal forces was the conventional amalgam plug design. If more retention and stability are required then other designs such as the stud attachment, the Ancrofix and Hader bar, transferred stress in a more favorable manner than other types tested.

Common failures in overdentures were related to poor case selection and inadequate maintenance. If proper patient selection, patient motivation, basic prosthodontic principles, home-care instruction and frequent recall are done than success of overdenture is high. Floss, periodontal aids, small brushes, rubber tips, must be utilized to minimise all plaque accumulation from the tooth surface and sulcus for the long life of overdenture prosthesis.

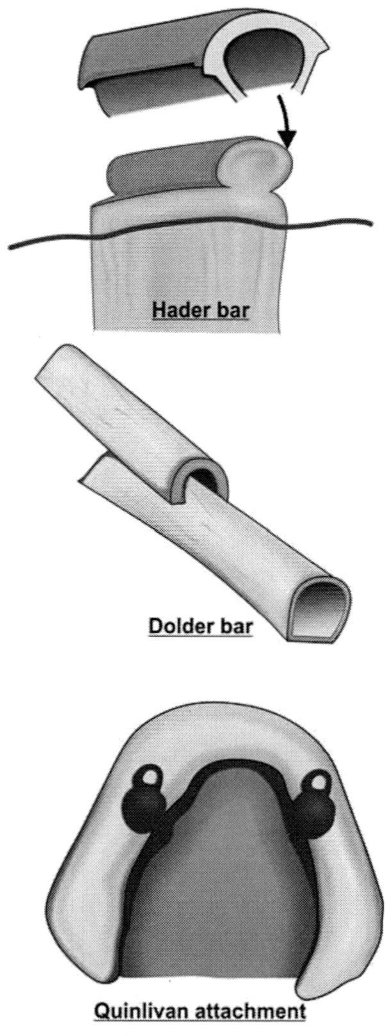


**Fig. 18:** Different types of attachments

## 32. Classify overdenture attachments and write in detail the popular attachments commonly employed.

### Classification

1. *According to shape, design and primary area of use:*

| ***Stud attachments*** | ***Bar attachments*** |
|---|---|
| Gerber attachment | Hader bar |
| Dalbo attachment | Dolder bar |
| Ceka attachment | Ackermann clip |
| Zest anchor | |
| Rothermann | |
| Schubiger | |
| Introfix | |
| Quinlivan | |

2. *Coronal :*
   a. Intracoronal
      i. Resilient
      ii. Non-resilient
   b. Extracoronal
3. Radicular :
   a. Telescope stud attachments
   b. Bar attachments
      i. Joints
      ii. Units
4. Accessory: Auxillary attachments
   a. Screw Units
   b. Pawl connectors
   c. Bolts
   d. Stabilizers/Balancers
   e. Interlocks
   f. Pins/Screws
5. Magnets
   Permanent magnets
   Induced magnets
   Open field magnets

| **Extracoronal** | **Intraradicular** |
|---|---|
| Gerber attachments | Zest anchor |
| Dalbo attachment | |
| Ceka attachment | |
| Schubiger attachment | |
| Quinlivan attachment | |
| Rothermann attachment | |
| Infrofix attachment. | |

## Extracoronal Attachment Systems

### *Dalbo Stud Unit*

a. Ball and socket
b. Rigid Dalbo.

**Features**—4 mm high with spherical shape male section easy to clean. The fingers of the socket are surrounded by nylon rings.

### *Gerber Attachment*

This allows vertical movement. Retention is obtained by a retaining spring in the female unit engaging a peripheral groove in the male section. The spring clip may be removed for adjustment by unscrewing.

### *Ceka system*

1. Rigid
2. Resilient.
   Rigid and Resilient designs share a common base, but the ceka extracoronal units are not identical. Therefore, it is not possible to change resilient for rigid constructions merely by changing, the retention portions. The vertical travel allowed by the resilient stud unit is 0.4 mm: The retention pin or male section is screwed on to the base ring.

### *Schubiger*

Consists of a short screw block for bar fixation. A larger one for fixed removable bridge work and an individual cap core system.
a. Solder base common to the Gerber
b. Sleeve in ceramic metal
c. A cap nut
d. Overall height is 2.8 mm.

## Intraradicular Stud Attachments

The advantages of this system lies in cost and space requirements. They do not require precious metal coping dowel or special laboratory procedures. They are relatively simple and quick.

### *Zest Anchor System*

A nylon male element is incorporated in the denture base and projects downward and engages a recess in the root preparation. Further the loads are applied at a point that is well apical to the gingival margin of the root. A variety of abutments may be employed including hemisected molar roots. Two sizes of zest anchor are available depending on the root length and diameter.

## Bar Attachments

The bar attachments help in splinting of the abutment teeth, retention and support of the appliance. Bar attachments are classified into two types bar units and bar joints.

- Bar unit has a rigid fixation where there is no movement between the bar and overlying sleeve and can be classified as tooth born.
- Bar joints permits rotational movement between sleeve and bar and derives more of residual ridge support.

### Types of Bar Attachments

- Hader bar
- Dolder bar attachment
- Bakers clips
- Ackermann clips and
- C.M. clip.

### Magnetic Denture Retention

Magnetic denture retention are of two types:

1. Those depending on the mutual repulsion or like magnetic pole (E.g. Friedman magnetic stabilizers).
   i. Less retentive when most needed (when jaws are apart).
   ii. Continued resorption.
2. Those depending on the mutual attraction of unlike poles.

Continuous attracting forces could cause the embedded bar magnets to move through the bone, erode the soft tissues and become exfoliated.

## 33. Enumerate various post-insertion problems in complete denture wearers, causes and management of them and add a note on laboratory remounting.

1. Post-insertion complaints are corrected in the one to three days adjustment period. This is the critical period in the denture wearing experience of the patient.
   The commonest complaint is **tissue irritation and ulceration**. In the upper denture soreness may develop on the borders, mucosa and crest of the residual ridge and slope of the residual ridge. The cause of this can be overextension, error in impressioning, tissue surface irritant, occlusion, pressures created by heavy contacts of opposing teeth in the same region, shifting of the denture bases from defective occlusal contacts.
   **Adjustment for overextension:** Locate the overextension and reduce and polish the overextended area.
   **Adjustment for defective occlusion** is done by first observing dentures in the mouth. Then the mandible is guided into centric relation by placing a thumb directly on the antero-inferior portion of the chin and directing the patient to open and close until the first feather touch of the back teeth occurs and close tight. If the teeth touch and slide there is an error in centric occlusion, remount dentures and if the same error is found on articulator, it is eliminated by selective grinding. If the error is too gross reset teeth.
   If the patient complains of burning or numbness in anterior part of the jaw, the incisive papilla needs to be relieved as the nasopalatine nerves are compressed.
   In the mandibular denture, tissue irritation and ulceration occur on lingual flange posteriorly due to tissue surface irritant, defective occlusion and loose tissue entrapment. Anteriorly too this occurs on the lingual flange. This is due to excessive loading from posterior occlusion shifting mandibular base forward. This needs to be corrected by checking balance for protrusive movement. If the patient complains of tingling or numbness at the corner of the mouth or lower lip, this is due to impingement on the mental nerve and this area in the lower denture needs to be relieved.
2. *Denture looseness:* This can be due to poor retention of mandibular denture due to improper impression technique, poor adaptation of bases, lack of seal in maxillary denture, excessive

thickness of distobuccal flange which interferes with normal movement of coronoid process, excessive thickness of height of flange of upper denture in region of buccal notch or distal to notch. Adjustment of denture looseness can be managed by reimpression, rechecking posterior palatal seal, and occlusion.

3. *Defective speech:* This is due to excessive opening of vertical dimension, deficient palatal contour, arch form incorrect anteriorly, posteriorly or both and increased tongue size. This can be managed by resetting to closed vertical dimension, repair by adding material or removing material, recontouring lingual surfaces and resetting teeth.
4. *Inability to eat:* Increased or decreased vertical dimension and incorrect centric relation. This is corrected by setting teeth to correct vertical dimension, selective grinding in case of occlusal errors.
5. *Gagging:* This is due to upper posterior border seal inadequate or too long. Managed by adding modelling compound which is later replaced with acrylic resin in case of short border and reducing length/depth in case of long border. In mandibular denture this can be due to posterior lingual flange extension. This is managed by reducing and polishing the extended area.
6. *Cheek biting:* This is due to incorrect arch form in posterior segment. This can be managed by providing horizontal overlap by resetting teeth of maxillary or mandibular denture or both. Or buccal contours of lower denture may be ground if excessive.
7. *Food catching:* This is due to poor finishing/contouring, occlusal interference, poor processing, and insufficient patient instruction. This can be managed by recontouring, polishing, correct occlusion, repair and replacement of teeth and re-educating the patient.
8. Faulty esthetics:
   1. The patient complains of a puffy look. This is due to expanded anterior or posterior arch.
   2. The patient complains of a collapsed appearance. This is due to a constricted arch form. These are managed by resetting teeth and remaking the denture.
   3. Lip wrinkles. This is usually anatomic, does not require treatment and needs only explanation to the patient.

## REMOUNTING

Remounting is done to check for any occlusal errors which could have taken place in the denture after the wax up and processing. These occlusal errors are corrected by selective grinding after remounting and verifying with interocclusal check records. Ideally a face bow index is made before separating the denture from cast. This helps to reseat the maxillary denture in the same relationship on the articulator.

### Advantages of Remounting

1. No patient participation.
2. Able to visualise the occlusion better.
3. Provides a stable working foundation without resilient tissues affecting the occlusion.
4. The absence of saliva makes possible more accurate markings with the articulating paper.
5. Objections from patients when they see their dentures being ground is avoided.

#### *Procedure*

Mandibular denture is oriented to the maxillary denture in centric relation by means of an interocclusal record.

### *Interocclusal Check Record*

Two thicknesses of softened passive type wax is placed on the occlusal surfaces of the mandibular teeth. The patient is instructed or guided to close into the wax when the jaws are in centric relation.

### *Verifying Record*

The teeth should not penetrate to make contact. Chill with cold air and remove. Trim the wax with slight indentations remaining, expose the facial side to visualise the seating of the maxillary denture.

### *Mounting*

Orient the mandibular denture to the maxillary denture by means of the interocclusal record and secure with sticky wax. After seating the mandibular cast in the denture, complete mounting by attaching to the mandibular member with plaster.

### *Rechecking Records*

Make another wax interocclusal record and check on the articulator after placing the dentures on the cast. While checking the condylar elements should be freed and place the teeth in the wax record indentations. The condylar elements should rest against the stops. Repeat with three records to confirm.

### *Selective Grinding Procedures*

In anatomic tooth forms to attain balanced occlusion, bilateral tooth contacts of the posterior teeth is required to evenly distribute the forces.

A cusp fossae marginal ridge relation of maximum intercuspation when the jaws are in terminal hinge position is needed to attain balance.

There should be no occlusal interference when jaw movements occur to and from centric and eccentric positions.

If selective grinding is done maximum intercuspation when the jaws are in centric relation, balanced centric occlusion is achieved.

If selective grinding done to make simultaneous cusp tip to cusp tip contact on both sides of the arch when the jaws are in a right or left lateral position, balanced occlusion in a static eccentric position exists.

When the anterior teeth make incisal edge to incisal edge contact in a straight protruded relation, and if the posterior teeth are altered to make cusp contacts at the same time balanced occlusion in protrusion exists.

The buccal cusps of the mandibular posterior teeth and the lingual cusps of the maxillary posterior teeth maintain the vertical dimension of jaw separation by contact in the fossae and on the marginal ridges of their antagonists. Generally the functional cusp of upper (lingual cusp) and functional cusp of lower (buccal cusp ) is never ground.

The non-functional cusps, deepening of fossae and the cuspal inclines are the ones that are altered to achieve balance.

## 34. Explain the various types of grafts used in ridge augmentation procedures.

- Bone graft materials are generally evaluated based on their osteogenic, osteoinductive, or osteoconductive potential.

- Osteogenesis refers to the formation or development of new bone by cells contained in the graft.
- Osteoinduction is a chemical process by which molecules contained in the graft (bone morphogentic proteins or BMPS) convert the neighboring cells into osteoblasts, which in turn form bone.
- Osteoconduction is a physical effect by which the matrix of the graft forms a scaffold that favors outside cells to penetrate the graft and form new bone.

## Classification of Graft Materials

### *Based on Original Source*

- Autograft—tissue transferred from one position to another within the same individual.
- Allograft—freeze-dried, fresh: tissue transferred from one individual to another genetically dissimilar individual of the same species.
- Xenograft—tissue transferred from one species to another species, e.g. Kielbone (oxbone).
- Alloplast—a synthetic graft or inert foreign body implanted into tissue.

## Autogenous Grafts

Autogenous grafts are harvested from the patient's own body and are superior at retaining cell viability.

Contain live osteoblasts and osteoprogenitor stem cells and heal by osteogenesis.

No histocompatibility differences and risk of disease transfer. Can be from intraoral and extraoral sites.

## Bone from Intraoral Sites

Intraoral grafts are osseous coagulum, bone blend, intraoral cancellous bone marrow transplants and bone swaging. The commonest sites intraorally are:

- Edentulous ridges
- Tori
- Maxillary tuberosity
- Healing bony wound or extraction sites
- Bone trephined from within the jaw without damaging the roots
- Bone removed during osteoplasty and osteotomy.

1. **Osseous Coagulum:**
   *Robinson* in 1969 described a technique using a mixture of bone dust (from cortical bone) and blood that he termed *osseous coagulum*. Advantage includes the ease of obtaining bone from already exposed surgical sites, and its disadvantages are its relatively low predictability and inability to procure adequate material for large defects.
2. **Bone Blend:**
   Bone is removed from a predetermined site, triturated in the capsule to a workable plastic like mass, and packed into bony defects.
3. **Intraoral Cancellous Bone Marrow Transplants:**
   Cancellous bone can be obtained from the maxillary tuberosity, edentulous areas, and healing sockets. After a ridge incision is made distally from the last molar, bone is removed with a curved and cutting rongeur.

4. **Bone swaging:**
   This technique requires the existence of an edentulous area adjacent to the defect from which the bone is pushed into contact with the root surface without fracturing the bone at its base.

## Bone from Extraoral Sites

Extraoral site is the illiac crest.
Iliac Autografts: The use of fresh or preserved iliac cancellous marrow bone has been extensively investigated in bony defects with various numbers of walls, furcations, and even supracrestally.

## Allografts

Allografts are bone taken from cortical bone within 12 hours of death, are later defatted, cut in pieces, washed in absolute alcohol, and deep frozen. The material may then be demineralized, and subsequently ground and sieved to a particle size of 250 to 750 mm and freeze dried. Finally, it is vacuum sealed in glass vials. The material is then treated with chemical agents or strong acids to effectively inactivate the virus, if still present.

**There are various types of allografts available, including**

1. Freeze-dried bone allograft (FDBA)
2. Demineralized freeze-dried bone allograft (DFDBA).

***Undecalcified freeze-dried bone allograft (FDBA)***

FDBA is an osteoconductive material, whereas decalcified FDBA (DFDBA) is an osteoinductive graft. DFDBA has a higher osteogenic potential than FDBA and is therefore preferred.

***Decalcified freeze-dried bone allografts (DFDBA)***

Demineralization in cold, diluted hydrochloric acid exposes the components of bone matrix that have been termed bone morphogenetic protein.

## Xenografts

A xenograft is a graft between different species.
Examples of xenografts are:

- Calf bone
- Kiel bone
- Anorganic bone
- Natural coral

*Calf bone:* Calf bone (Boplant), treated by detergent extraction, sterilized and freeze dried has been used for the treatment of osseous defects.

*Kiel bone:* Kiel bone is calf or ox bone denatured with 20% hydrogen peroxide, dried with acetone, and sterilized with ethylene oxide.

*Anorganic bone:* Anorganic bone is ox bone from which the organic material has been extracted by means of ethylenediamine; it is then sterilized by autoclaving.

Two products currently available are:

- Osteo Graf
- Bio-Oss

*Natural coral-Coralline calcium carbonate:* Biocoral (Inoteb, France) is a calcium carbonate obtained from a natural coral and is composed primarily of aragonite.
It is biocompatible and resorbable with a porous size of 100-200 μm, similar to the porosity of spongy bone.

## Alloplasts or Nonbone Graft Materials

- Sclera
- Dura
- Cartilage
- Cementum
- Dentin
- Plaster of Paris
- Plastic materials
- Bioceramics – Hydroxylapatite and Tricalcium phosphate
- Bioactive glasses
- Polymers
- Coral-derived materials.

*Sclera:* Sclera was originally used in periodontal procedures because it is a dense fibrous connective tissue with poor vascularity and minimal cellularity hence has a low incidence of antigenicity and other untoward reactions.

*Cartilage:* It can serve as a scaffold.

*Plaster of Paris:* Plaster of Paris (calcium sulfate) is biocompatible and porous, thereby allowing fluid exchange, which prevents flap necrosis.

*Plastic materials:*

HTR (Bioplant) polymer is a nonresorbable, microporous, biocompatible composite of polymethylmethacrylate (PMMA) and polyhydroxylethylmethacrylate (PHEMA) and calcium hydroxide.

The polymer resorbs slowly and is replaced by bone after approximately 4-5 years. It is osteophilic, and osteoconductive alloplastic bone substitute.

*Calcium phosphate biomaterials*

These materials are osteoconductive. Two types of calcium phosphate ceramics have been used:

a. Hydroxyapatite (HA) has a calcium-to-phosphate ratio of 1.67, similar to that found in bone material. HA is generally nonbioresorbable.
b. Tricalcium phosphate (TCP), with calcium-to-phosphate ratio of 1.5, is mineralogically B-whitlockite. TCP is at least partially bioresorbable.

***Bioactive glass***

Consists of phosphates, and silicon dioxide used in the form of irregular particles measuring 90 to 170 μm (*PerioGlas*) or 300 to 355 μm (*BioGran*). When this material comes into contact with tissue fluids, the surface of the particles becomes coated with hydroxycarbonateapatite, incorporates organic ground proteins, such as chondroitin sulfate and glycosaminoglycans, and attracts osteoblasts that rapidly form bone.

### *Coral-derived materials*

Two different coralline materials have been used in clinical periodontics: natural coral and coral derived- porous hydroxyapatite. Both are biocompatible but whereas natural coral hydroxyapatite resorbed slowly (several months), porous hydroxyapatite is not resorbed or takes years to do so.

## 35. Define palatal lift prosthesis and write in detail about its fabrication and post-insertion instructions.

Palatal lift prosthesis displaces the soft palate superiorly and posteriorly in order to assist the soft palate to affect closure with the peripheral pharyngeal tissues. First prosthesis was made by Gibbons and Bloomer in 1958.

### Uses

- Cleft palate, with palatal insufficiency and submucus cleft palate.
- Myasthenia gravis
- Bulbar poliomyelitis
- Cerebral palsy
- Injuries to soft palate (tonsillectomy, maxillary resections, etc.).

#### *Palatopharyngeal incompetence*

Defined as having normal anatomy but ineffective or absent motor function is treated with a palatal lift.

- Palatopharyngeal insufficiency
- Is caused by abnormal anatomy and is treated with a pharyngeal bulb prostheses or speech bulb.

#### *Advantages*

- Gag response is minimized- due to superior positioning and sustained pressure of the lift portion of the prostheses against the soft palate.
- Physiology of the tongue is not compromised due to superior position of palatal extension.
- The access to the nasopharynx for the obturator is facilitated.
- Lift portion can be developed sequentially to aid patient adaptation to the prostheses.

#### *Contraindications*

- Inadequate retention for the basic prostheses
- Palate is not displaceable
- Uncooperative patient.

### Diagnostic tools

- Video fluoroscopy
- Nasal endoscopy and
- Air flow measurements.

### Requirements

#### *Positioning*

- Position the weakened soft palate closer to posterior pharyngeal wall

- Complete closure of residual muscle activity
- Maintain nasal airway
- Complete pharyngeal closure for speech and swallowing.

### *Retention*

- The primary requirement for a successful palatal lift is retention.
- The lift is a posterior extension cantilevered from a removable denture base, the ability to keep the base portion in correct position is critical to success.

*Retentive aids*

- Teeth mainly I and II molars
- Tissue undercuts
- Retentive undercuts on teeth created by adding composite or orthodontic brackets
- Complete denture.

## Fabrication

### *1st Appointment*

- Accurate hydrocolloid impression of both arches.
- Upper impression must extend at least 2 cm posterior to fovea palatine.
- The cast is then surveyed and ideal position of clasps is decided.

### *2nd Appointment*

- Lift generation
- A retentive loop should be made at the same plane as the hard palate with a relief at the posterior end of lift portion extending approximately 2 cm.

## Step 1

- The oral portion with the loop is tried in the patient's mouth to ensure complete seating, and adjustments are made if necessary.

## Step 2

- Modeling compound is applied to the loop, shaped, flamed to create a smooth surface and then chilled before placing into the mouth.
- First addition of compound should cover the loop evenly and extend several millimeters beyond.
- Patient is allowed to wear the prostheses for a few minutes at this stage, to familiarize with it.

## Step 3

Small additions are made to the compound posteriorly until the soft palate is brought into light contact with the posterior pharyngeal wall.

## Step 4

- Lateral pharyngeal closure. Reduction of hypernasality is achieved with lateral extent of the lift.
- Addition of compound till there is reduction in size of lateral ports.
- With each addition, the patient is asked to breathe through the nose and attempt speech.

- Avoid addition of compound on the oral side of the lift, which may induce gag reflex if posterior tongue comes into contact with the lift.

### Step 5

- Assess improvement in speech. Ask them to say plosive sounds which increase intraoral pressure.
- Enlargement of lift is stopped when the speech professional is satisfied with the result.
- Reduce lateral aspect of lift if the patient is unable to breath, or if the downward force of the soft palate displaces the lift or retentive limit of clasps has been reached.

### Step 6

- The final step is to reduce 1-2 mm of the entire surface of the lift.
- Mouth temperature softening wax is applied in sufficient amount to replace the lost compound.
- The lift is tempered and reinserted.
- The patient is asked to speak, swallow water, and move his head in all directions to form the wax.
- The lift is then removed after 5 minutes and examined for areas of excess pressure.

### Insertion and Patient Instructions

1. Confirm effectiveness of lift during insertion appointment.
2. Check for excessive pressure with pressure-sensitive paste - reduce and polish areas of heavy pressure.
3. Check-up is done 2-3 days after delivery.
4. Check for mucosal irritation and relieve the areas.
5. If the lift completely occludes the nasal port, making the patient a mouth breather, the patient might prefer to wear it only during speech.
6. During eating - usage of lift is decided by the patient as many of them do not have a problem of food leakage.
7. Some do not tolerate the lift during eating as nasal airflow is necessary for olfactory portion of taste.
8. The prostheses should be removed during night.
   To give rest to the tissues
   To reduce the amount of time the abutment teeth are under orthodontic forces.

## 36. Classify the materials used for maxillofacial prosthesis and add a note on each of the materials.

Ideal requisites of maxillofacial material:

1. Material should have physical and mechanical properties similar to the human tissues such as variable consistency, dimensional stability, allow detail reproduction, high edge strength, high elasticity and light weight.
2. Material must be compatible with the human tissue, non-toxic, non-allergic easily cleaned, non-porous but permeable, odourless and resistant to microbial contamination.

3. Material must be capable of adherence to human tissue by adhesive or other mechanical means and permit easy removal of adhesive.
4. Material must be compatible with intrinsic and extrinsic means of coloring/staining.
5. Should have relatively simple polymerization process, not sensitive to minor processing variables and requiring molding procedures commonly used in dentistry.
6. Material should be easy to adjust, repair, reline and able to bond or laminate to other materials for better properties.
7. Completed prosthesis must have an acceptable service life of at least 4-5 years, must be capable of relining or readapting to the tissues surrounding the defect to prolong the service life.

Various materials used for maxillofacial prosthesis
- Vinyl polymers and copolymers
- Acrylic resin
- Latexes
- Silicones.

Commercially available newer materials:
1. Acrylic resin copolymer – Palamed-Kulzer
2. Vinyl polymers and copolymers:
   - Realistic – Prosthetic services, California
   - Mediplast – Std. Arts, Butler
3. Polyurethane elastomers – Epithane-3 Daro Products, Butler.
4. Silicone elastomer:
   - MDX 4-4210, Silastic 372, 373, Dow Corning Michigan.
   - Cosmosil, principality, UK
   - Elatosil M 3500, waker/chemic
   - Epsil – Dentamid
   - Silskin 2000 – Dupay Health Care.

### *Vinyl Polymers and Copolymers*

- The most widely used material for the fabrication of maxillofacial prosthesis.
- Vinyl are the derivatives of ethylene
- The vinyl chloride is polymerized in the presence of free radical catalyst to form polyvinyl chloride.
- The amount of vinyl acetate in the polymer varies from 5 to 20%.
- Flexible than natural rubber.
- Resistant to sunlight and aging.
- Vinyl acetate forms polyvinyl acetate on polymerization.
- Polyvinyl chloride is a clear, hard and odour less resin.
- It darkens when exposed to UV light and heat, hence requires heat and light stabilization agents.
- Polyvinyl acetate is stable to light and heat, but has an abnormal low softening point (35°– 40°).

## Types of Vinyls

### REALASTIC

- It is a polyvinyl chloride compound which solidifies into a flexible material when heated.
- These are esthetically satisfactory, but possess a short shelf life.
- Tinting can be accomplished both internally and externally using a variety of coloring agents.
- Ferrous pigments incorporated into the mixture provide a longer shelf life and provide best esthetic results.
- Metal molds are suggested because of their short shelf life.

### MEDIPLAS

- It is a heat curing plastisol of polyvinyl organic compound.
- Available in a variety of premixed base colors, which can be further tinted to match the patient's skin tone.
- The prosthesis becomes yellow when it is exposed to UV light, peroxide, ozone and tetra ethyl lead.
- Processing: Initial set - 100°C. Final set - 140°C for 10 mts.

### *Acrylic Resins*

These are used in fabrication of both intraoral and extraoral prosthesis.
Derivatives of ethylene, and these contain phenyl groups in their structural formula.
Obtained from acids (CH = CHCOOH), and methacrylic acids [CH2 = C(CH3)COOH].

### METHYLMETHACRYLATE

- It is a clear, transparent liquid at room temperature
- Melting point—48°C
- Boiling point—100.8°C,
- Density—0.945 g cubic cm
- Polymerization can be initiated by UV light, heat or chemicals.

## Advantages

1. The coloring can be done internally/externally.
2. Preferred for restoring defects which require minimal movements.
3. Useful in cases of rapidly changing defects where relining is mandatory.
4. Easily available, economical and familiar.

## Disadvantages

1. Rigid nature of the material → tendency to dislodge the prosthesis → irritation of underlying tissues.
2. Rigidity → difficulty in duplicating prosthesis.

### *Latexes*

- Soft, inexpensive material.

- Degenerate rapidly
- Color instability → infrequently used.
- Synthetic latex = tripolymer of butyl acrylate, methyl methacrylate and methyl methacrylamide.

***Silicones***

- Most commonly used materials for maxillofacial prosthesis.
- Poly-dimethyl-siloxane is called silicone
- Commercially available rubber form polymers have filters for additional strength, antioxidants and vulcanizing agents are added to transform raw mass into a rubbery resin during processing.

### Classification

1. Room temperature vulcanizing silicones (RTV).
2. High-temperature vulcanizing (HTV).

## RTV SILICONES

- Composed of comparatively short chains together with cross-linking agent (ethyl ortho silicate) with addition of a catalyst (stannous octoate).
- They are transparent/opaque white.
- Dry earth pigments added to color match before the introduction of catalyst.
- Can be cured in stone mold.
- Silica fillers increase strength and mask discoloration
- To enhance esthetics, a transparent RTV grade silicone (Dow corning MDX 4-4210) is recommended.
- Supplied as single paste systems colored by addition of dyed rayon fibers, dry earth pigments and/or paints.

## RTV SILICONES–CURING

- Dow corning manufactures different types of RTV silicones.
- Differences are in curing time and strength.
- Clear, translucent MDX 4-4210.
- Semi-transparent, such as silastic 399.
- Opaque and white, such as silastic 382.
- Supplied as semisolid/putty like materials.
- Require milling, packing under pressure, 30 min heat application cycle at 180°C.
- Pigments are milled into them → better strength and color stability.

## HTV SILICONES

They are considered superior to RTV silicones.
Disadvantages-Require a milling machine and metal molds
Due to high tensile strength, increased risks of damaging the mold.

## HTV SILICONES–CURING

- Translucent, milky white, semisolid materials.
- Dow corning manufactures 3 consistencies:
  MDX 4-4514, MDX 4-4515 and MDX 4-4516.
- MDX 4-4514 – extra oral prosthesis – Chalian et al (1972), Beder (1974) and Lontz et al (1974)
- Cut and rolled in the milling machine before packing into molds. Colors and fibers incorporated during rolling.

### Silastic 399

- Resembles white Vaseline.
- Supplied with 1 base paste and 2 catalyst.
- When mixing with catalyst 1, cross linking agent becomes milky, but working time will be longer.
- When mixing with catalyst 2, it sets up to translucent in 10-15 min.

### Silastic 382

- Medical grade silicone
- Thick white liquid and comes with a separate container of organometallic catalyst, which catalyses without the use of heat or pressure on combining with silicone.
- Working time varies from 2–6 min. depending on amount of catalyst.

### Silastic 6508

- Resembles sticky modeling clay in the raw state.
- Must be vulcanized at 260°F and formed in pressure molds
- Requires much more sophisticated handling.
- Tensile strength = 785 psi.

### Siphenylene

- An analene silicone polymer synthesized and formulated as a pourable, viscous RTV liquid.
- Consists of 3 unit kit – base resin, tetrapropoxy silicone (cross-linking agent) and a catalyst.
- High tensile strength and low modulus of elasticity.
- Feels like skin.
- Incorporation of fillers → ↑ tear strength.

### Dermasil

- Self curing silicone, clear base material and catalyst are used to initiate the reaction.
- Pigments added to base material to obtain proper shade.
- ↑ pigments → dull appearance of material.
- Fragile margins to be reinforced with nylon stocking material.

## POLYURETHANE ELASTOMERS

- Recent addition to materials used in maxillofacial prosthetics.
- Linkage/presence of urethane.
- Synthetic proportions of long chain linear polyesters/polyethers reacted with diisocyanates.

- Can be thermoplastic/thermosetting.
- Hard segments—extended diisocyanates.
- Soft segments—polyesters and ionocyanates.
- Catalyst—stannous octoate or dibutylin diacirate.
- Coloring agents—inorg. Colorants are preferred.
- When properly processed, they are chemically inert, resistant to solvents, odourless, abrasion resistant, have high tear and tensile strength.
- Do not harden with wear and are dimensionally stable.
- Can be colored easily (externally/internally).

## Dow corning MDX 4-4210

- Very useful silicone, but viscosity problems.
- Addition of Silskin (thickening agent) regulates viscosity.
- Recommended where soft silicone is required.
- The degree of softness can be varied with the addition of catalyst.
- Available in various color systems.

## Palamed

- Cross-linked copolymer of methacrylic and acrylics.
- Consists of powder and liquid, when mixed forms a dough-like material.
- The processed prosthesis will have a sponge like center and a continuous skin like covering.
- Proper packing of the molds is critical in obtaining satisfactory final prosthesis.
- It is necessary to use exact weight equivalent to Palamed to modeling materials.

## EPITHANE

- It is a polyurethane system.
- Consists of polyol components (mixture of polyesters), diisocyanate components and organic catalyst.
- Soft and more flexible
- Disadvantages—deterioration and skin reaction.

## COSMESIL–SILSKIN 2

- Cosmesil is a HTV silicone.
- Silskin is a RTV silicone.
- Available in elastomeric form and color systems.
- Curing temp. Cosmesil – 70°C for 2 hours.
- Silskin – bench press for 24 hours.

### *Role of Pigments in Maxillofacial Prosthesis*

Duplicating skin color and texture is difficult as color varies in different physiological, pathological (anemia) and emotional states which may lead to pallor/ flushing. Color depends on capillary blood flow, oxygenation, thickness of epidermis and presence of pigments (melanin and carotene).

### *Intrinsic Coloring*

- Metallic oxides/pigmented silicone concentrates are used and red fibers may be incorporated to simulate blood vessels.
- Coloring in RTV silicones (MDX 4-4210) is accomplished by adding various dry earth pigments.
- For accurate measurements, these pigments are mixed with RTV thinner in the ratio of 3 grains of pigments to 10 ml of thinner.

### *Extrinsic Coloring*

- Ouellete (1969) described spray coloring of silicone elastomer maxillofacial prosthesis.
- Pigments matching the patients' skin are mixed in proper proportions with clear elastomers and solvents which can be sprayed on to the prosthesis until the desired color is obtained.
- Tattooing using standard artist's oil paints by tattooing machine also can be done.
- The intrinsic coloring has more service life than extrinsic coloring.

### *Adhesives*

- Are polymeric compounds modified with solvents and tackifying fluids.
- Medicoadhesives may be used with polyvinyl chloride.
- Silicone and acrylic and epithane 3 adhesives have been recommended for polyvinyl chloride and silicone elastomers.

# SHORT NOTES

## 1. Diagnostic casts.

A diagnostic cast should be an accurate reproduction of the teeth and adjacent tissues, poured in dental stone because of its strength and abrasion resistance.

The impression for the diagnostic cast is made with irreversible hydrocolloid (alginate) in a perforated impression tray.

### IMPORTANCE OF DIAGNOSTIC CASTS

1. Diagnostic casts permit viewing of the occlusion from the lingual and buccal aspect.
2. To analyze the existing occlusion in case of needed occlusal adjustment and occlusal reconstruction.
3. Aids in diagnostic wax up to determine the occlusion before definitive treatment is begun.
4. Diagnostic casts helps to survey the dental arch as a whole.
5. Helps in surveying of the cast to determine existing soft tissue undercuts, parallelism of teeth as for overdenture cases.
6. Aids in mouth preparation decisions, as to the removal of soft tissue undercuts
7. Helps to show and discuss the case with patient regarding the treatment plans, needed corrections and problems if any.
8. Aids to select and fabricate trays.
9. If needed can duplicate diagnostic cast in case an undercut has to be blocked.
10. Diagnostic casts may be used as a constant reference.
11. In areas where alterations are required as in soft tissue or hard tissues, a rough alteration can be mocked on the duplicate cast to assess the outcome.

## 2. Types of denture-bearing areas (based on function).

### Primary Stress-bearing Areas in Maxillary Denture are

- Horizontal portion of hard palate
- Residual alveolar ridge.

The *residual ridge and most of the hard palate* are the primary stress-bearing areas in the upper jaw.

The *fibrous connective tissue* covering the crest of the residual alveolar ridge and the *compact bone* made up of haversian systems aids in supporting the denture due to its firmness and position.

### Primary and Secondary Retentive Areas

a. *The rugae area* in the anterior part of hard palate is at an angle to the occlusal plane of the residual ridge which helps in secondary retention provided it is not distorted in the impression procedure.
b. *The glandular region* the posterior part of the hard palate if covered by denture help in retention of the denture.

## Relief Areas

- Incisive papilla
- Ridge, cuspid eminence, malar bone
- Fovia palatines
- Midpalatine suture.

a. (Incisive papilla)
   The incisive papilla covering the incisive foramen is located behind and between the central incisors. If this area is not relieved it may cause interference with the blood and nerve supply.
b. (Median palatine raphe)
   As the mucosa in the median palatal suture is thin and attached to the periosteum, not relieving this area can cause soreness and rocking of the denture.

## Other Areas

a. Zygomatic process
   In long-term edentulous patients, the zygomatic or malar process located opposite the first molar region, need to be relieved. If not can to lead soreness of the underlying tissues and affects retention.
b. Posterior palatal area
   As the posterior palatine foramina are thickly covered by soft tissue they do not need to be relieved except in extreme cases of resorption.
c. Vibrating line of the palate
   It is an imaginary line drawn across the palate that marks the beginning of motion when the patient says "ah". It extends from one pterygomaxillary notch to the other and passes about 2 mm in front of the foveae palatinae. Ideally the distal end of the upper denture should end 1 or 2 mm posterior to the vibrating line, covering the tuberosities and extending into the hamular notches. Posterior palatal seal area is an area between the anterior and posterior vibrating lines which should be closely contacted by the denture. If a gap exists it jeopardises the retention of the denture.

## Denture-bearing Area in the Mandible (Fig. 1)

### *Relief Areas*

- Crest of alveolar ridge
- Mental foramen
- Mylohyoid ridge
- Torus mandibularis.

### *Supporting Structure*

- Primary stress-bearing area: Slopes of residual alveolar ridge.
- Secondary stress-bearing area: Rugae area.

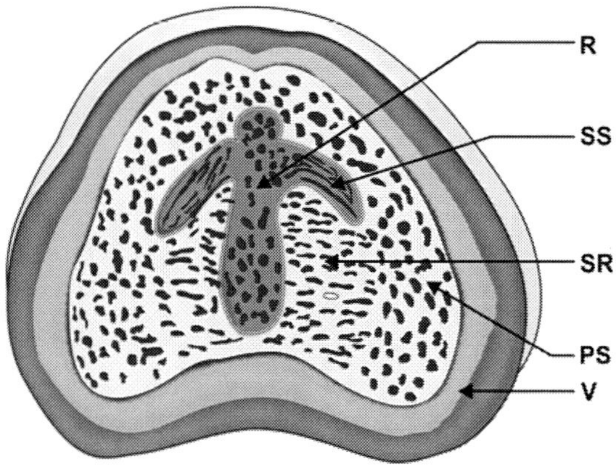


RS:Relief area
SS:Secondary stress-bearing area
SR:Secondary retentive area
PS:Primary stress bearing area
V:Valve Seal Area

**Fig. 1:** Areas of primary function of maxillary basal seat

## 3. Types of rugae.

Rugae are raised areas of dense connective tissue radiating from the median suture in the anterior one-third of the palate. Palatal rugae in mammals are transversely running crests, which are exclusively formed by the mucosa of the hard palate except where an ossified base can be distinguished.

**Definition:** Rugae are anatomical folds or wrinkles of irregular fibrous connective tissue located on the anterior third of the palate (GPT-8).

They are also called "plica palatinae" or "rugae palatine".

**Prosthodontic consideration:** This area is a secondary stress bearing area. It resists the anterior displacement of the denture.

### Classification

#### *Based on shape (Fig. 2)*

- Curved
- Wavy
- Straight
- Circular.

#### *Based on length*

- Primary rugae: 5 to 10 mm or more
- Secondary rugae: 3-5 mm
- Fragmentary rugae: Less than 3 mm.

***Based on unification***

Converge: Two rugae originate away from the center and unite towards it.
Diverge: Those rugae which originate from the center and diverge away.

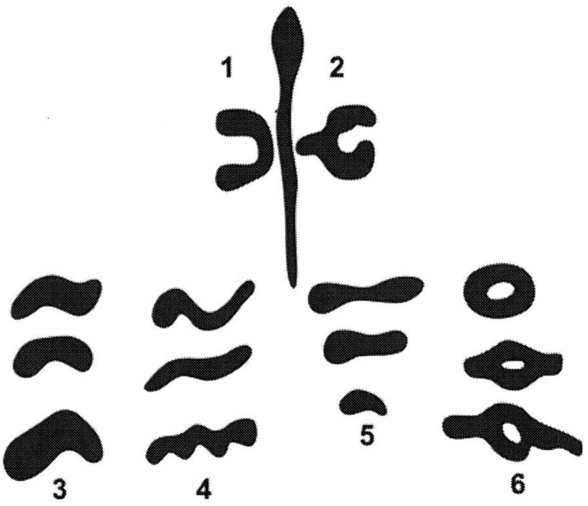


1. Diverge
2. Converge
3. Curve
4. Wavy
5. Straight
6. Circular

**Fig. 2:** Types of rugae

## Functions

- Palatal rugae have been shown to be highly individual and consistent in shape throughout life.
- The anatomical position of the rugae inside the oral cavity (surrounded by cheek, lips, tongue and the buccal pad of fat) also give some protection in cases of trauma or incineration.
- When identification of an individual by other methods is difficult, palatal rugae may be considered as an alternative source of information.
- It is assumed that the rugae facilitate food transport through the oral cavity, prevent loss of food from the mouth, and participate in food crushing.
- Because of the presence of tactile and gustatory receptors, rugae contribute to perception of taste, mechanical food qualities, and tongue position.

## 4. Classification of frenal attachment.

## House Classification

Class I—Frenum is located away from the crest of the ridge.
Class II—Frenum is located nearer to the crest of the ridge.
Class III—Frenum encroach on the crest of the ridge and may interfere with the denture seal.

### Labial Frenum

- It appears as a fold of mucous membrane extending from the mucus lining of the lip to or towards the crest of residual ridge on the labial surface
- It may be single/multiple
- It may be narrow/broad
- It contains no muscle fibers of significance
- Attachment is of three types
  - Close to crest of the ridge
  - Average
  - Distal to crest of the ridge.

#### *Clinical Consideration*

- Sufficient relief should be given during final impression procedure and in completed prosthesis because overriding of function of frenum will cause pain and dislodgement of denture.
- During impression procedure the lip should be stretched horizontal outwards for the proper recording of frenum.
- If frenum is attached close to the crest, frenectomy should be done to avoid decreased border seal.

### Buccal Frenum

Fold or folds of mucous membrane extending from mucous membrane reflection area to or towards the slope or crest of residual alveolar ridge.

**Significance:** Levator anguli oris (caninus muscle) lies beneath it, and hence influenced by other muscles of facial expression.

#### *Clinical Consideration*

During final impression procedure and in final prosthesis sufficient relief should be given for the movement of frenum because overriding of function of frenum will cause pain and dislodgement of denture.

a. During impression procedure the cheek should be reflected laterally and posteriorly.
b. If frenum is attached close to the crest of alveolar ridge, frenectomy is to be done.

## MANDIBULAR

### Labial Frenum

It is a fold of mucous membrane extending from mucous lining of mucous membrane of lips to or toward the crest of the residual alveolar ridge on the labial surface.

#### *Clinical Consideration*

During final impression procedure the lip has to be reflected anteriorly and horizontally.

During final impression procedure and in final prosthesis provision should be made in the form of notch to prevent overriding of function, which may result in laceration.

### Lingual Frenum

It is a mucobuccal fold that joins the alveolar mucosa to the tongue.

**Significance:** It overlies the genioglossus muscle, which takes origin from the superior genial spine on the mandible.

### *Clinical Consideration*

Sufficient relief should be given in the final impression and the final denture to prevent overriding of function of frenum.

During impression procedure touch the tip of the tongue to the incisive papilla region.

## 5. Muscles of mastication.

*The muscles are:*

- Masseter muscle.
- Temporalis muscle.
- Medial pterygoid muscle.
- Lateral pterygoid muscle.

### Masseter Muscle

**Shape** : Rectangular muscle.

**Origin** : From the zygomatic arch and extends downward to the lateral aspect of the lower border of the ramus of the mandible.

**Insertion** : Extends from the region of the second molar at the inferior border posteriorly to include the angle of the mandible.

### *Made up of Two Heads*

- Superior portion consists of fibers that run downward and slightly backward.
- Deep portion consists of fibers that run in vertical direction.

**Action**: When the fibers contract, mandible is elevated and teeth are brought into contact.

- The muscle provides force necessary to chew efficiently.
- Superficial portion also aid in protruding the mandible.
- When mandible is protruded and biting force is applied, the fibers of deep portion stabilize the condyle against the articular eminence.

**Nerve Supply:** Masseteric branch of anterior division of mandibular nerve.

### Temporalis Muscle

**Shape**: Large fan-shaped muscle.

**Origin**: Originates from the temporal fossa and the lateral surface of the skull.

**Insertion**: They extend downward between the zygomatic arch and the lateral surface of the skull to form a tendon that inserts on coronoid process and anterior border of the ascending ramus.

Can be divided into three portions according to fiber direction:

- **Anterior portion**: Fibers directed almost vertically.
- **Middle portion**: Fibers directed obliquely.
- **Posterior portion**: Fibers directed almost horizontally.

**Action :** When muscle contracts, it elevates the mandible and teeth are brought into contact.

- If only portions contract, mandible is moved according to the direction of those fibers that are activated.
- Because of angulation of fibers the muscle is capable of coordinating closing movements.
- When anterior portion contracts, mandible is raised vertically.
- When middle portion contracts, mandible elevates and retrudes.
- When posterior portion contracts, mandible retrudes.

**Nerve Supply**: Temporal branches from anterior division of mandibular nerve.

### Medial Pterygoid Muscle

**Origin**: The muscle originates from medial aspect of the lateral pterygoid plate.

**Insertion**: Extends downward, backward and outward to insert along the medial surface of mandibular angle.

**Action:** When fibers contract, mandible is elevated and the teeth are brought into contact. Muscle is active in protruding the mandible.

Unilateral contraction brings about a mediotrusive movement of mandible.

**Nerve Supply** : A branch from the trunk of mandibular nerve.

### Lateral Pterygoid Muscle

The muscle is described as two distinct and different muscles.

They are:

- Inferior lateral pterygoid muscle.
- Superior lateral pterygoid muscle.

### Inferior Lateral Pterygoid Muscle

**Origin:** Originates at the outer surface of lateral pterygoid plate and extends backward, upward and outward.

**Insertion:** Inserts on the neck of the condyle.

**Action:** When inferior muscle contracts, condyles pull down the articular eminences and mandible is protruded.

- Unilateral contraction creates mediotrusive movement of that condyle and causes lateral movement of mandible to opposite side.
- When this muscle functions with mandibular depressors, mandible is lowered and condyles glide forward and downward on the articular eminences.

### Superior Lateral Pterygoid

**Origin** : Originates at the infratemporal surface of the greater sphenoid wing, extending almost horizontally, backward and outward.

### Insertion

- Is on the articular capsule, the disc and the neck of the condyle.
- 60–70% fibers attach to the neck of the condyle.
- 30–40% fibers attach to the disc.
- Attachments are more predominant on medial aspect than on the lateral aspect.

### Action

- The muscle is active in conjunction with the elevator muscles.
- Active during power stroke and when the teeth are held together.

**Nerve Supply**: A branch from the anterior division of mandibular nerve.

## 6. Muscles of facial expression.

- Orbital group: Orbicularis oculi
  Procerus
  Corrugator supercili
- Nasal group : Compressor naris
  Dilator naris
  Depressor septi nasi
- Oral group
  ***Upper set:*** Risorius
  Zygomaticus major
  Zygomaticus minor
  Levator labii superioris
  Levator anguli oris
  Levator labii superioris alaeque nasi
  ***Lower set :*** Depressor anguli oris
  Depressor labii inferioris
  Mentalis
  ***Lateral set :*** Buccinator
  ***Circular set :*** Orbicular oris

### Orbicularis Oris

**Origin:** Intrinsic part: Superior incisivus, from maxilla
Extrinsic part: strata.
**Insertion:** Intrinsic part: Angle of mouth.
Extrinsic part: Lips and angle of the mouth.
**Nerve supply:** Motor nerve supply: Buccal branch of facial nerve.
Sensory nerve supply: Mandibular division of Trigeminal nerve.
**Action:** During deglutition, it seal lips/mouth.

#### *Clinical Significance*

In the upper lip it is supported by the six maxillary teeth and in lower lip the superior border is supported by the incisal edge of maxillary teeth when they are in occlusion.

When the muscles are relaxed, the lips become flaccid, it is important for the dentist to make the functional movements when making impression for the dentures.

### Mentalis

Conical, fasciculus, situated at the side of the frenulum of the lower lip.
**Origin:** It arises from the incisive fossa of the mandible.
**Insertion:**Inserted into the skin of the chin.

**Action**: It turns the lower lip outward and in contracting makes the lower labial vestibule shallow.

### *Clinical Significance*

This muscle can render the labial vestibule shallow and hence can dislodge the lower denture, particularly when anterior ridge is highly resorbed.

In certain cases surgical repositioning of mentalis muscle is indicated.

## Buccinator

### Origin

- Upper fibers arise from the outer surface of the maxillary alveolar process in molar region.
- Lower fibers arise from a corresponding area of the mandible
- Middle fibers arise from the pterygomandibular raphe.

### Insertion

- Upper fibers run in the upper lip to continue with the fibers to the opposite side.
- Lower fibers run in the lower lip to continue with the fibers of the opposite side.
- Middle fibers: The upper of these fibers run in the lower lip to continue with similar fibers of the opposite side. The lower of these fibers run in the upper lip similarly.

### Nerve Supply

- Motor nerve supply – Buccal branch of facial nerve.
- Sensory nerve supply – Mandibular division of trigeminal nerve.

### Action in Deglutition

Push food towards teeth during mastication, helps closing the mouth.

### *Clinical Significance*

In the lower jaw it becomes the part of the denture bearing areas.

The fibers of the muscle contract in line parallel with the occlusal plane so it does not directly dislodge the denture, but only when masseter is activated it pushes the buccinator medially against the denture borders in the area of retromolar pad. This is a dislodging force, and the denture border should be countered to accommodate this interaction between the buccinator and masseter muscles.

This counter in denture base is termed as masseteric groove, and if proper freedom is not given at the distobuccal flange it will displace the denture.

In the upper jaw, the position of attachment of the muscle determines the vertical height of distobuccal flange of the maxillary denture.

The action of buccinator muscle pulls the corners of the mouth laterally and posteriorly.

Major function of the muscle is to keep the cheeks taut, else during closure the muscles collapse and get in between the denture teeth, which is a major problem in senile individual with flaccid muscles.

## Common Facial Expressions and the Muscles Producing Them

1. Smiling and laughing – Zygomaticus major
2. Sadness – Levator labi superioris and levator anguli oris
3. Grief – Depressor anguli oris
4. Anger – Dialator naris and Depressor septi
5. Frowning – Corrugator supercilli and Procerus

6. Horror, terror and fright – Platysma
7. Surprise – Frontalis
8. Doubt – Mentalis
9. Grinning – Risorius
10. Contempt – Zygomaticus minor

## 7. TMJ ligaments.

These are composed of collagenous connective tissue and act predominantly as restraints to motion of the condyle and the disc.

### *Three Functional Ligaments*

1. Collateral ligaments
2. Capsular ligament
3. Temporomandibular ligament.

### *Two Accessory Ligaments*

1. Sphenomandibular ligament
2. Stylomandibular ligament.

## FUNCTIONAL LIGAMENTS

### Collateral Ligaments

- Short, paired (medial and lateral) structures attaching the disc to the lateral and medial poles of each condyle.
- Restrict movement of the disc away from condyle, allows smooth synchronous motion of the disc condyle complex.
- Vascular, innervated, fibroelastic in nature.
- The medial collateral ligament receives fibers from the inferior head of the lateral pterygoid muscle.

### Capsular Ligament

It encompass the joint, retaining the synovial fluid.

#### *Attachments*

- **Superiorly:** Temporal bone along the border of the fossa and the eminence
- **Inferiorly:** Neck of the condyle along the edge of the articular facet.
  Capsular ligament surrounds the joint spaces and disc attaching anteriorly, posteriorly, medially and laterally, where it blends with the collateral ligaments. They resist medial, lateral and inferior forces.
- Capsular ligament is well innervated, provides feedback regarding position and movement of the joint

### Temporomandibular (Lateral) Ligament

- Single structure that function in paired fashion with corresponding ligament on opposite TMJ.
- Can be separated into two distinct portions, which have different functions.
  **Outer oblique portion**—Descends from the outer aspect of articular tubercle and zygomatic process posteroinferiorly to outer surface of condylar neck.

**Inner horizontal portion**—Originates medial to the outer oblique portion of the ligament and outer surface of the articular tubercle and zygomatic process, runs horizontally backwards to attach to the lateral pole of the condyle and posterior aspect of the disc.

***Function***

- **Outer portion:** Limits amount of inferior distraction that the condyle may achieve in translatory and rotational movements.
- **Inner portion:** Limits posterior movements of the condyle during lateral movements (protects the retrodiscal tissues).
- Also called as *"check ligament"* of TMJ.

## ACCESSORY LIGAMENTS

### Sphenomandibular Ligament

- Arises from spine of sphenoid bone and descends into a fan-like insertion on mandibular lingula and lower portion of medial side of condylar neck.
- Important landmark during surgery as maxillary artery, auriculotemporal nerve and inferior alveolar nerve pass b/w the ligament and the mandibular neck.

***Function:*** Partly contributes to translation of the mandible.

### Stylomandibular Ligament

Dense thick band of deep cervical fascia extending from styloid process to posterior border of angle of mandible blends with the fascia of medial pterygoid muscle.
***Function:*** Similar to above, also limits excessive protrusion of the mandible.

### 8. Stability and support in complete denture.

## STABILITY

*Stability* is defined as, "The quality of a denture to be firm, steady, or constant, to resist displacement by functional stresses and not to be subject to change of position when forces are applied." -GPT.

Stability of the denture indicates its resistance to withstand horizontal forces.

## FACTORS AFFECTING STABILITY

1. Round, parallel ridges offer better stability than flat ridges.
2. Fibrous connective tissue that is firm aids in stability than flabby tissue.
3. An accurate impression with maximum coverage increases stability. Impressions should record the stress-bearing and nonstress-bearing areas under stress and relief respectively.
4. A well contoured occlusal rims with the occlusal plane oriented parallel to the ridge posteriorly and parallel to the interpupillary line anteriorly stabilises the denture.
5. If teeth are arranged in a well contoured occlusal rim, balanced occlusion and neutral zone is achieved easily which again aids in stability of the denture.
6. The polished surfaces should be contoured in regard with Neutral zone or action of various muscles tend to displace the denture. The neutral zone is defined as, "The potential space between the lips and cheeks on one side and the tongue on the other. Natural or artificial teeth in this zone are subject to equal and opposite forces from the surrounding musculature." -GPT

## SUPPORT

*Support* is defined as, "The resistance to vertical forces of mastication, occlusal forces and other forces applied in a direction towards the denture-bearing area."

**Factors affecting support**

1. Wide and maximum coverage of denture-bearing area distributes forces over a wide area which is termed as the "snowshoe" effect. This effect reduces the force per unit area.
2. If the primary stress bearing areas are stressed and if the incisive papillae, median palatine areas are relieved, it improves the support factor in a denture.
3. The peripheral tissues need to be accurately recorded to prevent over-extension of the denture and tissue irritation.

## 9. Closed mouth impression.

Closed mouth techniques record the tissues in their functional position.

In closed mouth technique pressure is applied by closing against occlusion rims or teeth that are attached to the impression trays by the patient.

Other muscle actions as swallowing, grinning, or pursing the lips are also done, while the impression material molds and records the tissue surface.

**Impression materials used for this technique are:**

a. Impression compound.
b. Waxes that flowed at mouth temperature.
c. Soft liners.

*Significance* of closed mouth technique as argued by Macmillan (1947) is that, this technique is capable of trimming the lingual borders of the lower denture during tongue movement.

**Disadvantages**

1. Soft tissues displaced by this impression technique tend to rebound to their undisplaced position when the forces are released. This unseats the denture.
2. As the denture is constantly held in a displaced position, the pressure limits the normal blood flow.
3. Excessive bone resorption as due to lack of proper blood flow
4. Inadequate retention.
5. Often the dentures made with closed mouth impressions are overextended and must be arbitrarily trimmed.

Soft liners are good for refitting complete dentures and also possess the advantage retaining compliance for many weeks.

## 10. Selective pressure techniques (Boucher, 1951).

The selective pressure technique is a combination of extension for maximum coverage with intimate contact with the movable, loosely attached tissues and light pressure in non-compressible areas.

*Principle of impression:* The mucosa over the ridge is able to withstand pressure, whereas the midline and incisive papillae are covered by thin layer of submucosal tissue which cannot withstand pressure.

### *Materials Used*

#### For Preliminary Impression

Impression compound relieved over the midline and incisive papilla areas in maxillary. In mandibular impression the only relief provided is on the crest of the ridge when the ridge is knife edged.

#### For Final Impression

Impression plaster or zinc oxide-eugenol impression paste as a wash impression which also records the relieved areas with minimal pressure and the ridge areas with pressure. Hence the midline and papilla sections of the denture will not make contact with the mucosa when the denture is not in function and when in function only applies mild pressure. The impression is refined with a minimum of pressure as escape holes are placed. This technique is common for maxillary arch.

#### Another Technique

A wax spacer is used to relieve the relief areas in a custom made tray. The borders of the tray are kept 2 mm short of sulcus depth. A border extension and refining with a low fusing impression material is done. After the borders have been refined, the wax spacer is removed, escape holes are placed and final impression is made with a free flowing zinc oxide-eugenol impression paste to record the supporting tissues in their undistorted positions. Minor corrections with waxes that flow at mouth temperature can be done. The impression is poured in stone immediately after the impression material sets.

### Disadvantages

1. Cannot be done on flabby ridges. This technique demands firm, healthy mucosal covering over the ridge.
2. Exceeding the movements will produce an under-extended denture.

### Advantages

1. Bone resorption is argued to be less compared to other techniques.
2. Good retention, support and stability.

## 11. Denture retention with note on physical factors.

Retention is defined as, "That quality inherent in the prosthesis which resists the force of gravity, adhesiveness of foods and the forces associated with the opening of the jaws."–GPT

It is the ability of the denture to resist displacement against its path of insertion.

### PHYSICAL FACTORS

1. Adhesion.
2. Cohesion.
3. Interfacial surface tension.
4. Capillarity or capillary attraction.
5. Atmospheric pressure and peripheral seal.

## 1. Adhesion

Adhesion is defined as "The physical attraction of unlike molecules to one another." –GPT

### *Factors Affecting Adhesion*

a. A thin film of saliva is essential in wetting the tissue surface of the denture and the mucosa. Thick ropy saliva displace denture by hydraulic pressure.
b. The amount of adhesion is proportional to the denture base area coverage. Some denture base materials help in wetting have better retention by adhesion.

## 2. Cohesion

Cohesion is defined as, "The physical attraction of like molecules for each other".

The factors that affect adhesion also affects cohesion. The cohesive forces act within the thin film of saliva. The greater the denture bearing area, more effective is cohesion.

## 3. Interfacial Surface Tension

It is defined as, "The tension or resistance to separation possessed by the film of liquid between two well-adapted surfaces." –GPT

These forces are found within the thin film of saliva, separating the denture base from the tissues which in turn resist the displacing forces. This force is dependant on the presence of air at the margins of liquid and solid contact (liquid air interface).

### *Factors Affecting Interfacial Surface Tension*

a. Consistency of Saliva (should be thin and even).
b. Perfect fit of the denture base.
c. Maximum coverage of basal seat area.
d. Good adhesive and cohesive forces, which aid to enhance interfacial surface tension.

## 4. Capillary Attraction

It is defined as, "That quality or state, because of surface tension causes elevation or depression of the surface of a liquid that is in contact with a solid."–GPT

Capillary attraction is a phenomenon in which a liquid tends to rise in a capillary tube by maximizing its contact along the walls of the tube at the interface between the liquid and glass.

### *Factors Affecting Capillary Attraction*

a. Good adaptation of denture base to soft tissue with maximum coverage.
b. Thin film of saliva.
c. When there is close adaptation between the denture and the mucosa.

## 5. Atmospheric Pressure and Peripheral Seal

Peripheral seal is the area of contact between the peripheral borders of the denture and the resilient-limiting structures. The peripheral seal prevents air entry between the denture and the soft tissue. When displacing forces act on the denture, a partial vacuum (natural suction) is produced between the denture and the soft tissues, which aids in retention.

Hence, atmospheric pressure is referred to as emergency retentive force or temporary restraining force.

### *Factors Affecting Atmospheric Pressure*

a. Good peripheral seal.
b. Perfect fit of denture.
c. Maximum coverage of basal seat.

## 12. Vibrating line.

Vibrating line of the palate is an imaginary line drawn across the palate that marks the beginning of motion of the vibrating in the soft palate when the patient says "ah".

The submucosa in the region of the vibrating line on the soft palate contains glandular tissue. The submucosa of the mucous membrane contained within the hamular notch is thick and made up of loose areolar tissue.

### *Divided as:*

- Anterior vibrating line.
- Posterior vibrating line.

### Anterior Vibrating Line

The anterior vibrating line is an imaginary line located at the junction of the attached tissues overlying the hard palate and the movable tissues of the immediately adjacent soft palate.

The anterior vibrating line is always on soft palatal tissues.

*Locating anterior vibrating line:* Is to have the patient do the Valsalva maneuver, in which both nostrils are held firmly while the patient blows gently through the nose. Another method is instruct the patient to say "ah" with short vigorous bursts. Due to the projection of the posterior nasal spine, the anterior vibrating line is not a straight line between both hamular processes.

### Posterior Librating Line

The posterior vibrating line is an imaginary line at the junction of the aponeurosis of the tensor veli palatini muscle and the muscular portion of the soft palate.

It demarcates between that part of the soft palate that has limited or shallow movement during function and the remainder of the soft palate that is displaced during functional movements.

*Locating posterior vibrating line:* The posterior vibrating line is visualized by instructing the patient to say "ah" in short bursts in a normal, unexaggerated fashion. The posterior vibrating line marks the most distal extension of the denture base.

### *Extent*

It extends from one pterygomaxillary notch to the other and about 2 mm in front of the foveae palatinae. The direction of the vibrating line depends on the shape of the palate.

In a mouth with a flat vault, the vibrating line is usually farther posterior with a gradual curvature, having a broad posterior palatal seal area.

The distal end of the upper denture should end 1 or 2 mm posterior to the vibrating line and cover the tuberosities and extend into the hamular notches.

### Posterior Palatal Seal Area

The posterior palatal seal area lies between anterior and posterior vibrating line and is cupids bow shaped. This area in the denture should adapt closely to the PPS for improved retention.

## 13. Fluid wax technique.

Fluid wax technique is one of the techniques that utilises waxes that flow at mouth temperatures to record posterior palatal seal area.

### Waxes used are.

a. Lowa wax ( white) developed by Dr. Earl S. Smith
b. Korecta wax No. 4 (orange) developed by Dr. O. C. Applegate
c. H-L physiologic paste (yellow-white) developed by Dr. C. S. Harkins
d. Adaptol (green) developed by Nathan G. Kaye.

### Procedure

a. After identifying the posterior palatal seal area in the mouth, the transfer markings are copied on to the final impression.
b. Any one of the four types of wax is selected depending on the dentist choice and is painted onto the impression surface within the outline of the seal area after melting.
c. After the wax is painted in the PPS region, the tray is reseated in the mouth and held in place under gentle pressure for four to six minutes.
d. A 30° flexion of the patient's head along with the tongue that is firmly positioned against the mandibular anterior teeth (handle) helps in molding the PPS region. The patient is asked to periodically rotate the head so that all functional positions of the soft palate are recorded.
e. The tray is removed from the mouth and if the wax has a glossy appearance the tissue contact is proper, if not, the procedure should be repeated.
f. The secondary impression is reinserted and held for three to five minutes under gentle pressure, followed by two to three minutes of firm pressure applied to the midpalatal area of the impression tray. During this time, the head and tongue positions must be maintained.

### Advantages

a. It is a physiologic technique displacing tissues within their physiologically acceptable limits.
b. Over compression of tissues is avoided.
c. Posterior palatal seal is incorporated into the trial denture base for added retention.
d. Mechanical scraping of the cast is avoided.

### Disadvantages

a. More time is necessary during the impression appointment.
b. Difficulty in handling the materials and added care during the boxing procedure.

### Fluid wax technique for adding a posterior palatal seal to already existing denture (Moghadam and Scandrett)

a. The locating, marking and placing the wax in the seal area are same.
b. After the wax has flown adequately, the denture is removed from the mouth and the anterior extent of the seal is marked on the denture.

c. Utility wax is placed vertically across the palate, separating the posterior two-third from the anterior region and extended around the posterior portion of the denture.
d. Dental stone is vibrated into the denture-wax surface outlined by the utility wax.
e. After the stone has set, the wax is eliminated, the denture cleaned and the area distal to the anterior vibrating line is ground.
f. After applying lubricant to the unground areas, including the polished surface, a separating medium is applied to the stone cast, denture is replaced on the stone cast and held firmly with rubber bands.
g. Acrylic is added till the space between denture and cast is filled. After waiting till the initial set has taken place, it is placed in a pressure pot with water (140°F) for 20 minutes under 30 psi pressure.
h. The cast and denture are separated, the excess acrylic is trimmed, and the border polished lightly.
i. Light cured resin can be used instead of acrylic resin.

## 14. Relevance of PpS.

The posterior palatal seal (PPS) is defined as, "The soft tissues along the junction of the hard and soft palates on which pressure within the physiologic limits of the tissues can be applied by a denture to aid in the retention of the denture." –GPT

### Importance of PPS

a. A positive contact is established posteriorly thereby preventing the final impression material from sliding down the pharynx.
b. For positioning the impression tray, accurately.
c. To create slight displacement of the soft palate.
d. To determine if adequate retention and seal can be achieved in the potential denture border.
e. Adequate border seal resist horizontal forces and lateral torquing of the maxillary denture.
f. The function of the posterior palatal seal in the completed maxillary prosthesis is to maintain contact with the anterior portion of the soft palate during functional movements as mastication, deglutition and phonation.
g. To aid the denture to achieve better retention.
h. The posterior palatal seal will reduce patient awareness of border of denture hence reducing gag reflex.

## 15. Functions of bite blocks/occlusal rims.

a. Helps to orient the occlusal plane.
b. Gives facial support.
c. Aids in accurate location of the midline of the arch.
d. Helps in positioning the incisors and cuspids.
e. Aids in locating the smile line (high lip line) and the speaking (low) lip line.
f. To establish accurate maxillomandibular jaw relations.
g. For arranging the artificial teeth to form the trial denture.
h. Helps to determine the length and width of the artificial teeth.

## Four factors in the fabrication of occlusion rims

1. Relationship of the natural teeth to the alveolar bone.
2. Relationship of occlusion rim to the edentulous ridge.
3. Fabrication technique.
4. Clinical guidelines.

## Relationship of the natural teeth to the alveolar bone and occlusal rim to ridge

- The natural maxillary anterior teeth are slightly forward of the alveolar bone and support the upper lip.
- The incisal edge of the incisor teeth appioximates the lower edge of the lip.
- The mandibular incisors are inclined forward and tend to support the lower lip. The incisal edge is approximately 1 to 2 mm behind the lingual surface of the maxillary incisors.
- The maxillary posterior teeth are positioned slightly buccal to the alveolar ridge and. the maxillary buccal cusps project 2 to 3 mm beyond the buccal cusps of the mandibular teeth.

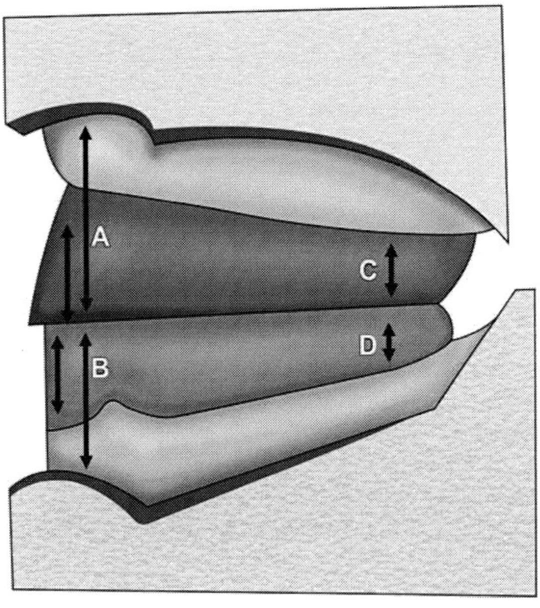


**A:** 20-22 mm
**B:** 16-17 mm
**C:** 5-7 mm
**D:** 3-6 mm

**Fig. 3:** Dimensions of maxillary and mandibular occlusal rims

## Fabrication Technique (Fig. 3)

- Maxillary height anterior region: 22 mm from the sulcus depth.
- Maxillary posterior height: 18 mm (length of the first maxillary molar crown).
- Mandibular anterior height: approximately 16 to 18 mm.
- Mandibular posterior height: a point representing one half the height of the retromolar pad.
- Width anteriorly for both rims: 3 to 5 mm wide.
- Width in posterior region: 8 to 10 mm.

## Clinical Guidelines

*Maxillary rim:* Anteriorly parallel to interpupillary line and occlusal rim should be 2 mm visible.

Posteriorly the upper rim one-quarter inch below Stensen's duct. The plane of occlusion is made parallel to ala-tragal line projected from the ala of the nose to the superior edge of the tragus of the ear (Camper's line).

Apart from the above factors as facial support, the length and width of the anterior teeth, the cuspid eminences, the smiling line, and the speaking (low) lip line.

*Mandibular rim:* Anteriorly should be at the level of lower lip and posteriorly one half the height the retromolar pad. From cuspid to cuspid, the rim is inclined slightly forward but remains within the border of the recording base. Posterior to the cuspid area, the rims should be located over the center of the crest of the ridge.

The final forming of the anterior portion of the maxillary occlusion rim are determined by the:
a. Nasolabial sulcus
b. Mentolabial sulcus
c. Philtrum
d. Commissure (corner) of the mouth.

## Nasolabial Sulcus and Mentolabial Sulcus

When proper lip support is not given there is a deepening of the nasolabial and mentolabial sulci with loss of definition in the philtrum and a drooping of the corners of the mouth.

If occlusal rims are over contoured the nasolabial and mentolabial folds and philtrum become shallow producing a "stretched look".

## 16. Occlusal plane.

### Procedure in adjusting the maxillary occlusal plane

a. Anteriorly the maxillary rim is reduced 1 to 2 mm below the lower edge of the lip "low lip line" and should be parallel to the interpupillary line.
b. Posteriorly the height in the first molar area is reduced about one-quarter inch below Stensen's duct.
c. The plane of occlusion is made parallel to the ala–tragal line (the ala of the nose to the superior edge of the tragus of the ear- Camper's line). When the occlusal plane is parallel to the ala-tragus line the closing force during clenching was greater than when it was altered plus or minus 5°.
d. The cuspid eminences are marked corresponding to lines placed at the corners of the mouth. These lines represent the location of the distal surface of the cuspid teeth.
e. From the occlusal view the occlusion rim is sloped slightly inward to create space, for buccal corridor, between the teeth and the cheeks.

## Mandibular Occlusal Plane

### *Anteriorly*

The occlusal plane is determined by the lower anterior teeth and the commissure of the mouth.

From cuspid to cuspid, the rim is inclined slightly forward remaining within the border of the recording base. Posterior to the cuspid area, the rims should be located over the center of the crest of the ridge.

The occlusal rim should terminate posteriorly at the junction of anterior one-third and posterior two-third of the retromolar pad. These landmarks orient the occlusal plane at the correct anteroposterior inclination which nearly parallel to the lower foundation plane. The parotid papilla was on the average 3.3 mm above the occlusal plane and it can be used as a guide for establishing the height of the occlusal plane.

If it is too high, the upper and lower posterior teeth can bite the papilla during function.

If the occlusal plane is too low, then the tongue can overlap the lower teeth and cause tongue biting.

#### *Buccally*

The teeth should not displace the buccal mucosa, but make passive contact with it so that the buccinator muscle will not forcibly move the lower denture by its action against the buccal surfaces of the teeth.

#### *Lingually*

The lower posterior teeth should not crowd the tongue or interfere with its normal function. The lingual cusps of the natural molars are approximately in vertical alignment with the mylohyoid ridge.

#### *Tongue Position*

At rest, after swallowing, the tip of the tongue touches the lingual surfaces of the lower anterior teeth.

The lateral border of the tongue will be at the level of the lingual contour of the lower natural posterior teeth.

The dorsal surface of the tongue is nearly level with the occlusal surfaces of the posterior teeth.

## 17. Atmospheric pressure.

### Introduction

- Stanitz (1945) states that there is differences in pressure between the atmosphere and the fluid film.
- Landa states that atmospheric pressure aids in retention of dentures.
- Oehl and Dresen acknowledged that atmospheric pressure acts only if the peripheral seal is correctly formed.
- Snyder showed that reduced atmospheric pressure decreased denture retention in a decompression chamber.
- Skinner and co-workers (1953) say that, "atmospheric pressure is an ordinary 'suction' and vacuum chamber does not have much influence on retention."
- Page and Moses considers atmospheric pressure to be of no importance in retention. Only interfacial surface tension helps in retention.

## Atmospheric Pressure and Peripheral Seal

Peripheral seal is the area of contact between the peripheral borders of the denture and the resilient-limiting structures. The peripheral seal prevents air entry between the denture the soft tissue. When displacing forces act on the denture, a partial vacuum (natural suction) is produced between the denture and the soft tissues, which aids in retention.

Hence, atmospheric pressure is referred to as emergency–retentive force or temporary restraining force.

## Factors Affecting Atmospheric Pressure

a. Good peripheral seal.
b. Perfect fit of denture.
c. Maximum coverage of basal seat.
d. Balanced occlusion.
e. Shape of the polished surfaces.

## 18. Cast metal bases/metal denture bases.

### Requirements for Cast Metal Bases

1. Metal bases should be thin but rigid.
2. Dense.
3. Accurate, having a positive fit on the master cast without rocking.
4. Biologically acceptable alloy.

### Advantages of Metal Bases Over Resin Bases (By Faber)

a. Prevention of acrylic warpage.
b. Lack of bulk with more strength.
c. Increased accuracy.
d. Less tissue change under the base.
e. Less porosity and therefore easier to clean and keep clean.
f. Thermal conductivity.
g. Less deformation in function.

### Disadvantages

a. High cost.
b. Greater weight.
c. Inability to be easily rebased.
d. Poor esthetic qualities.
e. Time-consuming construction.

### Materials for Cast Metal Bases

a. Gold alloys Types III and IV
   They contain copper, silver, palladium, platinum and some trace elements.
b. Chrome base alloys
   All the cast chrome alloys for RPD can be used, e.g. Ticonium, Vitalium and Nobelium etc.
c. Aluminum alloys
   - Pure aluminum with 29c to 4% magnesium and slight amounts of silicon is more common. The casting temperature of aluminum is between 704. 5° to 815. 5° C.
   - Anodized aluminum

### Design Principles

A pencil drawing indicating the amount of coverage, placement of finishing lines and type of resin retention on the master cast are used.

#### *Maxillary Bases*

The appropriate design covers the complete palate and ridge crest, but leaves the denture borders in resin. Covering the posterior palatal seal area in metal is also permitted and the resin periphery begins at the pterygomaxillary notch area.

#### *Mandibular Bases*

The mandibular cast base covers crest of the ridge with resin peripheries. This is preferred as easier to adjust and polish, though complete coverage of metal base can also be done.

#### *Resin Retention*

a. Retention mesh,
b. Non-relieved retention of beads,
c. Nail heads, and
d. Loops.

### Block out and relief

Soft-tissue undercuts under the bases need to be blocked out and placement of arbitrary relief areas are to be given. This block out reduces the number of sharp metal projections on the tissue surface to be removed during finishing.

### Casting Procedure

a. Vitalium and Nobelium needs higher temperature burnout, 982° to 1093°C. Cast all chrome base alloys in automatic induction casting machines.
b. For Aluminum 343.5 °C place the aluminum ingots in the induction crucible of the Electromatic Casting Machine. Use this crucible for aluminum only. Turn on the melt switch and probe the ingots with a quartz rod as they melt. When it is possible to push the top ingots into the mass, turn off the melt switch and allow the metal to cool.
c. Remove the mold from the furnace and place it in the cradle. Turn on the melt switch and watch the metal until it takes on the orange color of a harvest moon. At that point, throw the automatic cast switch and complete the casting. Keep the arm rotating for a full 3 minutes.
d. Remove the cast and allow it to bench cool for 10 minutes before quenching it in running water. Remove the bulk of the refractory material with a wax spatula or a similar hand instrument under running water. Do the final cleansing of the refractory cast by blasting it carefully with walnut-shell abrasives. Do not use a sand blaster because it will pit and dull the aluminum alloy.
e. As the aluminum alloy is soft, considerable care in fitting and finishing the casting is needed. The rest of the finishing is done with a slow-speed lathe or with a laboratory handpiece, finishing stones and burs.

## 19. Face-bow uses and types.

The face-bow is a caliper-like device used to record the relationship of the maxillae to the temporomandibular joints and to orient the maxillary cast to the articulator in the same relationship that exists between the maxillae and the opening and closing axis in the temporomandibular joints.

**Uses of face-bow**

a. It supports the casts while they are being attached to the articulator.
b. When cusp form teeth are used.
c. When balanced occlusion in the eccentric positions is desired.
d. When a definite cusp fossa or cusp tip to cusp incline relation is needed.
e. Interocclusal check records after face-bow transfer aid in verifying of jaw positions.
f. If the occlusal vertical dimension is changed and the alterations of tooth occlusal surfaces are necessary to accommodate the change.

**Types of Face-bow**

Arbitrary: Has two types: Ear piece face-bow and Facia type of face-bow.
Kinematic or hinge-bow.

## Arbitrary

a. The arbitrary face-bow is placed on the face with the condyle rods located approximately over the condyles.
b. Used in complete denture patients.
c. The condyle rods are positioned on a line extending from the outer canthus to the top of the tragus and 13 mm in front of the external auditory meatus locating the rods within 5 mm of the true center of the opening axis of the jaws. (Facia type) Hanau Model C. Without clamping the condyle rods, the dentist centers the device so equal readings are obtained on both sidebands, the wing nut of the clamp is tightened to hold the face-bow in place on the occlusal fork.
d. The rods of another are designed to fit into the external auditory meatuses. (Ear piece type, Whip Mix).
e. The fork of arbitrary face-bow is attached to the maxillary occlusion rim. Transverse axis of the articulator is 5/8 inch (15 mm anterior to the position of the ends of the face-bow).
f. This distance compensates for the distance between the external auditory meatus and the condyle.

## Kinematic Face-bow

a. The kinematic face-bow is so designed that the opening axis of the mandible can be located more accurately.
b. The fork of kinematic face-bows is attached to the mandibular occlusion rim.
c. As the patient retrudes the mandible and opens and closes the jaws, the movement of the points of the condyle rods are observed.
d. As the condyle rods of kinematic face-bows have sharp points, their motion can be observed more accurately.
e. When the points rotate only and do not translate, they are on the opening axis of the jaw.
f. At this position the mandible is in centric relation for the occlusal vertical dimension that has been established. After the hinge axis center is located it is marked on the face with indelible pencil. The face-bow is removed from the face-bow fork and the condyle rods are straightened and made parallel. The face-bow is now used in the regular manner by being fastened into place over the previously determined rotational points. This type of transfer will be exact in the positional relation of the cast, and will permit a recording medium as wax, zinc oxide-eugenol or plaster for interocclusal records without usual inaccuracy being produced. This is important when the interarch distance is to be increased or decreased.

g. Kinematic face-bow can aid in recording centric relation. The difficulty of attaching the lower occlusion rim to an edentulous mandible and movement of the recording base on the jaw makes determining the exact center of the opening axis difficult hence preventing its use for edentulous patients.
h. Aids in finding the appropriate vertical dimension clinically and does not change in the articulator.

## 20. Interocclusal distance (free way space).

### Definition

The interocclusal distance (formerly referred to as the "free way space") is the distance or gap existing between the occluding surfaces of maxillary and mandibular teeth when the mandible is in the physiologic rest position.

The difference between the occlusal vertical dimension and the rest vertical dimension is the interocclusal distance.

The interocclusal distance is 2 to 4 mm when observed at the position of the first premolars. It was observed that clinically recorded rest position and the electromyographically determined one have a range of 10 mm.

### Significance

1. In natural dentition it is essential to maintain the health of the periodontal tissues.
2. In complete denture patients failure to provide interocclusal distance will cause "clicking" of the dentures during speech, soreness of the tissues of the basal seat and rapid destruction of the residual alveolar ridges.
3. Interocclusal distance is important to record the correct vertical dimension of occlusion.

### Problems with Reduced Interocclusal Space

a. Esthetics: The chin appears too close to the nose and too far forward. The lips lose their fullness and the vermilion borders are reduced to approximate a line. The corners of the mouth turn down.
b. Muscular action: Decreases the action of the muscles, with a resultant loss of muscle tone.
c. Causes a crease to form at the corners of the mouth associated with angular cheilitis.
d. Leads to a *loss of the cubicle space* of the oral cavity.
e Pushes the tongue toward the throat. Displacing and encroaching adjacent tissues causing obstruction to the opening of the eustachian tubes interfering with ear function.
f. Trauma in the region of the TMJ fossa as obscure pain, discomfort, clicking sounds, headaches and neuralgia.
g. Excessive bone resorption: If adequate interocclusal distance is not provided it produces excessive interarch distance when the teeth are in occlusion. Hence the muscles will continue to exert force to overcome this obstacle and as a result the supporting tissues will be resorbed until the proper distance is returned.
h. Clicking of dentures: The premature contacting of the teeth results in a clicking noise.
i. Function: Proper functioning with the denture as chewing, Phonetics, swallowing are difficult.

### Methods of Establishing Interocclusal Space

a. Facial measurements
 Instruct the patient to stand or sit comfortably upright with the eyes looking straight ahead. Insert the maxillary record base with the attached contoured occlusion rim. With either an

indelible marker or a triangle of adhesive tape, place a point of reference on the end of the patient's nose and another on the point of the chin. Instruct the patient to wipe the lips with the tongue to swallow and to drop the shoulders. When mandible drops to rest position and then measure between the points with a millimeter ruler. Repeat the procedure until the measurements are consistent.

b. Tactile sense

   Then ask them to close slowly until the jaws reach a comfortable, relaxed position. The distance is measured between the points of reference and compared with the measurements made after swallowing.

c. Phonetics

   Have patients repeat "M" until they are aware of the contacting of the lips as "M" is pronounced. Repeat this procedure and ask that they stop all jaw movement when the lips touch. At this time measure between two points of reference.

   An adequate interocclusal distance is needed for the proper functioning of denture as well as the preservation of supporting tissues and health of the patient.

## 21. Silverman's closest speaking space

Vertical dimension can be measured by the speaking method with its speaking space. It is a phonetic method based upon the physiologic movement and position of the mandible during speech.

### Method

- The patient must sit erect without using the headrest, the eyes should look forward, and the occlusal surfaces of the upper posterior teeth should be parallel to the floor.
- The measurements must be taken under identical conditions of posture and vigor of speech.
- The patient must speak rapidly in a calm, relaxed and normal manner, without consciously controlling the muscular movement of the jaws.
- The patient closes into centric occlusion with the upper and lower teeth held together in maximum occlusal contact.
- The centric occlusion line is drawn with pencil on a lower anterior tooth at the horizontal level of the incisal edge of the opposing upper anterior tooth.
- The patient is then asked to pronounce the phonetic sound s, as in yes.
- While the s sound is made and held, the closest speaking line is drawn on the same lower anterior tooth on which the centric occlusion line was draw.
- The distance between the lower line (the centric occlusion line) and the upper line (the closest speaking line) is called the closest speaking space.
- The measurement of this closest speaking space is the measurement for vertical dimension.

### Significance

- Closest speaking space of each individual is constant throughout life.
- This system of determination of vertical dimension is based on physiologic function of muscles while used in speaking which is caused by maximum function of the muscle fibers involved.
- In addition to the s sound as yes, it has been found that all other sibilants generally cause the mandible to reach the closest speaking level (the closest speaking level of the lower jaw in relation to the upper jaw).

- The sibilants s, z, sh, eh, ch, and j, in such words as yes, buzz, fish, measure, church, and judge, produce the closest speaking level of the mandible in relation to the maxilla.
- Therefore, only the six sibilants of the forty-four phonetic sounds of the English language are used.
- The closest speaking line should first be located by use of the individual words like "Mississippi,"which has many sibilants.
- If there is a discrepancy in the position of the closest speaking line, it is due to the voluntary muscular control of the mandible by the patient when this line is drawn while the individual words are being spoken.
- This phonetic system of determining vertical dimension by the use of the six sibilants and the closest speaking space is different from centric relation and the free-way space.
- The rest position of the mandible and the free-way space establish vertical dimension when the muscles involved are completely relaxed.
- The speaking method, with its closest speaking space, measures vertical dimension when the mandible is in a speaking position and the muscles involved are in active function during actual speech.

## 22. Realeff.

Hanau described this factor as realeff, derived from resiliency and like effect.

### Factors in Realeff

A. The displacability and compressibility of the basal seat mucosa.
B. Realeff affects selective grinding procedures.
C. Because of Realeff "the teeth have a tendency to find premature contact of the distal inclines of the lower cusps with the mesial inclines of the upper cusps."

### Explanation for Realeff

This commonly occurs if the impressions and jaw relation records were made with a passive recording material such as plaster, softened wax or impression compound.

The cast obtained from the above technique is mounted and articulated in centric relation.

Maximum intercuspation or posterior tooth contact is developed in the articulator in centric relation.

When the same dentures are inserted in the patient's mouth and when the patient occludes into centric relation, the mucosa under the maxillary denture is displaced in a superior direction and the mucosa under the mandibular denture is displaced in an inferior direction.

This results in a change in maxillomandibular relation leading to the distal inclines of the mandibular posterior cusps having a tendency to find premature contact with the mesial inclines of the maxillary cusps.

### Correction Technique by Hanau

a. Initially "unstrained" jaw relation records with a passive material is made with no displacement of the mucosa.
b. Selective grinding is done first with unstrained mounting.
c. Next a "strained" jaw relation record is made with the jaws in terminal relation with a compressive impression material.

d. Selective grinding for strained record is done which results in an area of freedom of occlusion with the jaws in terminal relation (long centric or short protrusive occlusion).

## Precautions While Denture Making to Avoid Realeff

i. Sufficient time for tissue recovery in old patients (twenty-four hours for young persons and several days for the geriatric patient).
ii. To use low viscosity impression materials which will flow freely after the impression material is seated. Escape holes should be provided, especially in the maxillary arch.
iii. An impression should not be removed and inserted repeatedly if repeated placements are, needed. do border refinement at one appointment and make the refined impression the next day.
iv. Parafunctional habits produce light loads for long durations, whereas grinding, clenching produces heavy loads for short durations. These patients should be recognised early and treatment plan done accordingly.
v. Excessively thick mucosa should be evaluated and if surgical correction needed should be done.

## 23. Physiologic rest position

## Definition

"Physiologic rest position is the postural position of mandible when an individual is resting comfortably in an upright position and the associated muscles are in a state of minimal contractual activities" (GPT-6), otherwise termed as the vertical dimension of rest.

The vertical dimension of jaw separation at rest occurs when the maxillofacial musculature is in a state of tonic equilibrium during mastication, speaking, swallowing and breathing. These physiologic functions help in determining the vertical dimension of rest and occlusion.

**Vertical relations are classified as vertical dimensions of:**

1. Occlusion,
2. Rest and
3. Other positions.

The vertical dimension of rest (or physiologic rest position of the mandible) is established by muscles and gravity. Part of all voluntary muscles are always under some degree of contraction called tonus. This tonus helps to maintain muscles in postural position. The muscles involved in the activity of maintaining postural positions are called anti-gravity muscles.

## Muscles involved in Maintaining Postural Position of Mandible to Maxillae

a. Muscles of mastication (Masseter, temporalis, medial pterygoid and lateral pterygoid).
b. Suprahyoid and infrahyoid muscles (stylohyoid, sternohyoid, omohyoid, sternothyroid, thyrohyoid, posterior belly of digastric, suprahyoid muscles as anterior belly of digastric, mylohyoid.
c. Extrinsic muscles of tongue as genioglossus, hyoglossus.

The vertical dimension of rest is a postural relationship of the mandible to the maxillae and the teeth do not determine it. The mandible is said to be in its physiologic rest position when all the muscles that close and open the jaws are in a state of minimal tonic contraction sufficient only to maintain posture. Electromyographic studies conducted by Moyers, Hickey and others confirmed that antigravity muscles maintain the postural rest position. The rest position records vary in reclining position and upright position. In reclining position the rest position is less than in upright position. Hence while recording rest position the head should be upright and unsupported. According to Sicher the rest position is constant throughout life, unless changed by chronic illness.

## Recording the Vertical Dimension of Rest

Following are the different methods:

a. Facial measurements
   Instruct the patients to stand or sit comfortably upright with the eyes looking straight ahead. Insert the maxillary record base with the attached contoured occlusion rim. With either an indelible marker or a triangle of adhesive tape, place a point of reference on the end of the patients' nose and another on the point of the chin. Instruct the patients to wipe the lips with the tongue to swallow and to drop the shoulders. When mandible drops to rest position and then measure between the points with a millimeter ruler. Repeat the procedure until the measurements are consistent.
b. Tactile sense
   Then ask them to close slowly until the jaws reach a comfortable, relaxed position. The distance is measured between the points of reference and compared with the measurements made after swallowing.
c. Phonetics
   Have patients repeat "M" until they are aware of the contacting of the lips as "M" is pronounced. Repeat this procedure and stop all jaw movement when the lips touch. At this time measure between two points of reference
d. Preextraction records
   i. Profile photographs.
   ii. Measurements of anatomic landmarks on the photograph are compared with measurements using the same anatomic landmarks on the face.
   iii. Profile silhouettes.
   iv. Facial measurements.

## Niswonger's Method

The distance is measured and these measurements are compared with measurements made between these points when the occlusal rims are tried in.

## Importance of Physiologic Rest Position

1. It is a bone to bone relation in a vertical plane.
2. It is constant throughout life except in cases of illness.
3. It can be recorded and measured within acceptable limits.
4. It is used in determining the vertical dimension of occlusion.
5. It has to be recorded without delay.

## 24. Tooth supported complete denture.

## Definition

A tooth-supported complete denture is a dental prosthesis that replaces the lost or missing natural dentition and associated structures of the maxillae or mandible and receives partial support and stability from one or more modified natural teeth.

## Classification

Based on the method of abutment preparation.

- Noncoping
- Coping
- Attachments.

### Noncoping Abutments

In noncoping, selected root abutments are reduced to a coronal height of 2 to 3 mm and then contoured to a convex or dome-shaped surface. These abutments commonly require endodontic therapy and are prepared conservatively to receive an amalgam or composite type restoration.

### Abutments with Copings

Cast metal copings with a dome-shaped surface and a chamfer finish line at the gingival margin are fabricated and cemented.

Two types of copings are prepared:

1. Short coping.
2. Long coping.

### Abutments with Attachments

Attachments are used to improve retention of the denture base and generally are secured to the abutment by a cast coping.

## Indications

For young patients who face the loss of the remaining natural teeth.

## Advantages

1. The retained natural tooth in overdenture aids in providing tensile stimulation to the residual alveolar ridge, hence preserving residual alveolar ridge.
2. Preservation of proprioceptive response.
3. The modified teeth provide a definite vertical stop for the denture base.
4. Horizontal and torquing forces are minimized.
5. Stability and support are increased.
6. The retention of only one tooth frequently makes for a more favorable prognosis.
7. Less post insertion problems.
8. Convertibility: Can be easily relined or rebased into a conventional complete denture.

## Disadvantages of an Overdenture

1. Caries susceptibility of the abutment teeth.
2. Periodontal disease can cause failure in overdenture functioning.
3. Bony undercuts adjacent to the overlaid teeth (usually buccally), prevent close adaptation of the denture flange to the underlying tissue.
4. If undercuts are blocked it causes spacing between denture and tissue creating a food trap.
5. Esthetics, bony under cuts cause over contouring of denture resulting in improper lip fullness.
6. Under contouring leads to improper retention and stability.
7. Encroachment of the interocclusal distance when internal attachment is used.

## 25. Osseointegration.

Osseointegration is defined as, "A process whereby clinically asymptomatic rigid fixation of alloplastic materials is achieved and maintained in bone during functional loading."

Bone implants have an interface that consists mainly of bone tissue.

### Osseointegrated Interface

Osseointegrated implant is an implant in which the bone will grow into surface irregularities of the implant forming three-dimensional stabilization. This is a biomechanical process.
If instead of biomechanical process a strong chemical bonds develop between bone and implant materials, such implants are called "biointegrated" (Ceramic implants).

### Factors Determining Failure of Osseointegrated Implants

1. Functional loads: An adequate load results in a very strong interface, if the implant is overloaded during its incorporation or during interfacial organization the implant interface is disturbed leading to implant loosening.
2. When ions from the implant leak out, the surrounding bone gets disturbed.
3. Micromovements of implants.
4. Implant surface too smooth, resulting in primary failures; or too rough, with a risk of adverse bone reactions and secondary loss of integration.
5. Irradiated host bone.
6. Improper surgical technique.
7. Implant biocompatibility.

### Implant Biomaterials

- Pure Titanium (In compromised bone beds Cp titanium is the safest alternative).
- Titanium - 6Aluminum - 4Vanadium (Ti-6Al-4V) alloy.
- Niobium.
- Hydroxyapatite (calcium phosphate ceramic material).
- Hydroxyapatite coated titanium implants.
- Plasma sprayed Titanium implants.

### Ideal Implant Design for Osseointegration

- Cylindrical implants: Threaded or non-threaded, Coated or uncoated.
- Threaded/coated oral implants have shown better osseointegration.
- Implant surface: The ideal implant roughness needed for osseointegration was found to be between 1 and 1.5.

### Factors Affecting Implant Bed

a. Age: Extreme young age is a relative contraindication to the insertion of implants.
b. Previous irradiation: Implants that are inserted immediately before irradiation will show a high failure rate, but after irradiation had better results.
c. Smoking: Yielded to significantly lower success rates with oral implants.
d. Surgical technique:
Minimal tissue violence at surgery: Careful cooling while surgical drilling, low rotatory rates, sharp instruments and the use of a graded series of drills is essential for proper osseointegration.

e. The insertion torque of threaded screw-type implant should be of moderate level. If high, can lead to stress concentrations around the threads, with subsequent bone resorption.
f. Loading conditions.
g. Two-stage implant insertion.
h. At the first stage the implant is inserted in the bone and the soft tissues are sutured back.

At a second surgical procedure 3 to 6 months later, the buried implant is exposed and connected to the oral cavity via a transepithelial abutment.

The above factors helps the dentist to assess the success of osseointegration and in turn the implant.

## 26. Obturators

**Broad classification is based on**

a. Stages of treatment
b. The material used
c. Location of restoration
d. Movements.

### A. Based on the Stages of Treatment

#### Surgical Obturators

It is defined as, "A temporary prosthesis used to restore the continuity of the hard palate immediately after surgery or traumatic loss of a portion or all of the hard palate and/or contiguous alveolar structures (i.e., gingival tissue, teeth)." – GPT

- Immediate surgical obturator: Inserted at the time of surgery
- Delayed surgical obturator: Inserted 7–10 days after surgery.

#### Interim obturators or Tentative Obturators

It is defined as, "A prosthesis that is made several weeks or months following the surgical resection of a portion of one or both maxillae. It frequently includes replacement of teeth in the defect area. This prosthesis, when used, replaces the surgical obturator that is placed immediately following the resection and may be subsequently replaced with a definitive obturator." –GPT

#### Definitive Obturators

It is defined as, "A prosthesis that artificially replaces part or all of the maxilla and the associated teeth lost due to surgery or trauma." –GPT

### B. Based on the Material Used

a. Metal obturators
b. Resin obturators
c. Silicone obturators
D. Combination of metal and resin.

### C. Based on the Location of Restoration

a. Palatal obturator
b. Meatal obturator.

## D. Based on the Movements

a. Hinge type - Slight vertical movement.
b. Fixed type - Utilises soft tissue undercuts.
c. Meatus type - Used in extensive clefts, does not extend to Passovants pad.

Main function of any type of obturator is to aid the patient in speech, mastication and swallowing. In case of surgical obturators they act as a template, preventing infection, also can aid as carriers in medication, hence reducing the pain of patient.

The common complaint of these patients if not treated with an obturator is food and water coming through the nose and difficulty in speech. These patients also avoid social functions. Obturator therapy helps them to recover back their normal self in all ways.

## Obturator Therapy is Required for

a. Congenital defects as cleft palate.
b. After surgery in patients who had carcinoma.
c. After surgery to retain surgical grafts.
d. Accident cases with palatal defects.
e. Diseases as myasthenia gravis, bulbar poliomyelitis, cerebral palsy, palatal lift prosthesis is made.

## Palatal Obturator Procedure

*Preliminary impression:* Alginate impression with proper extension recording all undercut areas.

Custom tray oriented into the defect.

*Border molding:* The velo-pharyngeal extension recorded by asking the patient to swallow, flexing the head from side to side, placing the chin down onto the chest and some time asking the patient to pronounce certain syllables.

*Final impression* with elastic impression material.

*Jaw relation*: Acrylic denture bases are preferred.

*Teeth arrangement* depending on the existing occlusion.

*Insertion and instructions to patient.*

## Surgical Obturators

a. Before surgery an impression is taken and cast is poured in dental stone on which a mock surgery is performed.
b. A clear acrylic plate with clasps is made on this cast and inserted after surgery in dentulous patients.
c. In case the patient is edentulous, obturator is wired into the alveolar ridge and the zygomatic arch.
d. This clear acrylic plate is retained for 7 to 10 days after surgery.
e. After 7 to 10 days a delayed surgical obturator is inserted. If this obturator therapy need to be prolonged then lining of the obturator can be done.
f. This obturator is retained for 3 to 4 months post-surgically until the wound heals.

## Meatal Obturator

This obturator aids in closing the defect between nasal structures and the posterior border of hard palate in extensive soft palate defects. The closure is established against the conchae and the roof of nasal cavity.

### *Disadvantage*

Nasal resonance will be altered.

## 27. Conventional immediate complete dentures

The "Glossary of Prosthodontic Terms" defines an immediate denture as "the complete or removable partial denture constructed for insertion immediately following the removal of natural teeth."

### Advantages

1. No time will he or she be without teeth.
2. The digestive function is uninterrupted.
3. The general appearance of the patient is less affected because there is only a minimal change in muscle tone and the occlusal vertical dimension can be maintained.
4. Centric relation is also easier to record.
5. As the ridges are subjected to early function, less resorption will take place and the resultant ridges are better preserved and adapted to supporting a complete denture.
6. The healing period is faster and less painful as immediate denture acts as a protective covering over the wound.
7. The artificial teeth of the same size and shade as that of the natural teeth can be set in the identical positions occupied by the natural teeth.

### Disadvantages

1. After insertion the alveolar bone and soft tissue will remodel in and around the extraction sites, as the healing proceeds and resorption occurs hence the denture will not fit well.
2. Immediate complete denture treatment is more costly.
3. There can be no anterior try in hence the esthetics of the immediate denture cannot be evaluated until the insertion appointment.

### Treatment Procedures

The posterior teeth are removed at the initial appointment except the first premolars.

After six to eight weeks when ridges heal completely impression procedures are performed.

The immediate denture is fabricated during several appointments prior to the extraction of the remaining anterior teeth and inserted at the second surgery appointment.

#### *Steps*

*Initial impressions:* With irreversible hydrocolloid (alginate) in a stock tray.

*Tray fabrication:* The remaining teeth are covered with a double thickness of baseplate wax and other undercut areas are blocked out with wax. An acrylic tray is made.

*Border molding:* With stick compound.

*Final impression:* Perforations are placed in the tray and an appropriate adhesive light bodied polysulfide rubber is used for the final impression. If the remaining teeth are mobile preventive measures include blocking out undercuts and interproximal areas with soft wax and lightly coating the teeth with petrolatum is done. In case of extreme mobility a vacuum formed resin stent is used.

## Alternative Two Step Impression Procedure

*Preliminary impression* with alginate.

*A special tray fabricated* in which border molding is done on the borders of the special tray and edentulous area is recorded using zinc oxide-eugenol impression paste.

*A pick up impression* using alginate is made. The impression is poured with vacuum mixed dental stone.

## Tooth Selection and Arrangement of Posterior Teeth

The posterior teeth are arranged on the recording base. The teeth are set so as to provide multiple bilateral posterior contacts in centric relation. There should be no anterior contact in centric relation. Bilateral balancing contacts should be provided in lateral and protrusive excursions.

## Posterior Try in

Centric relation and occlusal vertical dimension are verified. The position of the posterior palatal seal is verified and scribed in the maxillary master cast.

## Arrangement of Anterior Teeth

The anterior denture teeth are arranged after the posterior try in appointment. The anterior teeth are removed one at a time at the level of the gingival margin with a rotary instrument or sharp knife and the remaining ridge is smoothed with a hand instrument. Denture teeth are placed alternatively and selectively ground to the ridge lap portion of the tooth. Modifications in anterior arrangement is done as to the patients liking. The wax up of the denture is completed to provide proper contour and thickness of the denture base. After wax boil out the cast can be modified as needed and the denture is processed using conventional techniques.

## 28. Fully adjustable articulators.

Initially the term *Fully Adjustable* was used and this meant that Articulators in this category can duplicate all mandibular movements. As studies proved that it cannot duplicate all mandibular movements, hence the fully adjustable and semi-adjustable were classified as *adjustable articulators.*

The difference between the Semi and Fully adjustable articulators are that fully adjustable ones.

1. Accept three-dimensional dynamic registrations and utilize a face-bow transfer.
2. The condylar pathways, or cams, are formed by registrations engraved by the patient.
3. The immediate Bennett movement and Progressive Bennett movement can be determined.
4. They have curvilinear condylar guidances.

*These articulators are classified as:*

1. *Mechanical adjustments:* Hanau 166-1 radial shift, Whip mix 8340, Whip mix DB 2200 are few examples.
2. *Preformed Fossae:* Denar Anamark, Panadent SL, TMJ Delux.
3. *Custom created:* Denar D5A, Stuart Gnathologic Computer and TMJ Stereographic.

All articulators in this class are arcon instruments with adjustable intercondylar distances. The condylar housings can be adjusted in the horizontal, sagittal and frontal planes. Each has a Bennett guide adjustment. They all accept arbitrary or hinge axis face-bow transfers. They are often referred to as gnathologic instruments, because of their full adjustability.

### Hanau 166-1 Radial Shift

- Horizontal guidances have ¾ inch curvature adjustable in inclination from 0 to 60 degrees.
- Lateral condylar guidance has a radial curve (immediate side shift) adjustable from 0 to 3 mm.
- Progressive side shift adjustable from 0 to 30 degrees.
- Condylar elements are fixed at 110.

### Panadent: By Lee and Lundeen

- In this there are five analog fossa features with a precurrent side shift of 0.5, 1.0, 1.5, 2.0, 2.5 mm.
- A hinged centric latch mechanism holds two members together and permits 180 degree range of opening.
- Fixed intercondylar distance of 110 mm.
- Dynalinks are elastic elements preventing separation of two frames during lateral excursive movements and also aids in returning to centric relation afterwards.

### TMJ Stereographic by Kenneth Swanson in 1965 (Class 4)

An intraoral registration generated by studs in autopolymerizing resin similar to chew in technique this is called a "stereographic" recording.

The stereographic recording is then placed on the articulator and used to mold fossae in autopolymerizing resin which is supposed to produce an accurate analog of the patient's temporomandibular joint function.

### Stuart Gnathologic Computer by Charles Stuart in 1955

Gnathology refers to the study of occlusion and occlusal rehabilitation through the use of pantographs and fully adjustable articulators.

The Bennett guides are situated in the middle of the posterior aspect of the instrument similar to the Gysi Trubyte articulator.

The Bennett guides can be angulated and customized.

Numerous plastic condylar inserts are available and they can be customized by grinding if necessary.

### Denar D5A Modification of D4A by Niles Guichet 1968

Condylar guidances are adjustable in three planes.

Intercondylar element adjustments from 90 to 150 mm.

Is similar to the D4A except for refinements in machining and in the centric latch mechanism located at the rear of the articulator.

Plastic condylar inserts are available that can be custom ground.

The Bennett adjustment is located in the medial wall of the condylar housing and has provisions for both immediate side shift (straight) and progressive side shift (angular) adjustments. Instruments in this class will accept three-dimensional dynamic registrations and utilize a face-bow transfer. The condylar pathways can be selectively angled and customized.

The three-dimensional dynamic registration procedure utilized in this class is the pantographic tracing procedure. The tracings produced by the pantograph are called pantograms.

The Pantronic is an electronic pantograph which provides a computer printout of numerical condylar measurements. In addition, several electronic tracings can be made consecutively and the condylar measurements compared immediately via the computer printout.

## 29. Semi-adjustable articulators.

Instruments in this class accept a face-bow transfer and a protrusive interocclusal record. They have Rectilinear guidances.

Articulators belonging to this class are:

- Hanau 183 Wide-Vue
- Dentatus
- Kinoscope by Hanau
- Ney articulator by De Pietro in 1960
- Trubyte articulator by Gysi
- SAM.

### Hanau Model H

- The most popular instrument of this class was the Hanau Model H, by Rudolph Hanau, in 1923.
- This is a non-arcon articulator.
- This articulator accepts a face-bow transfer and the horizontal condylar inclinations are set by a protrusive interocclusal record.
- The condyles are on the upper member.
- The Bennett angle (L) was calculated from the horizontal condylar inclination (H) by means of Hanau's equation, $L = (H/8) + 12$.
- If the $H = 30°$, then the Bennett angle would be 16.

### Dentatus (1944)

- Designed in Sweden.
- In this articulator the upper and lower members can be standardized with a "gauge block", so that casts can be transferred from one articulator to another and still maintain the same relationship.
- In Dentatus the horizontal condylar inclination are set by protrusive interocclusal record.
- The Bennett angle on both sides are set by left and right lateral records correspondingly. The rest are same as for Hanau H.

### Trubyte articulator by Gysi

- It is a non-arcon instrument with a fixed intercondylar distance.
- The horizontal condylar inclinations are individually adjustable and individual Bennett adjustments are located near the center of the intercondylar axis.
- The incisal guide table is adjusted to the patient's Gothic arch angle. This instrument accepts some lateral interocclusal records.

### Kinoscope by Hanau in 1927

It has double condylar posts on each side. The inner condylar posts have the horizontal condylar guides and are adjusted mediolaterally to produce mechanical equivalents of intercondylar distance. The Bennett angle is adjusted by rotating eccentric cones against the horizontal axis shaft.

### Ney articulator by De Pietro in 1960

It was a true arcon instrument. This is the first articulator to have condylar housings that contained adjustable rear, medial and top walls in one assembly. The intercondylar distance is adjustable.

### Hanau 130-21 by Richard Beu and James Janik in 1964

It has a split horizontal axis that can be adjusted vertically and horizontally, adjustable intercondylar distance, adjustable Bennett guides and adjustable horizontal condylar path guides. It is utilized with protrusive and lateral interocclusal records.

### Teledyne articulator by Richard Beu

It is an arcon instrument with adjustable medial and rear walls and adjustable horizontal condylar guidances.

## 30. Requirements of an articulator and difference in arcon and non-arcon types.

1. The articulator must accurately maintain the correct horizontal and vertical relationship of the patient's casts.
2. The patient's casts must be easily removable and attachable to the articulator without losing their correct horizontal and vertical relationship.
3. The articulator should have an incisal guide pin with a positive stop that is adjustable and calibrated. For control over the patient's occlusal vertical dimension by the dentist and laboratory technician.
4. The articulator should be able to open and close in a hinge-like fashion.
5. The articulator should accept a face-bow transfer utilizing an anterior reference point. The face-bow transfer relates the maxillary cast to the horizontal axis of the articulator in the same manner that the patient's maxilla relates to the opening axis of the temporomandibular joints. This allows minor changes in the patient's vertical dimension without grossly changing the patient's occlusion at the centric position. Also, the anterior reference point transfer facilitates the arrangement of the anterior teeth to the desired labiolingual inclination.
6. The construction should be accurate, rigid and of a noncorrosive material. The moving parts should resist wear. The adjustments should be able to move freely and be definitely secured.
7. The design should be such that there is adequate distance between the upper and lower members and that vision is not obscured from the rear. The articulator should be stable on the laboratory bench.

### Additional Articulator Requirements

These articulator requirements are necessary if dentures are to be fabricated with balanced occlusion.

1. The condylar guides should allow right lateral, left lateral and protrusive movements.
2. The condylar guides should be adjustable horizontally.
3. The articulator should have provisions for adjustment of Bennett movement.
4. The incisal guide table should be a mechanical table that can be adjusted in the sagittal and frontal planes or a table that can be customized with autopolymerizing resin or by grinding.

Optional articulator capabilities are adjustable intercondylar distance and an immediate Bennett adjustment. The articulator may either be arcon or non-arcon.

The primary advantage of an arcon articulator for complete denture construction would be for the visualization of condylar movement (the Hanau H2, Hanau Arcon H2, Hanau Radial Shift, Hanau Wide Vue, Whip-Mix and Denar Mark II). Any one of these articulators can be used with success.

Only Denar Mark II and Whip-Mix can be transferred from one articulator to another without losing their horizontal and vertical relationships in the above series mentioned. the rest of the models require, a separate articulator for every set of complete dentures under construction for lab procedures.

Bergstrom designed an instrument in 1950 called the Arcon, derived the name Arcon from ARticulator and CONdyle.

The term arcon is commonly used to indicate an instrument that has its condyles on the lower member and the condylar guides on the upper member. Instruments that have the condyles on the upper member and condylar guides on the lower member, are called condylar instruments or nonarcon instruments.

*Advantage of an arcon articulator* is that the condyles move in a relationship to their condylar housings that is similar to the way the condyles move in relationship to the glenoid fossae in the skull.

## 31. Condylar guidance and incisal guidance.

### Condylar Guidance (Posterior Determinant)

*Condylar guidance* is defined as, "Mandibular guidance generated by the condyle and articular disc traversing the contour of the glenoid fossa".—GPT

It is the path of movement taken by the condyle in the glenoid fossa.

The glenoid fossa and the condyle are the articulating surfaces of the temporomandibular joint.

The condyle moves along the surface of glenoid fossa during mandibular movement so the glenoid fossa determines the path of movement of the condyle.

The slope of the glenoid fossa is a 'S' bend. Hence the condyle also moves along a 'S' shaped path. This shape of the glenoid fossa, which determines the path of movement of the condyle, is called the condylar guidance.

The condylar guidance can be measured using a protrusive interocclusal record.

*Protrusive interocclusal record* is defined as, "The influence of the contacting surfaces of the mandibular and maxillary anterior teeth during mandibular movements". –GPT

### Importance of Condylar Guidance

A steep condylar path needs a steep compensating curve for occlusal balance.

If a lesser compensating curve is substituted for a steep condylar guidance it would result in a steep incisal guidance resulting in loss of molar balancing contacts.

### Setting the Condylar Guidance in the Articulator (Hanau)

Protrusive record is placed on the mandibular occlusal rims and the condylar thumb nuts on the articulator are made loose so that the upper member of the articulator can be easily guided into the imprint of the protrusive record perfectly. Rotate the right and left guidances back and forth to accurately seat the upper and lower rims into the protrusive record. After checking the value on both sides of the condylar guidance on the articulator, tighten the thumbnut. Approximate value is with in +30 degrees and almost the same value on both sides.

## Incisal Guidance

When the mandible is protruded the incisal edge of the lower anteriors slide along the slope of the lingual surface of the upper anterior teeth before reaching edge to edge contact.

The lingual surface of the maxillary anteriors guide the mandible during protrusive movement and is called the Incisal guidance.

*Incisal guide angle* is defined as, "The angle formed in the horizontal plane by drawing a line in the sagittal plane between the incisal edges of the maxillary and mandibular central incisors when the teeth are in centric occlusion". –GPT

## Importance of Incisal Guidance

In complete denture patients incisal guidance is not present and it is arbitrarily set using a standard incisal guide value while arranging the anterior teeth. It is modified during esthetic anterior try-in. If the incisal guidance is steep, it requires steep cusps, a steep occlusal plane, or a steep compensating curve to effect an occlusal balance.

A steep inclined plane is detrimental to the stability and equilibrium of the denture base hence the incisal guidance should be as flat as esthetics and phonetics will permit.

When the arrangement of the anterior teeth necessitates a vertical overlap, a compensating horizontal overlap should be set to prevent dominant incisal guidance (anterior interference) from upsetting the occlusal balance on the posterior teeth.

## Preparation of Anteroposterior Guides

The occlusion rims should be removed to evaluate the interridge space and arch form. A mark is placed on the occlusal rim as a projection of a line running from the incisal tip of the mandibular canine to the apex of the retromolar pad.

This reference line is checked in relation to the arch form as in the palatal surfaces of the upper incisors. This is known as the protrusive incisal path or incisal guidance.

The angle formed by this protrusive path to the horizontal plane is called as the incisal guide angle.

If the incisal guidance is steep, steep cusps or a steep occlusal plane or a steep compensatory curve is needed to produce balanced occlusion.

## Setting up the Incisal Guidance

The upper six and lower six teeth are set by esthetics, function and phonetics.

Lock articulator in centric. Occlusal rims are seated in vertical and centric relation. Incisal pin is placed at zero horizontal incisal guide and the lateral wings are also placed at zero with the chisel end of the pin resting on the center of the incisal table. Lock the thumb screw. Loosen the locknut for protrusion and release the centric locks.

Guide the upper cast into straight protrusion with the lingual edge of upper central incisors in contact with the incisal edges of the lower incisors. The incisal guide is rotated antero- posteriorly to make contact with the incisal pin. Tighten locknut to maintain angulation.

The upper cast guided into right lateral canine to canine and the lateral wing on that side is elevated to contact the incisal pin and lateral wing locknut adjusted thence is tightened. Repeat with the other side. Normal value within 5 degrees.

### Factors Affecting Incisal and Condylar Guidance

As occlusal plane, condylar guidance, incisal guidance, compensatory curves and cuspal inclination are all interrelated, any alteration to one of the factors affects the rest also.

## 32. Programming a semiadjustable articulator

- Maxillary cast is mounted to the upper member of the semi-adjustable articulator using a face-bow.
- A split cast is made. Tentative jaw relation is registered. Mandibular cast is mounted to the lower member of the articulator using tentative centric record. This is further verified using a graphic tracer.
- Extraoral tracer consists of central bearing point and plate. Tracer unit consists of stylus and table. The central bearing plate and central bearing point are attached to the occlusal rims in such a way that the height – the established vertical dimension is maintained and at the same time a uniform gap is provided.
- The central bearing plate is submerged into the maxillary occlusal rim but the shape of which is kept unaltered.
- Height of the mandibular occlusal rim is reduced by 4 mm and is maintained parallel to the maxillary occlusal rim. The plate carrying the central bearing point is kept flush with the modified mandibular occlusal rim.
- The height of the central bearing point is adjusted to make a point contact with the central bearing plate attached to the maxillary occlusal rim.
- Central bearing point is positioned at the approximation of occlusal rims in the protrusive position.
- After the tracing unit is attached, the stylus movement is checked whether it is contained with in the table.
- Assembly is now transferred to the patient's mouth and once consistency at centric relation point is obtained, the patient is asked to make excursive movements.
- First the patient is asked to make right lateral and come back to centric then left lateral and back to centric.
- A thin layer of contrast medium using okelson spray, marker pen, wax or mixture of zinc oxide and spirit is applied on the tracing table and the patient is asked to perform the jaw movements.
- It has an arrow point that represents the centric relation. The excursive movements – protrusive, right lateral and left lateral movements of the mandible will be represented by straight lines. However, the tracing obtained from the protrusive movement need not always be a straight line because it is controlled by both the joints.
- With a calliper an arc is drawn on the tracing which will cut at 6 mm distance on all the lines from the centric point. The number of records to be obtained is based on the type of the articulator used.
- If Hanau wide vue articulator is used, two records are to be made, one at the centric and the second at the protrusive point which was marked before. Articulators like Dentatus require records made on the lateral tracings also.
- While making the record, the stylus has to be held at the desired points and for that a plastic template is used. A transparent plastic sheet is selected and trimmed according to the dimensions of the tracing table and it is fixed over the tracings made.

- The points at which the records are to be made are marked on the plastic plate and a fine hole is drilled. This hole will hold the stylus at the desired point, for example at centric and at 6 mm protrusion.
- Now the occlusion rims are to be modified by closing the gaps between the central bearing plates and the rim. On the wax rim, triangular locating notches extending to the buccal surfaces are prepared both on the maxilla and mandible.
- Petroleum jelly is smeared on the wax and metal surface to act as a separating medium between wax and plaster. Patient is asked to hold the stylus first at the centric position and an accelerated mix of plaster is injected between the upper and lower occlusal rims.
- Excess material flowing out should be wiped. Once the plaster is set, the assembly can be removed and the record is carefully separated out. Record can be considered as accurate if the central bearing point makes clear perforation in the plaster record.

## Programming

- First the centric record has to be placed and it has to be found out whether it matches with tentative centric relation.
- For this purpose the bases with the tracing assembly is brought back to the casts mounted in the articulator. After keeping the interocclusal record, the upper cast and the lower cast are to be secured and for that retentive pins have to be incorporated on both sides.
- Fine holes can be drilled on the casts and on each side 2 pins on the upper and 2 pins on the lower can be fixed. While fixing on the maxillary pins, care should be taken to drill the holes well below the split. Before securing the pins the split has to separate. With a thread the lower cast, the lower base, the plaster record, the upper base and the upper cast should be secured into a singular block.
- The incisal guide pin and the stylus have to be raised at this point and they need not make contact with the respective tables .
- The upper member of the articulator with the upper split of the cast should now be approximated. At this point it is desirable to release the centric lock.
- When it is approximated, both the parts of the split cast must approximate closely. While it is closed, if the condylar spheres are making contact with the respective stops it can be considered that the tentative centric is matching with graphic tracing.
- If it is not matching it is desirable to go back to the check bite and re-register the tentative centric and repeat the entire process. If the centric matches the articulator can be programmed. Up to this stage, the articulator simulated the patient in the opening and closing movement.
- The articulator has the capability to make translatory movements for which the horizontal condylar path has to be adjusted similar to the condylar path inclination present in the patient. For this purpose the protrusive record is used. In the place of the centric record, protrusive record is positioned and the casts are secured.
- The centric lock, as well as the thumbscrew present behind the condylar housing will be released so that both the condylar elements and the condylar paths can be moved. The upper member with the upper split cast is approximated. If there is a gap, the brass disc containing the condylar path can be moved so that the split completely gets obliterated.
- When it is obliterated, hold the upper member and the lower member of the articulator tight and note down the condylar path set by itself. The path is fixed at this point.
- The lateral condylar path in Hanau articulator is adjusted using the formula which will approximately be 15 degrees.

- From now onwards the articulator will function as a simulator of the patient's jaw with movement capability both in opening and in translation.

## 33. Gnathology.

Gnathology is defined in the "Glossary of Prosthodontic Terms" as a science that deals with the masticatory apparatus as a whole, including morphology, anatomy, histology, physiology, pathology and therapeutics.

Gnathology refers to the study of occlusion and occlusal rehabilitation through the use of pantographs and fully adjustable articulators.

### Gnathologic Instruments

Gnathologic instruments are arcon instruments with adjustable intercondylar distances, in which the condylar housings can be adjusted in the horizontal, sagittal frontal planes, has a Bennett guide adjustment and which accepts arbitrary or hinge axis face-bow transfers and are fully adjustable.

### Features of Gnathologic Instruments

Instruments in this class will accept three-dimensional dynamic registrations and utilize a face-bow transfer.

The condylar pathways can be selectively angled and customized.

The three-dimensional dynamic registration procedure is done by pantographic tracings called pantograms.

Six styli and tracing tables are attached to the maxilla and mandible by means of face-bows and clutches attached to the mandible and maxilla. Two tracing tables are located adjacent to each condylar area in the horizontal and vertical planes. Two additional tracing tables are located anteriorly in the horizontal plane. Mandibular movement then produces pantograms on the tracing tables.

The mandibular position and pathways recorded on the tracing tables are the most posterior position of the mandible to the maxilla, the right and left lateral border pathways of the mandible and the protrusive pathway of the mandible. All are repeatable except for the protrusive pathway.

These tracings are then transferred to the articulator in the same relationship in which they exist in the patient.

The Pantronic by Denar in 1982 is an electronic pantograph which provides a computer printout of numerical condylar measurements hence eliminating the time-consuming procedure of transferring the tracings to the articulator. Pantronic also aids in recording several electronic tracings consecutively and the condylar measurements can be compared immediately via the computer printout.

### Examples of Gnathologic Instruments

- Gnathoscope, designed by Charles Stuart in 1955.
- Denar (D4A) designed by Niles Guichet in 1968.

- D5A modification of D4A.
- Simulator, designed by Ernest Granger.

### Gnathoscope

The Bennett guides are situated in the middle of the posterior aspect of the instrument similar to the Gysi Trubyte articulator.

The Bennett guides can be angulated and customized.

Many plastic condylar inserts are available and they can be customized by grinding if necessary.

### Denar D4A and D5A

Denar D4A and D5A are fully adjustable articulators.

The D5A is quite similar to the D4A except for refinements in machining and in the centric latch mechanism located at the rear of the articulator.

Plastic condylar inserts are available that can be custom ground.

The Bennett adjustment is located in the medial wall of the condylar housing and can record immediate side shift (straight) and progressive side shift (angular) adjustments.

### Simulator

It is same as any other fully adjustable articulator except that the Bennett guide can be set by adjustment only and cannot be customized.

## 34. Curve of Spee.

### Anteroposterior Compensating Curves

They compensate for the curve of Spee seen in natural dentition and is incorporated in a anteroposterior direction.

Curve of Spee is defined as, "Anatomic curvature of the occlusal alignment of teeth beginning at the tip of the lower canine and following the buccal cusps of the natural premolars and molars, continuing to the anterior border of the ramus as described by Graf von Spee". –GPT

### Significance

This imaginary curve starting from the canine joining the buccal cusps of the mandibular posterior teeth and passing through the head of the condyle helps in maintaining balance during protrusion of the mandible. Aiding in the stability of denture in various mandibular movements.

### Incorporation of Curve of Spee (Fig. 4)

The curve of Spee is incorporated in a properly oriented plane of occlusion starting with the canine and joining the buccal cusps of the mandibular posterior teeth by raising it at the distal and continuing this initiated curve with further rise in the second molar.

The radii of the curve depends on the angle of the incisal guidance and the condylar guidance.

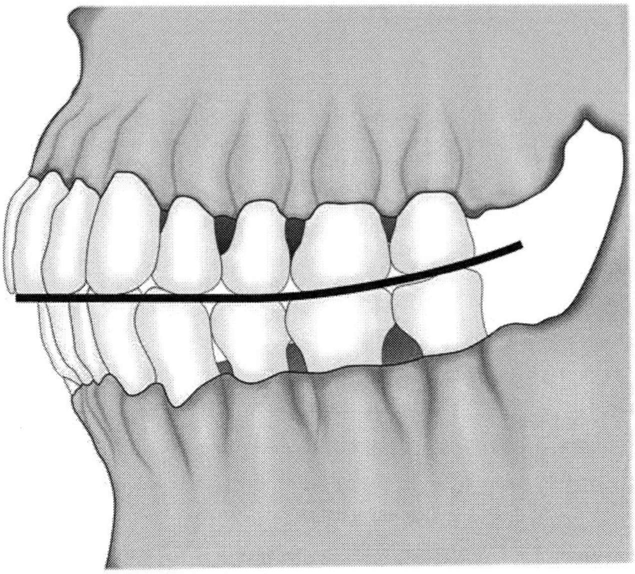

**Fig. 4:** Curve of Spee

## 35. Compensatory curve/compensating curves

Compensating curve is defined as, "The anteroposterior and lateral curvatures in the alignment of the occluding surfaces and incisal edges of artificial teeth, which are used to develop balanced occlusion." –GPT

### Types of Compensating Curves (Fig. 5)

- Anteroposterior curves
- Lateral curves.

In complete dentures compensating curves similar to curve of Spee, Wilson's curve and Monson's curve are incorporated to produce balanced occlusion. Ideally these curves are present in natural dentition.

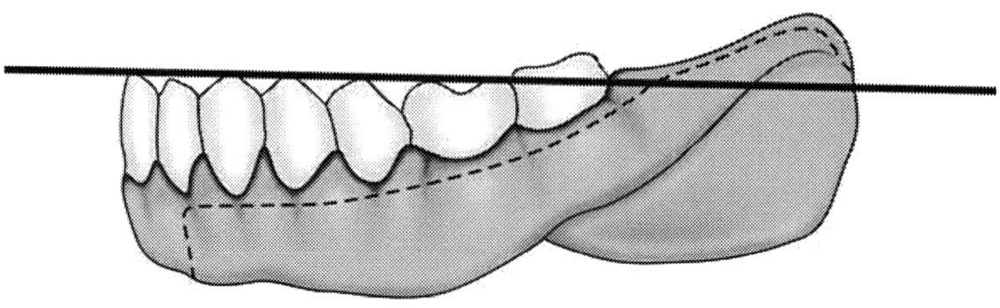

**Fig. 5:** Compensatory curve of lower posterior teeth in relation to a straight line

### Anteroposterior Compensating Curves

They compensate for the Curve of Spee seen in natural dentition and incorporated in a anteroposterior direction.

*Curve of Spee* is defined as, "Anatomic curvature of the occlusal alignment of teeth beginning at the tip of the lower canine and following the buccal cusps of the natural premolars and molars, continuing to the anterior border of the ramus as described by Graf von Spee". -GPT It is an imaginary curve joining the buccal cusps of the mandibular posterior teeth starting from the canine passing through the head of the condyle.

*Significance:* In protrusion the posterior teeth arranged incorporating this curve will remain in contact without disocclusion as in Christensen's phenomenon.

## Lateral Compensating Curves

Seen transversely from one side of the arch to the other.

*Monson's curve* is defined as, "The curve of occlusion in which each cusp and incisal edge touches or conforms to a segment of the sphere of 8 inches in diameter with its center in the region of the Glabella". -GPT

This curve runs across the palatal and buccal cusps of the maxillary molars. During lateral movement the mandibular lingual cusps on the working side should slide along the inner inclines of the maxillary buccal cusp. In the balancing side the mandibular buccal cusps should contact the inner inclines of the maxillary palatal cusp. This relationship forms a lateral balance.

*Wilson's curve* is defined as, "A curve of occlusion which is convex upwards". -GPT

This curve runs opposite to the direction of the Monson's curve. This curve is followed when the first premolars are arranged. The premolars are arranged according to this curve so that they do not produce any interference to lateral movements.

*Reverse curve* is defined as, "A curve of occlusion which in transverse cross-section conforms to a line which is convex upward". -GPT It was originally developed to improve the stability of the denture. The reverse curve was modified by Max. Pleasure to form the pleasure curve.

*Pleasure curve* is defined as, "A curve of occlusion which in transverse cross-section conforms to a line which is convex upward except for the last molars". -GPT

It was proposed by Max Pleasure. He proposed this curve to balance the occlusion and increase the stability of the denture. Hence the first molar is horizontal, the second premolar is lingually tilted and second molar is buccally tilted. This curve runs from the palatal cusp of the first premolar to the distobuccal cusp of the second molar.

## Factors Affecting Compensating Curves

- Condylar guidance
- Incisal guidance
- Occlusal plane
- Cuspal inclination.

**Condylar guidance:** Condylar guidance can be defined as, "Mandibular guidance generated by the condyle and articular disc traversing the contour of the glenoid fossa". —GPT A steep condylar path needs a steep compensating curve for occlusal balance. If a lesser compensating curve is substituted for a steep condylar guidance it would result in a steep incisal guidance resulting in loss of molar balancing contacts.

**Cuspal angulation:** Cusp angle is defined as, "The angle made by the average slope of a cusp with the cusp plane measured mesiodistally or buccolingually". -GPT

The mesiodistal cusps lock the occlusion, such that repositioning of teeth does not occur due to settling of the base. If locking need to be prevented then mesiodistal cusps are reduced during occlusal reshaping. When mesiodistal cusps are reduced the buccolingual cusps are considered as a factor for balanced occlusion.

In cases with a deep bite (steep incisal guidance), teeth with high cuspal inclines are required to produce posterior contact during protrusion.

Inclination of the posterior teeth and their vertical relationship to the occlusal plane results in a curve that is in harmony with the movement of the mandible as guided posteriorly by the condylar path.

**Incisal guidance:** It is defined as, "The influence of the contacting surfaces of the mandibular and maxillary anterior teeth during mandibular movements". –GPT

Incisal guidance is expressed in degrees of angulation from the horizontal by a line drawn in the sagittal plane between the incisal edges of the upper and lower incisor teeth when closed in centric occlusion. If the incisal guidance is steep, it needs steep cusps, a steep occlusal plane, a steep compensating curve to produce occlusal balance. Ideally the incisal guidance should be as flat as esthetics and phonetics will permit. If the anterior teeth necessitates a vertical overlap, a compensating horizontal overlap should be set to prevent anterior interference.

**Occlusal plane:** It is defined as, "An imaginary surface which is related anatomically to the cranium and which theoretically touches the incisal edges of the incisors and the tips of the occluding surfaces of the posterior teeth. It is not a plane in the true sense of the word but represents the mean curvature of the surface". –GPT

It is established anteriorly by the height of the lower canine, almost coinciding with the commissure of the mouth and posteriorly by the height of the retromolar pad. It is usually parallel to the ala-tragus line or Camper's line. Tilt of the plane of occlusion beyond 10° is not advisable.

If the occlusal plane is too low, tongue interference can cause tongue biting. At rest, after swallowing, the tongue with its tip should gently touch the lingual surfaces of the lower anterior teeth, the tongue assumes a position in which its lateral border, at the junction of the keratinized and non-keratinized mucosa, is at the level of the lingual contour of the lower natural posterior teeth. The dorsal surface of the tongue is nearly level with the occlusal surfaces of the posterior teeth.

## Incorporation of Compensating Curve

The compensating curve incorporated in a properly oriented plane of occlusion starts with the first molar by raising it at the distal and continuing this initiated curve with further rise in the second molar. The radii of the curve needed to achieve balance depends on the angle of the incisal guidance and the condylar guidance. It is easier to set the correct compensating curve when the lowers are set first because the determining factors of the incisal guidance and condylar inclination can be readily analyzed and related to the mandibular cast, which is in a fixed relationship to them on the articulator.

This is accomplished by setting as shallow an incisal guide angle as phonetics, esthetics and function of the anterior teeth will permit.

## Significance of Compensating Curves

- To provide balancing occlusal contacts for protrusive mandibular positions.
- Enhances retention, stability of the denture.

- As the forces distributed are uniform while compensatory curves are incorporated the residual ridge resorption is decreased.
- Masticatory efficiency is improved.

## 36. Spa factor/dentogenic concept.

(Frush and Fisher 1955 to 1957)

This concept by Frush and Fisher aids tooth selection based on the age, sex and personality of the patient.

### Age and Tooth Color

The color of the natural teeth darkens with age as the pulp chamber becomes smaller with deposition of secondary dentin in it; this makes the tooth more opaque.

As age progress the lips lose their curves and the teeth wear at the incisal edges and interproximal surfaces, making the tooth surface smoother and more reflective.

The labial surfaces seem flatter and the outline form appears squarer.

#### *Color of the Teeth*

Color has four qualities: hue, saturation (chroma), brilliance (value) and translucency. All these are involved in the selection of teeth.

- *Hue* is the specific color produced by a specific wavelength of light (bluish, greenish, or reddish yellow).
  The hue of teeth must be in harmony with the color (hue) of the patient's face.
- *Saturation* (chroma) is the amount of color per unit area of an object (Some teeth appear more yellow than others).
- *Brilliance* (value) is the lightness or darkness of an object. Variations in brilliance are produced by dilution of the color (the hue) by white or black. The amount of white or black in the teeth determines their lightness or darkness.

  People with fair complexions generally have teeth with less color and the colors are less saturated: thus the teeth are lighter and in harmony with the colors of the face.

  People with dark complexions generally have darker teeth that are in harmony with the coloring of the face.
- *Translucency:* Permitting some light to pass through by diffusing it.
  When the mouth is nearly closed, the teeth will appear darker.

  When the mouth is open, light is reflected through the teeth from the oral cavity and teeth will appear lighter.

#### *Selection of Shade*

The color of the teeth should be observed in natural light. White light after 10 o'clock in the morning and before two in the afternoon is ideal. The teeth should also be observed in artificial light, since denture patients are seen in this light also.

The tooth and the shade guide should be viewed from a distance of six or eight feet and in different angles. The "squint test" can be used to evaluate colors of teeth with the complexion of the face.

Staring at a blue card for 30 seconds will help to make a more accurate observation of the yellow color.

### *Select the Shade by Three Methods*

1. Outside the mouth along the side of the nose to identify hue, brilliance and saturation.
2. Under the lips with only the incisal edge exposed to reveal the effect of the color of teeth.
3. Under the lips with only the cervical end covered and the mouth open to simulate exposure of the teeth as in a smile.

Basic considerations are the harmony of tooth color with the color of the patient's face, hair, eyes and the teeth should be inconspicuous. Harmony should exist between the color of the teeth and the color of the skin.

### Sex

Curved facial features are associated with femininity and square features are associated with masculinity

### Personality

Self-consciousness is possible with either natural or artificial teeth. An unselfconscious person may have had natural teeth pleasant in appearance or dentures with natural appearing artificial teeth. The dentist has to arrange the artificial teeth in a manner to encourage the development of an attractive personality.

## 37. Monson's curve.

It is a lateral compensatory curve. Seen transversely from one side of the arch to the other.

*Monson's curve* is defined as, "The curve of occlusion in which each cusp and incisal edge touches or conforms to a segment of the sphere of eight inches in diameter with its center in the region of the Glabella".–GPT (Fig. 6).

### *Lateral Plane of the Teeth*

The lower natural teeth are inclined slightly to the lingual, creating a transverse curve of the occlusal surfaces from side to side. This is called the Monson curve, which has about an eight inches diameter for normal dentition. This lingual inclination gives prominence to the lower buccal cusps in the transverse horizontal plane, bringing buccal cusps into heavy occlusal contact with the uppers in lateral working position.

The lingualized occlusion necessitates that occlusal surfaces be horizontal in a transverse plane unlike in natural teeth with lingual inclination.

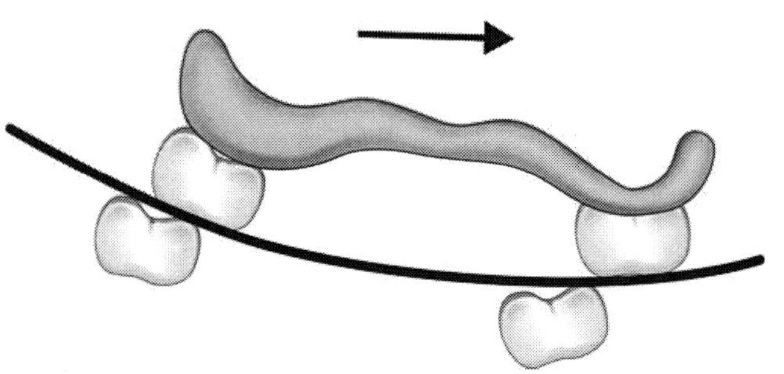

**Fig. 6:** Monson's curve

## 38. Sears posterior teeth.

It is a type of non-anatomic tooth form. It was the first type of non-anatomic tooth form designed by Victor Sears in 1922 and in 1927. It was otherwise called the channel tooth.

### Features of Sears Teeth

1. Deep channels that ran mesiodistally on the entire length of maxillary occlusal surfaces of the four posterior teeth.
2. The lower posteriors were half the buccolingual width of standard anatomic teeth and was designed as a single central uninterrupted ridge that ran the entire length of the occlusal table.
3. The uninterrupted ridge of the lower posterior teeth articulated with the central channel of the maxillary teeth.

### Advantages

1. Unlimited protrusive glide with inclines that limited lateral glide.
2. Suppose to increase the chewing efficiency.
3. Denture in balance with wide mandibular movements than for anatomic tooth forms.

### Modification of Sears Tooth Forms

Avery brothers in 1930 introduced modified form, the opposite of Sears, called the "scissor-bite" technique.

### Features of Modified Tooth Form

1. The posterior occlusal surfaces were locked anteroposteriorly by grinding steps on the surface of the teeth, with the angle determined by the inclination of the condylar path.
2. Sears teeth were modified to be free in lateral excursion.
3. The occlusion of these teeth was meant to shear food in lateral excursions.
4. These teeth were not marketed commercially.

## 39. Denture cleansing agents.

Denture cleansing agents help clean denture from plaque accumulation, stains and maintain oral hygiene in turn.

Cleansing of the denture can be done by:

- Chemical cleaning agents
- Mechanical cleaning methods
- Sonic cleaners.

### Chemical Cleaning Agents

These are commercially available and also can be prepared at home. The cleaning agents used for tissue lined dentures are available separately. Both the commercially available once and home made once are safe and effective.

Home made cleaning solution (The State University of New York at Buffalo School of Dental Medicine formulated this).

This is only to be used for complete acrylic dentures with resin or porcelain teeth. Not to be used for prosthesis containing chrome cobalt or other metals as the sodium hypochlorite may pit or corrode the metal.

**The formula is:**

- 1 tablespoon (15 cc) sodium hypochlorite (household bleach)
- 1 teaspoon (4 cc) Calgon
- 4 ounces (114 cc) water
- Sodium hypochlorite is a bleaching agent. The weak sodium hypochlorite solution is also an effective germicidal agent.
- Calgon, a water softener, provides a detergent action loosening food deposits.
- After using chemical agents, the patients are instructed to brush their dentures with a soft brush under running water.
- This eliminates all the chemical cleaner and removes the soften and loosen deposits from the denture base and teeth.
- If calculus is present, overnight soaking with 4 ounces (114 cc) white vinegar is required. The safe concentration of acetic acid decalcifies calculus deposits. Only occasional soaking in white vinegar is necessary to control calculus build-up and formation.

## Mechanical Cleaning

The use of a brush, soap or denture cleaning paste and water is a common method of cleaning complete dentures. Gentle brushing with a soft denture brush and a nonabrasive detergent is an excellent mechanical cleaning method.

### *Disadvantages*

Abrasion of tooth and denture base (if stiff brush and harsh cleaner is used).

## Sonic cleaners

They clean dentures by employing vibratory energy.

### *Advantages*

1. Effective in removing calculus in a variety of cleaning situations.
2. Effective in helping to remove cigarette and coffee stains.
3. Soft liners: Cannot be chemically cleaned as it distorts the liner causing color changes, internal porosities, surface roughness and loss of resiliency.

## Cleaning Procedure

Wash under cold running water with soft cotton, the external surface can be brushed the normal way.

## 40. Remount procedure.

This is done to check for any occlusal errors which could have taken place in the denture after the wax up and processing. These occlusal errors are corrected by selective grinding after remounting and verifying with interocclusal check records. Ideally a face-bow index is made before separating the denture from cast. This helps to reseat the maxillary denture in the same relationship on the articulator.

### Advantages of Remounting

1. No patient participation.
2. Able to visualize the occlusion better.
3. Provides a stable working foundation without resilient tissues affecting the occlusion.
4. The absence of saliva makes possible more accurate markings with the articulating paper.
5. Objections from patients when they see their dentures being ground is avoided.

### Procedure

Mandibular denture is oriented to the maxillary denture in centric relation by means of an interocclusal record.

#### *Interocclusal Check Record*

Two thicknesses of softened passive type wax is placed on the occlusal surfaces of the mandibular teeth. The patient is instructed or guided to close into the wax when the jaws are in centric relation.

#### *Verifying Record*

The teeth should not penetrate to make contact. Chill with cold air and remove. Trim the wax with slight indentations remaining, expose the facial side to visualize the seating of the maxillary denture.

#### *Mounting*

Orient the mandibular denture to the maxillary denture by means of the interocclusal record and secure with sticky wax. After seating the mandibular cast in the denture, complete mounting by attaching to the mandibular member with plaster.

#### *Rechecking Records*

Make another wax interocclusal record and check on the articulator after placing the dentures on the cast. While checking the condylar elements should be freed and place the teeth in the wax record indentations. The condylar elements should rest against the stops. Repeat with three records to confirm.

## 41. Selective grinding.

In anatomic tooth forms to attain balanced occlusion, bilateral tooth contacts of the posterior teeth is required to evenly distribute the forces.

A cusp fossae marginal ridge relation of maximum intercuspation when the jaws are in terminal hinge position is needed to attain balance.

There should be no occlusal interference when jaw movements occur to and from centric and eccentric positions.

If selective grinding is done maximum intercuspation when the jaws are in centric relation, balanced centric occlusion is achieved.

If selective grinding done to make simultaneous cusp tip to cusp tip contact on both sides of the arch when the jaws are in a right or left lateral position, balanced occlusion in a static eccentric position exists.

When the anterior teeth make incisal edge to incisal edge contact in a straight protruded relation and if the posterior teeth are altered to make cusp contacts at the same time balanced occlusion in protrusion exists.

The buccal cusps of the mandibular posterior teeth and the lingual cusps of the maxillary posterior teeth maintain the vertical dimension of jaw separation by contact in the fossae and on the marginal ridges of their antagonists. Generally, the functional cusp of upper (lingual cusp) and functional cusp of lower (buccal cusp ) is never ground.

The non-functional cusps, deepening of fossae and the cuspal inclines are the ones that are altered to achieve balance.

## 42. Relining and rebasing.

### Definition

*Relining* is the process of adding some material to the tissue side of a denture to fill the space between the tissue and the denture base.

*Rebasing* is a process of replacing all the base material of a denture. The purpose of such a process is to fill the space between the tissue and the denture base without changing the position of the teeth and the relation of the dentures.

### Indications for Relining and Rebasing

1. Immediate dentures after three to six months when the extraction sockets have healed and remodelled.
2. Extensive ridge resorption with loose fitting denture especially when patient is happy with esthetic aspect.
3. Poor patients who cannot afford the cost of having new dentures constructed.
4. Geriatric or chronically ill patients.

### For a Denture to be Relined or Rebased

1. Healthy oral tissue.
2. Correct occlusal vertical dimension.
3. Centric occlusion should coincide with centric relation.
4. Adequate interocclusal distance.
5. Satisfactory esthetics (The size, shapes, shade and arrangement of the artificial teeth must be satisfactory).
6. Coverage of denture bases should be adequate.
7. The denture base extensions should be adequate as to distribute masticatory forces to a large area as possible.
8. Satisfactory speech.

### Contraindications

1. When centric relation record is not accurate.
2. When interocclusal distance is not proper.
3. Excessive bone resorption.
4. When abused soft tissues are present.
5. When the patient complains of temporomandibular joint problems.
6. When the denture base is under extended.
7. Poor esthetics.
8. Major speech problem.
9. In severe osseous undercuts.

### Relining Techniques

There are two major relining techniques:

- Open-mouth technique
- Closed-mouth technique

In an open-mouth technique major emphasis is given to making separate impressions, with independent attention given to recording jaw relations.

In a closed-mouth relining technique a habitual centric occlusion is usually accepted. This centric occlusion may or may not be the same as centric relation.

### Tissue Preparation

1. Excessive hypertrophic tissue should be surgically removed. The dentures can be used as a surgical splint.
2. The oral mucosa should be free of areas of irritation.
3. Removal of the dentures from the mouth during sleep is a must for several weeks before treatment commences.
4. The dentures should be left out of the mouth at least two to three days before making the final impression.
5. Daily massage of the soft tissues is helpful to stimulate their blood supply.

### Denture Preparation

1. Pressure areas on the tissue surface of the dentures should be relieved.
2. Minor occlusal disharmony is corrected by selective grinding.
3. Small border inadequacies are corrected.
4. A correct posterior palatal seal area should be established before the final impression. Stick compound and autopolymerizing acrylic resin can be used for this purpose.

### Principal Pitfalls

The principal pitfalls that must be avoided in any technique to refit a complete denture are as follows:

1. Do not increase the occlusal vertical dimension.
2. Multiple even contacts (maximum intercuspation) should be present in centric relation.
3. Do not permit the maxillary denture to move forward during impression making.
4. Ensure that centric relation and centric occlusion are identical.
5. Ensure that an accurate posterior palatal seal has been established.
6. An equal thickness of final impression material should be used.

#### *Chairside Technique*

Both the static technique and the functional impression technique are good techniques in cases for simple situations and complicated situations as excessive tissue changes. Chairside technique was uncommon due to chemical burn on the mucosa; a bad odour; lack of color stability of the lined acrylic and if the denture was not positioned correctly, the material was difficult to remove. Use of visible light-cured (VLC) resin system as substitute to the liner was a better choice of material than acrylic because of its many advantages.

*Advantages* are good fit, strength, ability to polymerise without residual components, ease of fabrication and manipulation, patient acceptance, ability to bond with other denture base resins and low bacterial adherence.

## 43. Selective grinding procedures.

The displacability of the basal seat mucosa (realeff) must be considered when the teeth are altered by selective grinding procedures.

Selective grinding procedures are done to correct the occlusal discrepancies which has taken place after the denture is waxed up and processed.

Selective grinding of anatomic teeth is done to achieve:

1. Balanced occlusion when the jaws are in centric relation.
2. Balanced occlusion in eccentric relations.
3. On working side: By having all of the posterior teeth and the cuspids in contact.
4. On balancing side: Only the posterior teeth should contact.
5. Protrusive balance: The anterior teeth should make incisal edge-to-edge contact with the tips of the buccal and lingual cusps of the posterior teeth in contact.

### Procedure

#### *Locating the Area of Premature Contact*

1. The horizontal and lateral condylar inclinations are set with the protrusive interocclusal relation record.
2. The horizontal condylar elements are released to allow freedom of the articulator in eccentric positions.
3. The incisal guide pin is raised and secured above the height of the guide table.
4. Areas of tooth contact in the centric and eccentric positions are evaluated.
5. The articulator is closed with the condylar elements against the centric relation stops until the posterior teeth are in contact and anterior teeth out of contact.
6. If the rest of tooth are out of occlusion when the lingual cusps of the maxillary posterior teeth and the buccal cusps of the mandibular posterior teeth occlude then premature contact exist.

#### *Recording the Premature Contact*

After securing the right condylar element in the centric position place the lingual cusps of the maxillary posterior teeth in balancing relation with the buccal cusps of the mandibular posterior teeth.

#### *Possible Prematurities*

a. If the balancing side is not in the correct relation, the error appears on either balancing or working side.
b. If the balancing contact is excessive, the working side teeth will be out of contact.
c. If the working side contact is excessive, the balancing side will not contact.
d. If the teeth on the working side are too long, there will be no contact on the balancing side.
e. If a single tooth is high on the working side, there will be no contact on the balancing and the working side.

Repeat the procedure with the left side as the working side and record all the premature contacts on both sides with articulating tape.

Place the tape on the occlusal surfaces and the incisal edges of all the mandibular teeth.

## Steps in Selective Grinding Procedures

Return the incisal guide pin to the table and:

1. If the cusp is high in centric and eccentric position, reduce the cusp.
2. If the cusp is high in centric and not in the eccentric position, deepen the fossae or the marginal ridges.

## For Balanced Grinding Occlusion

Working side reduce the inner inclines of:

1. The buccal cusps of the maxillary teeth and
2. The lingual cusps of the mandibular teeth.

Balancing side reduce the inner inclines of the mandibular buccal cusps.

Protrusive balance reduce the distal inclines of the maxillary cusps and the mesial inclines of the mandibular cusps.

## Refining

After the occlusal corrections are done refine the occlusal anatomy using the mounted inverted cone points and polish all the ground surfaces with pumice on a wet rag wheel.

## Selective Grinding of Non-Anatomic Teeth

1. The steps of recording and marking the occlusal discrepancies are the same.
2. A mounted wheel is used to grind the occlusal surfaces of the teeth until simultaneous even contacting areas on the right and left are developed without anterior tooth contact.
3. The altered surfaces are polished with wet pumice on a wet rag wheel.

*Stripping method for the occlusal equilibration of zero degree teeth: by Dr. Gronas in 1970*

This is a carborundum stripping technique to eliminate cuspal interferences.

A 220 grit paper is used to modify porcelain teeth and a fine 320 grit paper is used for acrylic resin teeth.

### *Procedure*

Adjusting for Centric Occlusion

1. Locate the premature contacts as in selective grinding procedures and reduce gross interferences with a stone or bur until a flat occlusal plane is obtained in centric and eccentric positions.
2. After the gross reduction is done if any, carborundum strip of the appropriate width with the abrasive side against the teeth are placed, the articulator is closed in centric relation.
3. With light pressure to the upper member of the articulator the strip is pulled briskly between the teeth without altering the vertical dimension of occlusion.
4. Reduction of the contacts with the strips is continued by stripping an equal number of times with the abrasive side alternated up and down until uniform bilateral contacts on the posterior teeth are obtained.
5. This procedure is repeated in the eccentric position.
6. Finish the reduction with finer grits of sandpaper strips to produce a smooth flat surface.

## 44. Impression trays.

Defined as a device which is used to carry, confine and control the impression material for making an impression.

### Types

1. *Stock trays*
   a. Edentulous trays
      i. Perforated
      ii. Non-perforated
   b. Dentulous
      i. Perforated
      ii. Non-perforated
      iii. Rimlocked
2. *Custom trays* or *Special trays*
   To make corrective or final wash impression.

### Materials Used

- Shellac
- Tray compound
- Acrylic resin (with spacer and stops)
- Metallic (Chrome-Cobalt).

### Functions of Impression Trays

1. To support the impression material while in contact with oral tissues.
2. For various impression techniques as Selective pressure technique.
3. To support the impression material so that cast can be poured.

### For Successful Impression Knowledge of the Following is Necessary

1. Oral anatomy
2. Impression materials
3. Impression technique
4. Operator skill.

### Custom Made Tray

#### *Ideal Requirements*

1. Material should be rigid and dimensionally stable.
2. Accurately and closely adapting to oral tissues.
3. Impression material should adhere to the tray.
4. There should be sufficient space between vestibular sulcus and tray border.
5. Should be strong enough to carry impression material.

## 45. Repair.

It is the procedure by which the fractured parts are assembled and joined using the same denture base material.

**Types of fracture**

- Tooth fracture
- Denture fracture.

## Tooth Fracture

Can be anterior tooth or posterior tooth. The tooth material as plastic tooth or porcelain tooth can be replaced.

## Anterior Tooth Replacement

1. Keeping the labiogingival margin intact the fractured tooth is removed using round bur.
2. If it is a porcelain tooth, heat with a torch and remove with a No. 7 wax spatula in the ridge lap area.
3. Another tooth of appropriate shade and size is selected and positioned in place with sticky wax.
4. Plaster index is made on the labial surface of tooth to be restored including the adjacent tooth.
5. After the plaster index sets, its removed and indentations are placed in the replacement area.
6. Resin is added on to the lingual aspect of the tooth and this tooth is fixed in place with the help of index.
7. Place in pressure pot for 30 minutes at 20 psi pressure and cure.
8. Remove and polish with pumice and wet rag wheel.

## Posterior Tooth Replacement

1. The casts have to be mounted in centric relation and after checking the occlusion the tooth to be replaced has to be sealed to the opposite tooth in occlusion with sticky wax.
2. The area from which the tooth was removed have to be intended with round bur.
3. Close the articulator, check the occlusion and fill the space with resin between the cervical aspect of tooth and denture after applying monomer to the tooth.
4. After the final cure, polish the denture and check the occlusion.
5. If required a face-bow record and transfer is made.
6. Right, left lateral records and a straight protrusive record can be made before mounting the casts.
7. The records are then used to mount casts on articulator and adjust the condylar inclinations and Bennett shift.

## Denture Fracture

### Types

a. Non-separated fracture or Midline fracture
b. Complex fracture (Fractured into two or more parts)
c. Fractured dentures with missing section.

## Procedure for Repair

1. Denture is held together with sticky wax and small wooden sticks.

2. A cast of model plaster is poured after undercuts inside the denture are blocked out.
3. The denture is removed from the cast, free of sticky wax and 2–3 mm of acrylic from the midline fracture area is removed.
4. A long rounded bevel is made on each side of the opening about 5 mm wide along the entire midline and onto the labial surface.
5. The plaster cast is painted with a separating solution and the two pieces of the denture are placed back on the cast.
6. The repair acrylic is applied by wetting the pieces to be repaired with monomer and dusting on the polymer and adding more monomer until the fracture area is covered.
7. Curing of acrylic: Placed in a pressure pot at 30 pounds per square inch pressure for about 30 minutes.
8. The denture is then removed from the pressure pot, trimmed and polished. The steps for repair of the mandibular denture are the same as those for the maxillary denture.

### Cast Strengthener for Repeated Mandibular Denture Fractures

- A cobalt-chromium cast strengthener is used along with heat cure acrylic resin.
- Strengthener is placed on cast before wax-up.
- After wax up the strengthener is imbedded in waxed up denture.
- This waxed-up denture is processed in the usual manner.
- During boil-out of the wax, the strengthener is cleaned and placed back on the cast in position and the denture is packed.

### Light-Cured Resin Repairs

- The resin is cured with a visible light source that emits intense light in the 400–500 nm range.
- The pieces of the broken denture are assembled and stabilized with sticky wax.
- A cast is made and it is coated with a separating agent.
- The borders of the fractured sections are prepared.
- The edges are coated with monomer and the light-cured resin is adapted to the fracture area.
- Light from the visible light source (or a hand-held unit) is applied to the repair area for five to ten minutes.
- Minimal finishing and polishing are required.

### Advantages

1. Convenient to use.
2. Neat to work and no free monomer.
3. Less time needed to complete the repair.
4. Easy control of the position of the repair material.

## 46. Differences between natural and artificial occlusion.

### Complete Denture Occlusion

Supported by Soft and hard tissues.

### Soft Tissues

They vary in thickness, resiliency and tolerance to pressure and are in a state of constant change. They respond rapidly to external stimuli such as pressure, scuffing, heat and cold and to internal stimuli such as the amount of contained fluids, nutrients, salts and blood pressure. These changes in soft tissues affect the position of the bases and the occlusion they carry.

## Hard Tissues

### *Reaction of Bone to Pressure and Tension*

If the force on a tooth is principally in line with its long axis, there is apposition of bone.

Lateral forces tangential to the long axis of a tooth cause bone resorption, tooth migration and mobility.

*In natural teeth* these lateral forces are countered by avascular tissues such as teeth, joints and discs that are covered and protected by specialized fibrous tissue, fibrocartilage, or hyaline cartilage.

In natural dentition when stress is applied to bone it stimulates the osteoblasts and the osteoclasts to remodel bone.

*In complete denture occlusion*: The stresses of pressure and tension on bone are transmitted through the residual ridge. If pressure is against the periosteum, the blood supply is disturbed and leads to bone resorption.

Blood supply is from two sources: from the periosteum and from its internal system of arteries.

Arteries from the external periosteal network enter the bone; interference as direct pressure or inflammation by a denture base lead to bone necrosis and resorption.

## Differences Between Natural and Artificial Occlusion

Occlusion of natural and artificial teeth vary to a great extent. It is important for one to know about these differences in order to understand the need of balanced occlusion in a complete denture which is discussed later.

### *Natural Teeth*

1. Natural teeth are retained by periodontal tissues with proprioceptive feedback.
2. Natural teeth function independently and can withstand occlusal forces by proper dissipation of these forces.
3. Malocclusion in natural teeth is well adjusted to and is normal without deteriorating effects.
4. Non-vertical forces are well tolerated and only affects the teeth involved
5. Incising does not affect the posterior teeth.
6. Second molar region is the ideal area for heavy mastication for better leverage and power.
7. Bilateral balance is not found in natural dentition.
8. Proprioceptive impulses help to avoid occlusal interference and establish a stable habitual occlusion away from centric relation.

### *Artificial Teeth*

1. Artificial teeth are placed on bases seated on resilient tissues.
2. The artificial teeth move as a unit.
3. Artificial teeth function as a unit on their base with distribution of forces on the entire denture base coverage area.
4. Malocclusions pose immediate response involving the entire tissue support.
5. Non-vertical forces damage the supporting tissues.

6. Incising will displace the denture from its basal seat.
7. Placing load only on the second molar region can shift the denture base.
8. Bilateral balance is important to produce stability and retention of the denture.
9. As there is no feedback and as the denture relation is in centric relation. Any occlusal interferences in this position can displace the denture.

## 47. Theories of occlusion.

**Occlusion**: It is the static contact of teeth that exist after the jaw movements have stopped. It is the contact relationship of the upper and lower teeth.

All occlusal forms should at least have a tripod contact in centric relation. Balanced occlusion should have tripod contact even in eccentric relation.

### Concepts of Occlusion/Theories of Occlusion

1. Spherical concept of occlusion (Monson)
2. Bonwill's theory of occlusion
3. Conical theory of occlusion
4. Organic concept of occlusion
5. Neutrocentric concept of occlusion
6. Centric occlusion
7. Balanced occlusion.

### Spherical Concept of Occlusion (Monson in 1918)

It is defined as the lower teeth moving over the surface of the upper teeth as over the surface of a sphere with a diameter of 8 inches (20 cm).

Center of the sphere being the center of glabella and the surface of the sphere passes through the glenoid fossa. This theory was based on the findings of Von Spee.

Instruments based on this theory was Maxillomandibular instrument and Hageman balancer.

Based on this concept, the anteroposterior and mesiodistal inclines of the artificial teeth should be arranged in harmony with a spherical surface.

### Bonwill's Theory of Occlusion/Theory of Equilateral Triangle (WGA Bonwill)

Bonwill's theory of occlusion proposed that the teeth move in relation to each other as guided by the condylar controls and the incisal point. In this theory there is a 4 inch distance between the condyles and between the condyles and incisor point.

Instrument based on this theory is mean value articulator.

It permits lateral movements but as the condylar guidances are not adjustable they move in a horizontal plane.

### Conical Theory of Occlusion

Conical theory of occlusion proposed that the lower teeth move over the surfaces of upper teeth as over the surface of a cone generating an angle of 45° with the central axis of the cone tipped 45° to the occlusal plane.

Instrument based on this theory – Hall automatic articulator by RE Hall. This requires a 45° cusp teeth to confirm to this concept of occlusion.

## Organic Concept of Occlusion

The aim of Organic Concept of Occlusion is to relate the occlusal surfaces of teeth to be in harmony with the muscles and joints during function.

Organic occlusion employs cusp form posterior teeth that are not arranged in protrusive and bilateral balance.

The shapes of the teeth are altered to have cusps suitable for the patient.

The movement of the condyle determines the direction of the ridges and grooves of the teeth.

Mandibular movements determine the cusp height, fossa, depth of the fissure and concavity of the lingual surfaces. The muscles and joints determine the mandibular position of occlusion without tooth guidance.

*Three phases of organic occlusion are:*

1. The posterior teeth should protect the anterior teeth in centric occlusal position.
2. Maxillary incisors should have vertical overlap sufficient to provide separation of posterior tooth during incisal edge-to-edge contact.
3. In excessive lateral mandibular movements the cuspids should prevent contact of all other teeth.

## Neutrocentric Concept of Occlusion

The term neutrocentric denotes an occlusion that eliminates the anteroposterior and buccolingual inclines in order to direct the forces to the posterior teeth.

In this concept the plane of occlusion should be flat and parallel to the residual alveolar ridge and not dictated by the horizontal condylar guidances. This is similar to the monoplane occlusion used to set non-anatomic teeth.

The neutrocentric concept of occlusion maintains that the anteroposterior plane of occlusion should be parallel with the plane of the denture foundation and not inclined to form compensating curves.

In a mediolateral direction the teeth are set flat with no medial or lateral inclination.

The horizontal condylar guidances and the lateral condylar guidances of the articulator are set at zero as the teeth are not arranged for balancing contacts.

The condylar elements of the articulator may be secured to function in the opening and closing movements. To direct force toward the center of the support.

The buccolingual width of the teeth is reduced and the number of teeth is reduced to direct the forces in the molar and bicuspid area of support.

## Balanced Occlusion

Balanced occlusion is the simultaneous contacting of the maxillary and mandibular teeth on the right and left and in the anterior and posterior occlusal areas when the jaws are in either centric or eccentric relation.

Balanced occlusion is associated with cusp form posterior teeth.

Teeth arranged in balanced occlusion provides stabilizing forces to the denture bases on their basal seat when the teeth make contact and the jaws are in centric or eccentric relation.

### Centric Occlusion

It is the maximum intercuspation between the maxillary and mandibular teeth. Either centric occlusion can be made to coincide with centric relation or a range of tooth contact in this area called freedom in centric can be given. In centric occlusion only the working occlusal units are in contact. The first bicuspids, the cuspids and the incisors have at least 1 millimeter clearance when the teeth are in centric occlusion. In the mediolateral direction the buccal surfaces of the posterior teeth that extend over the lateral half of the residual alveolar ridge are ground to have at least 1 millimeter clearance with their antagonists.

## 48. Requirements of complete denture occlusion

- Stability of occlusion at centric relation position.
- Balanced bilateral occlusal contacts for all eccentric mandibular movements.
- Unlocking the cusps mesiodistally to allow settling of the bases due to tissue deformation and bone resorption.
- Control of horizontal force by buccolingual cusp height reduction.
- Anterior incisal clearance during all posterior masticatory function.
- Minimum occlusal contact areas for reduced pressure.
- Generous sluice-ways (Anatomic tooth forms).

The **requirements of complete denture occlusion** is divided into three units as:

a. Incising,
b. Working,
c. Balancing.

### Requirements for Incising Units

1. Sharp enough to cut efficiently.
2. During mastication incising units should be out of contact.
3. Contact only in protrusive incising function.
4. Horizontal overlap to allow for base settling without interference.
5. Should have flat incisal guidance as possible as esthetics and phonetics permit.

### Requirements for Working Occlusal Units

1. Efficient in cutting and grinding.
2. Decreased buccal-lingual width to minimize the work force to the denture foundation.
3. Plane of occlusion as parallel as possible to the mean foundation plane.
4. Placed over the ridge crest in the masticating area for lever balance.
5. Should have a surface to receive and transmit the force of occlusion vertically.
6. Should center the workload near the anteroposterior center of the dentuer.
7. Should function as a group with simultaneous harmonious contacts.

### Requirements for Balancing Occlusal Units

1. Should contact on the second molars when the incising units contact in function.
2. Should contact at the end of the chewing cycle when the working units contact.
3. Should have smooth gliding contacts for lateral and protrusive excursions.

## 49. Sears axioms for artificial occlusion

These axioms were published by Sears 1973 and have guided the planning of complete denture occlusion for many years:

1. The smaller the area of occlusal surface acting on food, the smaller will be the crushing force on food transmitted to the supporting structures.
2. Vertical force applied to an inclined occlusal surface causes nonvertical force on the denture base.
3. Vertical force applied to a denture base supported by yielding tissue causes the base to shift when the force is not centered on the base.
4. Vertical force applied lateral to the ridge crest creates tipping forces on the base.
5. Vertical forces applied to inclined supporting tissues will cause non-vertical forces on the denture base.

These axioms aid the dentist in the final outcome of success in complete denture as it helps to increase the stability, function and comfort of the denture.

## 50. Endosteal implants

An endosteal implant is an alloplastic material surgically inserted into residual ridge, primarily to serve as prosthodontic foundation.

Endo means Within and Osteal means Bone.

The other types are sub-periosteal and intramucosal implants.

### Commonly Available as:

Pin, needle, screw, cylinder
Plate or blade or Blade vent implant.

### Depending on Design it is Divided as:

a. Cylindrical-Microscopic retention, bonding to bone.
b. Screw root forms.
c. Combination root forms (both cylinder and screw design).

### Classified as:

a. Immediate function or of later function as loaded after a healing time.
b. Totally submerged or partially submerged.
c. Function with a direct bone interface or Functions with a peri-implant connective tissue ligament.
d. Final prostheses can be removed destructively or non-destructively.

### Endosteal Implants

Three methods of placing endosteal implant.

1. The implant can be immediately loaded with a provisional prosthesis.
2. It can be fully submerged and allowed to heal for a number of months (Branemark screws, sinus-lift blades).
3. It can be semi-submerged and allowed to heal out of function.

## Blade or Plate-Form Implants (by Linkow 1970)

*Types*: Latticework design and closed bottoms.

These two types can be:

a. Coated with materials such as hydroxyapatite or
b. Plasma sprayed titanium.

Their ease of insertion led to extensive use.

### *Three Insertion Techniques*

1. A blade can be inserted and placed into immediate function with a temporary prosthesis or left out of function.
2. After the implant is allowed to heal undisturbed for several weeks, the healing head is replaced by final abutment head.
3. Implant is inserted and fully submerged beneath the mucosa for extended healing. A covering cap is threaded into the abutment neck receptor site. A second surgical procedure is done to expose the covering cap and replace it with the final abutment head.

The S implants of Tatum are wide blades with horizontal loading platforms. They can be used in broad alveolar ridges.

If the ridges are shallow, a lateral approach, rotating a portion of the wall of the sinus upward, maintaining the membrane intact and adding autogenous or synthetic bone is done followed by implant placement.

## Screw, Root and Pin-Form Implants

### *Types*

a. Smooth
b. Threaded: These types can either be coated or uncoated
c. Hollow submergable or nonsubmergable
d. Solid
e. Perforated.

### *Parts of Screw Type*

Implant body fixture, First stage cover, Second stage permucosal extension, Abutment, Hygiene screw, Transfer coping, Analog, Coping and coping screw.

Smooth tantalum pin implant of Scybalum was the earliest type in this. The most commonly used material is pure titanium. Concept of submerged healing prior to loading and the use of attachment mechanisms permit a wide range of stress-breaking and non-destructive removal of prostheses.

## 51. Subperiosteal implants

Implants placed on top of resorbed alveolar ridges are called sub-periosteal.

*Types:* Total or full subperiosteal implants. They can be non-coated or coated with hydroxyapatite.

Materials for subperiosteal implants are surgical vitalium, titanium, or titanium alloy, wironium, bionium and nickel-free cobalt-chromium alloy.

## Parts of Subperiosteal Implants

Part below the periosteum is called **Substructure.**

It consists of:

1. *Primary struts* which consist of a peripheral (lay on extended areas of cortical bone) and abutment struts (connects labial, lingual struts and vertical permucosal post on the crest of ridge).
2. *Secondary struts* help to distribute forces from primary abutment struts.
3. *Permucosal attachment* acts as prosthetic retainer.

   The part of implant above the tissue is called **Mesostructure.**

It consists of:

1. *Mesobar*
2. *Superstructure* which attaches to mesostructure.

## Procedure

An impression of the residual maxilla or mandible with a bone-bite registered at centric relation and the proper vertical dimension is made.

A cast is then made and the implant designed and fabricated.

A more extended two-stage procedure, where the implant is inserted 20-30 days after the initial bone impressioning with the help of a CAT-scan bone model.

## Technique of Subperiosteal Implants

### *Preliminary*

1. The normal prosthetic procedure for constructing complete upper and lower dentures is carried out until the dentures have reached the trial stage.
2. The lower denture being retained in the wax stage.
3. The first molars and the canines are removed from the wax lower denture and an instrument pushed through the wax in the areas occupied by these teeth until it penetrates the surface of the ridge of the cast.
4. These marks on the cast locate the positions of the abutments of the implant. A template is replaced on the cast and holes are drilled through it in the areas marked for the future abutments.
5. Two impression trays are made on the cast and they will be used to take the impression of the bone surface when the mucoperiosteum has been reflected.
6. An acrylic record block is also constructed to occlude with the finished upper denture. Rims are only built in the premolar and molar regions and wire staples are inserted into the acrylic in the premolar regions to facilitate its manipulation.
7. This record block will be used lined with gutta-percha to record the jaw relationship when the mucosa has been reflected to enable the cast of the bone impression to be correctly related to the upper denture.

*There are two surgical stages*

The first consists of the reflection of the mucoperiosteum, two impressions of the surface of the bone and the recording of the occlusion taken with the record block fitting the bone.

The second stage, is about three to six weeks after the first, consists of the reflection of the mucoperiosteum and the insertion of the implant substructure after completing the lab procedures.

In the **lab procedures,** care should be taken to prepare the abutment posts with a neck of 2.5 to 3 mm diameter and with a depth slightly greater than the thickness of the mucosa. The diameter of the base of the abutment posts should be about 4 mm in the canine regions and 6 mm in the molar regions and each post should have a 5° taper. Casting of the pattern is made with a nickel-free cobalt-chromium alloy. The implant is positioned on the cast, thimbles waxed to the abutment posts and joined by wax bars. The whole wax pattern cast in cobalt-chromium to form the superstructure.

The cast superstructure is seated on the abutment posts and the lower denture waxed around it.

*Reasons for failures are:*

1. Inaccurate fit of the cast frame work.
2. Incorrect outline and inadequate extension of the substructure.
3. Uneven pressure.
4. Careless surgical technique.
5. Compromised general health of the patient and careless oral hygiene.

## 52. Impression technique for flabby tissues.

If flabby tissues cannot be treated by any surgical procedures due to certain clinical situations other methods as tissue conditioning should be tried before going in for impression procedures. The patient's existing denture can be relined with a tissue-conditioning material to promote tissue healing.

### Hypermobile Ridge Tissue

This condition results from resorption of the alveolar bone under an ill-fitting denture from constant unbalanced occlusal forces in a localized area.

If the movable tissue is localized and does not interfere with the stability of the denture, then a nonpressure, mucostatic impression technique can be done.

If the tissue is excessive and pendulous and interferes with the stability of the denture then, surgical removal is recommended.

### Impression Technique

#### *Preliminary Impression*

With alginate impressions that should be poured immediately.

Thirty minutes is the maximum time which should elapse between making the impression and pouring it.

### Impression plaster/anti-expansion solution

#### *Composition:*

- Impression plaster is based on calcined calcium sulphate hemihydrate
- Alazarin red–colouring agent–0.04%
- The impression plaster is mixed to anti-expansion solution containing

- Potassium sulphate–4% (reduces expansion to 0.05% acts as an accelerator also)
- Borax–0. 4% (Retarder)
- This setting reaction is associated with an expansion of 0.3–0.6%
- The plaster is mixed with water or an anti-expansion solution in the ratio of 100 gram to 50–60 ml
- Setting time 3 min.

### *Special Plasters*

- Special plasters are obtainable for impressions which contain potassium sulphate and borax in the solid form and so have only to be mixed with water.
- *Another type* contains starch which makes a very smooth mix with the added advantage that it is slightly sticky and so will adhere to the tray and is easy to remove from the cast by boiling, water which causes the starch granules to swell and so disintegrate the whole impression.

## Impression for Flabby Ridges

### *Mixing Plaster for Impressions*

About 20 mL of anti-expansion solution in a dry bowl, quickly sift plaster and allow it to stand for 30 s without disturbance. After half a minute when the entire plaster is moistened throughout, stirs two or three times with a spatula for a homogeneous mass.

### *Individual Trays*

Cold-cure acrylic tray with handle measuring 2 cm from the sulcus is made. The lower tray should have a finger stand in the first molar region on both sides.

Check and trim the trays for plaster impressions.

After the impression is made the green stick compound should be seen through the plaster impression. This can ensure that the impression plaster has determined the height of the sulcus appropriate to the width already decided by the buccal trim.

### *Puddling of Plaster*

Instead of using firm direct pressure, the hand is wriggled and puddled into the mass with a gentle vibratory movement so that the plaster flows around the tissue surface. This method is referred to as puddling.

## Failures with Plaster Impressions

1. Using a tray of the wrong design.
2. Failure to reduce the depth of the flanges of the tray.
3. Insufficient plaster in the tray.
4. Too much plaster in the tray.
5. Seating the tray after the plaster begins to set.
6. Incorrect centring of the tray.
7. Direct pressure and not puddling the tray into position.

The patient is often pre-medicated with atropine to reduce salivary flow so that the surface of the impression, made in low-viscosity impression paste, is in very close and intimate contact with the mucosa.

In order to maintain the mucostatic theme, the denture base is finished without encroaching on muscle tissue and so the periphery is much shallower and thinner than with other techniques.

## Displaceable Maxillary Ridge

An anterior ridge which is displaceable, in the upper with the incisive papilla lying towards the front of the flabby ridge and the bunched pairs of palatal rugae on the crest of the ridge.

## Impression Techniques

### *Mucocompression without Displacement*

This is a two-stage technique designed to compress the flabby tissue so that the compression throughout the whole of the maxillary denture-bearing area is as uniform as possible.

*Preliminary impression:* Made with alginate and a cast is poured. A special tray is made with chemically activated resin.

The borders are refined and border molding with green stick compound is done.

*Final impression:* With Zinc oxide eugenol impression paste.

After the paste sets, the tray is trimmed of corresponding to the flabby portion. This appears as a window in the tray.

*The second stage:* Impression plaster is painted on to the flabby portion with a brush. The tray is removed after the plaster sets and poured in dental stone after applying separating media at the region of plaster impression.

## 53. Vestibuloplasty.

Vestibuloplasty is the surgical procedure designed to restore alveolar ridge heights by lowering muscle attachment on the buccal, labial and lingual aspects of the residual ridges.

## Procedures

- Transpositional flap vestibuloplasty for anterior mandible
- Maxillary submucosal vestibuloplasty
- Floor of mouth lowering
- Epithelial graft vestibuloplasty
- Secondary epithelialization procedures.

### *Transpositional Flap Vestibuloplasty/Lip Switch*

*Indication*—To increase the vestibular depth in anterior mandible when there is 15 mm bone height.

*Procedure*—A submucosal dissection from the inner aspect of the lower lip to mucogingival junction followed by a supraperiosteal dissection to replace the muscle and soft tissue attachments to the desired vestibular depth.

A periosteal incision is made near the crest of the ridge and the periosteum is lifted off the bone and it is sutured to the raw lip bed. The mucosal flap is adapted to the exposed bone to the depth of the vestibule and fixed with sutures or stent.

### ***Maxillary Submucosal Vestibuloplasty*** (described by Mcintosh and Obwegeiser)

*Indication*—When there is good underlying bone but not available due to high frenal and muscle attachments.

To ensure the depth a mouth mirror is placed in the vestibule and checked for shortening of the lip, if the lip does not shorten then the case can be considered for submucosal vestibuloplasty.

*Procedure:* A vertical midline incision is made on the anterior maxilla and a subperiosteal tunnel is created by dissecting the tissue away from the periosteum. The intervening submucosal tissue is then repositioned superiorly and it is secured in place with postoperative stent. The stent is worn for one week. The healing period is 3 weeks. In the mean time a new prosthesis is fabricated to the new vestibular depth and inserted to prevent relapse.

### *Floor of Mouth Lowering*

*Procedure:* Crestal incision is made lingual to the attached gingiva and supraperiosteal dissection is done to the desired depth and sutured to the periosteum. The denuded periosteum is allowed to heal by secondary epithelialization or an epithelial graft is placed.

### *Vestibuloplasty with Split Thickness Skin or Palatal Mucosal Graft*

Vestibuloplasty with grafting increases the sulcus depth and the amount of attached tissue. There is very little postoperative loss of vestibular depth.

*Procedure:* The skin graft is harvested from caudal part of iliac crest or inner aspect of the thigh with a dermatome. Intraorally an incision is made at the mucogingival junction and a supraperiosteal dissection is done. The detached tissue is sutured to the depth of periosteum and the graft is maintained by a stent held by circum mandibular wiring.

## 54. Leon William classification (1914) (Fig. 7)

It was classified by Leon William to aid in the selection of anterior teeth for complete denture prosthesis.

He claimed that the shape of the upper central incisor bears a definite relationship to the shape of the face.

### Classification

- Square
- Tapering
- Ovoid.

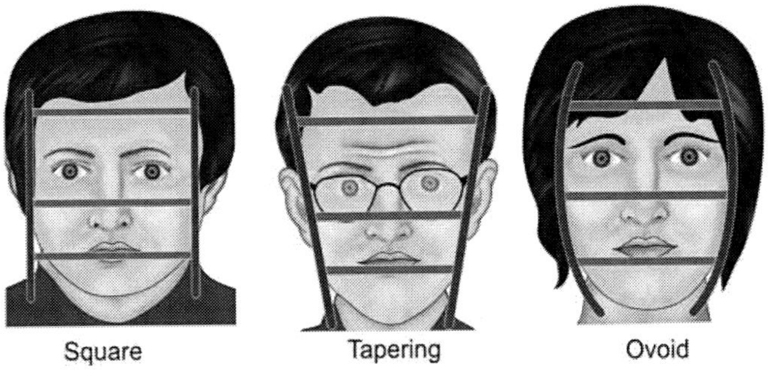


**Fig. 7:** Leon William classification

## Locating the Teeth Shape

If one of these teeth were enlarged and the incisal edge placed above the brows with the neck of the tooth on the chin, then the outline of the tooth would coincide with that of the face.

Two lines, one on either side of the face, running about 2.5 cm in front of the tragus of the ear.

## Classification of Patients

A complete denture prosthesis patient can present themselves to the dentist in any of the three classes stated below:

1. Those whose upper anterior teeth are still remaining but will soon be extracted due to various reasons. This group can be considered for Immediate Dentures.
2. Those who are already complete denture wearers. The period of time these patients wore complete dentures are important as longer the period, the patient and his immediate circle of relations and friends, would have been satisfied with the appearance of the dentures. When remaking dentures for these patients it is not advisable to make very marked alterations in an individual's appearance.
3. The third category of patients are those who present for the first time edentulous and requiring dentures, who have lost their dentures or who are dissatisfied with the existing dentures.

The Leon William classification for selection of anterior teeth will be considered depending on the:

- Shape
- Size
- Color.

## Shape

From the observation of many patients it was found that there was some relationship between the shape of the edentulous upper arch and the upper teeth.

## The findings were that

1. A V-shaped arch is associated with incisors which are narrower at the neck than at the incisal edge.
2. A squarish arch with almost parallel-sided incisors.
3. A round arch with ovoid teeth.

## 55. Instructions to complete denture patient.

They should be educated not to make comparison of chewing, speech patterns or compare to the experience of other denture wearers.

1. *Adaptability to new dentures:*
   - Younger the patient, the more adaptable to dentures.
2. *Appearance with new dentures:*
   - Appearance with new dentures will become more natural with time as initially the dentures will feel strange and bulky in the mouth.
   - Patients should be instructed to refrain from exhibiting their dentures until they are more confident or they may become unfairly critical of the dentures.

3. *Mastication with new dentures:*
   - As learning to chew with new dentures requires at least 6 to 8 weeks patients are made aware that this learning period is to be expected and the muscles of the tongue, cheeks and lips must be trained to maintain the dentures in position on the residual ridges during mastication.
   - Patients are instructed to chew soft food cut into small pieces and the chewing is best done on both sides of the mouth at the same time.
4. *Position of the tongue:*
   - Ideal position is to position the tongue on the lingual surfaces of the lower anterior teeth. This will help develop stability for the lower denture
5. *Speaking with new dentures:*
   - Initially the additional bulk over the palate and the linguogingival border of the anterior teeth would cause a speech defect, especially in the production of "S" sounds. But as the tongue is very adaptable it doesn't cause, phonetic changes that are too great to be readily compensated.
6. *Oral hygiene with dentures*
   - Patients must be convinced of the importance of maintaining good oral hygiene. Plaque, stain and calculus accumulate on dentures and oral mucosa of edentulous patients.
   - Patients should be instructed to rinse their dentures and their mouths after meals. Leaving the dentures in the cleanser (Kleenite) overnight is needed for effective killing of micro-organisms and removal of all stain.
   - After the dentures are removed from the soaking cleanser, they should be brushed gently with a soft brush and rinsed thoroughly.
7. *Preserving the residual ridges:*
   - Patients must be cautioned not to do any adjustments to the dentures.
   - Patients should be told that dentures must be left out of the mouth at night to provide needed rest from the stresses they create on the residual ridges. When dentures are left out of the mouth, they should be placed in a container filled with water to prevent drying and possible dimensional changes.
8. *Periodic recall of patients:*
   - As the tissues supporting dentures change with time, depending on local and general factors all edentulous patients should be examined by a dentist at least once a year and should be placed on a recall list.
9. *Educational material for patients*
   - Written instructions or other formal educational material is helpful to educate the patient and to follow instructions without doubt.

## 56. Notes on.

## A. Christensen's Phenomenon

## B. Buccal Corridor

### A. Christensen's phenomenon

Protrusive movement of the mandible which is created by the downward and forward movement of the condyles riding along the articular eminence removes the posterior teeth from contact in the natural dentition.This shifts the occlusal pressure to premolars and is known as the Christensen's phenomenon.

If complete dentures are not balanced in the protrusive excursion, the resulting posterior disocclusion and pressure in the premolar area can cause dislodgement of the denture bases. A fully balanced denture will negate this phenomenon.

### *Sagittal Christensen Phenomenon*

The Sagittal Christensen phenomenon means that when the patient protrude, a reversely open, wedge-shaped gap occurs at the molars.

### *Transverse Christensen Phenomenon*

The Transverse Christensen phenomenon means that when the patient performs laterotrusion, on the non-working side, a reversely open, wedge-shaped gap occurs at the molars. The same occurs during canine guidance in natural teeth.

## B. Buccal Corridor

The area between the corners of the mouth during smile formation and the buccal surfaces of the maxillary teeth (particularly the bicuspids and molars) form a space known as the buccal corridor.

The greater and more pronounced this negative space becomes, the more these posterior teeth are concealed, restricting the full breadth of the smile.

A full and symmetric buccal corridor is an important element of an esthetic smile. The buccal corridor should not be completely eliminated because a hint of negative space imparts depth to the smile.

### *Factors Influencing the Appearance of the Buccal Corridor*

- Width of the smile and the maxillary arch
- Tonicity of facial muscles
- Individual smiling characteristics
- The position of the labial surfaces of the maxillary bicuspids
- The predominance of the cuspids, particularly at the distal facial line angle
- Any discrepancy between the value of the bicuspids and the six anterior teeth
- This negative space is often accentuated when smile rejuvenation is limited to the maxillary six anterior teeth
- When the hue and value of newly restored teeth do not blend with the untreated teeth, an unwanted exaggeration of the sense of depth, darkness, and the prominence of the buccal corridor occurs.

## 57. Lingualized occlusion (Alfred gysi in 1927).

Lingualized occlusion uses the maxillary lingual cusp as the dominant functional element, occluding against corresponding position of mandibular tooth.

### Types

- Balanced lingualized occlusion
- Nonbalanced lingualized occlusion: This type of occlusion involves the use of a large upper palatal cusp against a wide lower central fossa. In this scheme, the buccal cusps of the upper and lower teeth do not contact each other.

### Advantages

1. Reduces the damaging forces while maintaining chewing efficiency.
2. Allows easier accommodation to unpredictable changes taking place in the basal seat because it provides an area of closure.
3. Simplicity.
4. Flexibility.

### Incorporation of Lingualized Occlusion in Arrangement (Fig. 8)

a. The height of anterior teeth are determined by aesthetics and phonetics.
b. Buccolingually the lingual cusps of the mandibular teeth are located within a line drawn from the distal of canine to the buccal and lingual sides of the retromolar pad.
c. A 20° template is used to set a shallow anteroposterior and mediolateral compensatory curves.
d. The maxillary posterior teeth are set with the palatal cusp in the central groove of the mandibular tooth. The maxillary buccal cusp are elevated off the occlusal plane more as one moves posteriorly.
e. Sometimes the mandibular fossa and the inclines of the maxillary palatal cusp needs selective grinding to accommodate for uniform contacts in working, balancing and protrusive movements.

Payne proposed the use of 30° anatomical teeth which were reshaped to obtain lingual occlusion.

### Myerson's Lingualized Integration (MLI)

- Myerson proposed specialized tooth molds namely control contact (CC) mold and maximum contact (MC) mold.
- The remaining teeth are common for both these molds.
- MC mold are used for patients who can reproduce accurate centric position
- CC mold for patients with variations in centric position. The 'MC' mold maxillary posteriors have taller cusps with anatomical appearance compared to the 'CC mold.
- These teeth provide maximal inter-cuspation, and a natural and pleasing appearance.

### Non-balanced Lingualized Occlusion (Payne)

Here the arrangement is same as for the anatomical form except that Maxillary teeth with blunt cusp and mandibular teeth with limited occlusal anatomy is used to allow more anteroposterior freedom.

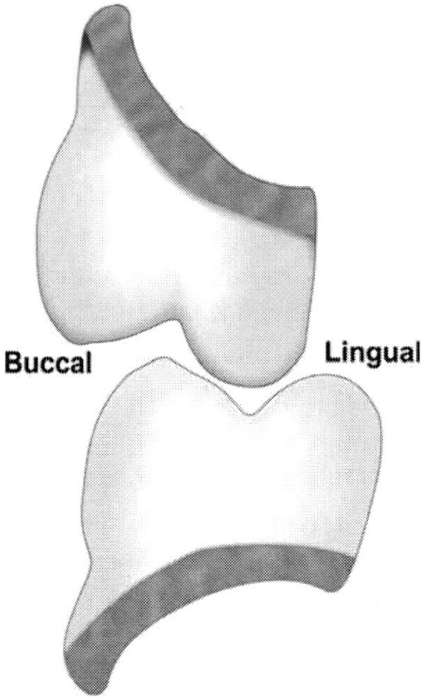


**Fig. 8:** Lingualized occlusion

## 58. Neutrocentric concept.

The term neutrocentric concept of occlusion denotes any occlusion that eliminates anteroposterior or mediolateral inclines of the teeth and directs the forces of occlusion to the posterior teeth.

### DeVan's "neutrocentric Concepts (1954)

1. The teeth should have flat occlusal surfaces.
2. The teeth should have flat planes in all directions with no inclination to the underlying denture foundation.
3. Balance was not required as the resulting inclines would create instability of the dentures.

#### *Incorporating Neutrocentric Concept*

1. The anteroposterior plane of occlusion should be parallel with the plane of the denture foundation.
2. The teeth are arranged on a flat plane, which do not form compensating curves.
3. In a mediolateral direction the teeth are set flat with no medial or lateral inclination.
4. The posterior teeth are placed in as mediolateral a relation in reference to the residual ridge as the tongue function will allow.
5. Articulator settings:
   - As incising is avoided with no cusps projecting above or below the occlusal plane, the horizontal condylar guidances can be set at zero.
   - As the teeth are not arranged in balancing contacts in eccentric relations the lateral condylar guidances of the articulator can be set at zero.
   - The condylar elements are secured to function in the opening and closing movements.

### Factors in Tooth Selection

1. Zero degree tooth.
2. Buccolingual width of the teeth is reduced.
3. Number of teeth is reduced to direct the forces in the molar and bicuspid area.
4. Tooth is not placed on the ridge incline in the second molar area.

### Patient Instruction

Not to incise with the incisors.

## 59. Try in.

Try in is done for the waxed dentures in the patient's mouth before finishing them to verify occlusion and other factors.

### Factors to Check at Trial

#### *Lower Denture*

1. Peripheral outline:
   The Buccal, Labial, Lingual and Posterior flanges are checked for under extension and over extension.
2. Stability
3. Tongue space
4. Height of the occlusal plane.

#### *Upper Denture*

1. Peripheral outline:
   The buccal, labial and posterior flanges are checked for under extension and over extension.
2. Stability
3. Retention (efficiency of posterior palatal seal).

#### *Both Dentures Together*

**In occlusion**

1. Centric relation
2. Vertical dimension of occlusion
3. Uniform bilateral contact
4. Balanced occlusion
5. Appearance.

#### *In anterior try in*

1. Midline
2. Anterior plane
3. Shape of the teeth
4. Size of the teeth
5. Shade of the teeth
6. Profile and lip form
7. Smile line
8. Approval of appearance by the patient.

## Lower Denture

### *A. Checking for Extension*

1. *The buccal and labial periphery:*
   Hold the denture in place with light pressure on the occlusal surfaces and move the cheek on one side upwards and inwards, if the denture rises from the ridge. It is over extended and needs trimming.
   Shape of the buccal aspect of the denture: A gentle convexity in the molar region and concave in the premolar region.
2. *The lingual periphery:*

Hold the denture in place with light pressure and ask the patient:

a. to protrude his tongue sufficiently to moisten his lips.
b. to put the tip of his tongue up to the back of his palate. If in any of these actions the denture lifts, it is over extended and needs trimming.

3. *Posterior extension:*
   The heels of the lower denture are extended as high up the ascending ramus of the mandible.
4. *Under-extension:*
   If the denture is found to be under-extended in any part of the periphery, an inaccuracy in the impression has taken place which must be retaken.

### *B. Stability*

After applying pressure in the premolar and molar regions of each side alternately, the pressure on one side should not tilt the denture on the opposite side.

### *C. Tongue Space*

The ideal place for the artificial teeth placement is the neutral zone. The area in the mouth where the forces of the tongue pressing outward are neutralized by the forces of lips and cheeks pressing inward.

If the tongue is cramped, the denture will begin to rise immediately when the tongue is raised.

*The causes of lack of tongue space are:*

a. Posterior teeth set inside the ridge.
b. Molar teeth which are too broad buccolingually.
c. Molar teeth leaning inwards.
d. Setting the upper teeth over the ridge almost invariably leads to the occluding lower teeth lying too far lingually.

### *D. Height of the Occlusal Plane*

## Upper Denture

### *A. Checking for Extension*

Checking of peripheral extension in buccal and labial aspects are same as for checking in lower denture.

### *B. Stability*

Same as for checking in lower denture.

### *C. Retention*

Retention is checked by seating the denture with a finger on the vault of the palate and then attempting to remove the denture at right angles to the occlusal plane.

Load is applied upwards and outwards in one canine region to check the retentive force in the contralateral corner of the denture as the tuberosity vestibular space and pterygomaxillary notch. Check the other side in the same way.

## Both Dentures Together

### *Anterior plane:*

- Check the midline
- Shape of the teeth
- Size of the teeth
- Shade and blend of the teeth
- Profile and lip form.

### *Posteriorly:*

a. *Check centric relation:*
   Hold the lower denture in position on the ridge and ask the patient to relax, and instruct to close on patients back teeth gently and maintain them in occlusion. If the registration is accurate, the teeth will interdigitate in the mouth in exactly the same manner as they do on the articulator.
b. *Vertical height:*
   Ask the patient to relax with the lips closed. While observing the point of the chin, ask the patient to close the teeth together; the chin should move upwards, a small definite amount. Counter check with phonetic test as Silverman's closest speaking test.
c. *Evenness of occlusal contact:*
   If the horizontal and vertical relationships are correct, the occluding teeth should occlude evenly and with equally distributed pressure all round.

   *Uneven contacts are due to:*
   1. Pressure on the blocks being heavier on one side than the other when the records were made.
   2. Sealing error in the casts and blocks together when mounting them on the articulator.
   3. Warpage of the base-plates.
d. *Balanced occlusion and articulation:*
   In the mouth check for evenness of occlusal pressure in the retruded contact position with Mylar tape and then test for occlusal balance with gentle lateral and protrusive movements. With the teeth in a working position of occlusion, insert a thin blade between the teeth on the balancing side and attempt to separate them. The thin blade should not separate of easily. Minor errors of cuspal interference are best left until the dentures have been finished and fitted.

## 60. Advantages of interim dentures.

1. The appearance of the patient without teeth during the complete denture procedure is avoided.

2. The patient can carry on with the social activities as usual.
3. In patients with severe periodontal disease where the need for preservation of residual ridge resorption is more.
4. Immediate dentures with proper exodontic treatment has minimum of trauma, with less residual ridge resorption.
5. The placement of interim dentures for patients who have been without posterior teeth for a long time can help to attain progressive occlusal adjustment and conditioning lining, to help the basal seat tissues, muscles and joints return to normal and healthy condition.
6. Occlusal vertical dimension can be altered by grinding or adding acrylic resin to the occlusal surfaces of the teeth when required.
7. For patients with posterior stops prior to extraction, the placement of the interim dentures preserves the health of the joints, muscles and oral physiology and aids the patient in avoiding, the edentulous state problems as in diet, speech and appearance.
8. Interim dentures can be worn during the construction of new dentures and can act as spare dentures later on.
9. Interim dentures are good temporary substitutes and can be worn to maintain the oral tissues during rebasing or repairing of the second dentures.
10. The patient's vertical dimension and muscle function will be maintained, along with proper lip support and other appearance factors.
11. The cost of the interim denture can be compared with the cost of refitting immediate dentures which usually is necessary during the first year. .

    The gingival and interseptal tissue should be retained to provide good cushioning for the denture. Interim dentures should not be made for patients with numerous and heavy undercuts. Interim dentures are ideally suited for solving the periodontal problem because maximum alveolar contour can be maintained.

## 61. Classification of soft palate.

### House's Classification of Soft Palate

It depends on the amount of posterior tissue that will accept posterior palatal seal:

- ***Class 1:*** More than 5 mm of movable tissue available for post-damming, ideal for retention.
- ***Class 2:*** 1–5 mm of movable tissue available for post-damming, good retention is usually possible.
- ***Class 3:*** Less than 1 mm movable tissue available for post damming, retention is usually poor.

### House's Classification of Palatal Throat Forms

- ***Class I***: Large and normal in form, relatively with an immovable band of tissue 5 to 12 mm distal to a line drawn across the distal edge of the tuberosities.
- ***Class II***: Medium sized and normal in form, with a relatively immovable resilient band of tissues 3 to 5 mm distal to a line drawn across the distal edge of the tuberosities.
- ***Class III***: Usually accompanies a small maxilla. The curtain of soft tissue turns down abruptly 3 to 5 mm anterior to a line drawn across the palate at the distal edge of the tuberosities.

### *Soft Palate and Palatal Throat Form*

The relationship between the soft palate and the hard palate is called the palatal throat form. On this basis, soft palates can be classified as:

- ***Class I***: It is horizontal and demonstrates little muscular movements. In this case more tissue coverage is possible for posterior palatal seal.
- ***Class II***: soft palate makes a 45 degree angle to the hard palate. Tissue coverage for posterior palatal seal is less than that of a class I condition.
- ***Class III***: Soft palate makes a 70 degree angle to the hard palate. Tissue coverage for posterior palatal seal is minimum.

## 62. Masseteric notch.

**Masseteric Notch Area:** It is immediately lateral to retromolar pad and continuous anteriorly to buccal vestibular sulcus.

### Significance

When masseter is activated, it pushes the buccinator medially against the denture borders in the area of retromolar pad.

Due to the contraction of masseter, a depression is formed at the distobuccal corner of retromolar pad.

This is a dislodging force, and the denture border should be contoured to accommodate this interaction between the buccinator and masseter muscles. This counter in denture base is termed as masseteric groove.

### Clinical Consideration.

a. During wide mouth opening the denture borders can cut into the tissue if the denture base is not properly shaped in that area.
b. During impression procedure in the area of masseteric notch downward pressure is applied and the patient is asked to close the mouth against the pressure.
c. Overextension of denture causes laceration.

## 63. Modiolus

The modiolus is a strong knot of muscle that alters the position of the angle of the mouth. The main muscles that converge at the modiolus are:

- Buccinator
- Orbicularis oris
- Zygomaticus major
- Levator anguli oris and
- Depressor anguli oris.

Free movement of this knot of muscle must be ensured if the lower denture is to be stable. The modiolus determines the position of the premolar teeth and the shape of the polished surface in that region. This produces a narrowing of the denture so that the polished surface does not hinder the movements of the modiolus during function.

## 64. Retromolar pad

**Location:** The retromolar pad is a triangular soft pad of tissue at the posterior end of the alveolar arch just at the inferior medial attachment of the mediotemporal tendon at the distal end of the lower ridge. The distal end of the mandibular denture region is bounded by the anterior border of the ramus.

### Contents

1. Glandular tissue.
2. Fibers of the temporalis tendon.
3. Buccinator fibers enter it from the buccal side.
4. Fibers of the superior pharyngeal constrictor enter it from the lingual.
5. The pterygomandibular raphe enters the pad at its superoposterior inside corner.

### Significance of Retromolar Pad

1. The actions of contents within the retromolar pad limits the extent of the denture.
2. The contents within also prevents placement of extra pressure on the retromolar pad during impression procedures or when reducing the posterior borders of the pad on the cast.
3. Retromolar pad must be covered by the denture to perfect the border seal in this region.
4. Retromolar pad posteriorly defines the posterior limit of the denture.
5. The height of the pad can be used as a guide in determining the plane of occlusion for dentures. The occlusal plane should lie at the junction of the upper and middle thirds of the retromolar pad.
6. It aids in the stability of the denture by adding another plane to resist movement of the base. Retromolar region is fairly constant, as alveolar resorption is less in this region hence, the distal end of the denture should cover as much of the pad as possible.

#### *Adjusting Special Tray*

The retromolar pad is encapsulated by the tray, without being pushed buccally or lingually. Trimming the inner surface of the tray can provide relief in this area.

#### *Border Molding*

The tray is placed in the mouth, after the area directly over the pad is softened with a Hanau torch, resculptured with the broad rounded end of a wax spatula, tempered and checked again in the mouth until the desired relief is attained.

The retromolar pad area is completed by the addition of tracing stick compound to the border, which is well tempered, the tray stabilized and the patient is instructed to open wide several times which will clear any raphe interference at the distal aspect of the denture.

The occlusal surfaces of the natural molar teeth is slightly above the height of the retro-molar pad.

The distal extension on the retromolar pad is limited by the anterior border of the ramus, the temporal tendon, the buccinator muscle and the pterygomandibular raphe.

## 65. Tongue and lateral throat form.

### TONGUE

The tongue is a powerful group of muscles and it is in constant contact with the denture at rest and during function. During rest the two critical areas for the tongue are the anterior lingual flange and posterior to the molar teeth. The polished surfaces must be correctly shaped to allow for the tongue to lie unhindered in these areas. During function, the position of the anterior and posterior teeth are critical. If the anterior or posterior teeth are set lingually the tongue will be cramped and the denture will be displaced during function. There must be sufficient tongue space to allow for movement. The occlusal plane is also important for stability. It should not be too high as to 'wall in' the tongue but should allow it to lie on the occlusal surface during rest.

## Classification of Tongue

### *Position of the Tongue—Wright Classification*

- **Class I** (favorable): Tongue lies in the floor of the mouth with the tip forward and slightly below the lower incisal edges
- **Class II** (unfavorable): Tongue is flattened and broadened but tip is in normal position.
- **Class III** (unfavorable): Tongue is retracted and depressed into the floor of the mouth, providing no border seal.

### *Tongue Sizes—House Classification*

**Class I:** Normal in size, development and function. Sufficient teeth are present to maintain this normal form and function.
**Class II:** Teeth have been absent long enough to permit a change in the form and function of the tongue.
**Class III:** Excessively large tongue. All teeth are absent for an extended period of time, allowing for abnormal development of the size of the tongue. Insufficient denture can sometimes lead to the development of Class III tongue.

## Size of the Tongue

*Macroglossia:* Prolonged edentulous state leads to an enlarged tongue. This will lead to difficulty in impression making and denture instability.
*Microglossia:* A small tongue could jeopardize the lingual seal.
*Ankyloglossia:* An ankylosed tongue has restricted movements and pose problem in impression making and denture retention. Normal attachment of frenum is 8.03 mm below gingival sulcus. In tongue-tie, it is 3 or 4 mm.

## Management

A groove can be made in the lower denture to program the tongue by asking the patient to consciously position the tongue over the groove in case of microglossia.
Tongue movements during functional impression:

- During mandibular edentulous impression making, the tongue is protruded and pressed against the anterior palate to activate the mylohyoid muscle, which determines the length and slope of the lingual flange.
- During maxillary edentulous impression, the tip of the tongue should touch the handle of the tray. This pulls palatoglossus anterior and molds posterior border of the impression and prevents flow of the material into the throat.

## Tongue Space

- If it is too lingual can lead to reduced tongue space and cause altered speech and dislodgement of denture.
- If the vertical dimension is too less, space for the tongue will reduce and the tongue falls back leading to gagging reflex.

**Adaptability of Tongue**

- The tongue responds to the loss of posterior teeth and alveolar bones by changing its size to bring the lateral borders contact the buccal mucosa.
- When a denture is introduced, the intrinsic musculature conform to the shape of the tongue in the space available. Retraining of the tongue activity also occurs.

**Retention of Denture**

- The tongue fits the lingual surfaces of the lingual flanges and provides the border seal on the lingual side.
- The base of the tongue is guided on top of the lingual flange. This provides the border seal at the back of the mandibular denture.

**Speech**

- Due to the extreme adaptability of the tongue most patients master speech within weeks of using new denture.
- However, if the denture is not technically sculpted, speech defect can occur especially with 's' sounds. A rugae pattern in the denture can aid the tongue in the production of 's' and 'ch' sounds.

## LATERAL THROAT FORM

### Neil Classification

- Class I- deep lateral throat form
- Class II- moderate lateral throat form
- Class III- shallow lateral throat form.

### Boundaries

| | |
|---|---|
| • Anteriorly | • Mylohyoid muscle |
| • Posterolaterally | • Superior constrictor |
| • Posteromedially | • Palatoglossus |
| • Medially | • Tongue |
| • Laterally | • Pear-shaped pad |

Located posterior to mylohyoid ridge and bounded posteriorly by the fibers of superior constrictor of pharynx.

### Significance

The distolingual portion of the flange is influenced by the glossopalatine and superior constrictor muscles, which on stretching constitute the retromylohyoid curtain.

Constitutes the most important bracing potential in the mandibular foundation.

### Clinical Consideration

This area has to be recorded very critically for stability of mandibular denture.

### 66. Alveololingual sulcus.

## ALVEOLOLINGUAL SULCUS

It is the space between the residual ridge and the tongue. It can be divided into 3 regions:

- Anterior region

- Middle region
- Posterior region.

### Anterior Region

- It extends from the lingual frenum to where the mylohyoid curves down below the level of the sulcus.
- Here a depression can be palpated – "premylohyoid fossa".
- It is also affected by the action of genioglossus muscle.

### Middle Region

- It extends from the premylohyoid fossa to the distal end of the mylohyoid ridge, covering medially from the body of the mandible.
- The middle of the lingual flange is made to slope towards the tongue, so that it extends over the mylohyoid muscle and also the functional movement of the muscle.

### Posterior Region

It is called as retromylohyoid space or lateral throat form. It starts from the mylohyoid ridge to retromylohyoid curtain, bounded by anterior tonsillar pillar (palatoglossus) fold, superior constrictor muscle of the pharynx and retromolar pad.

## THEORIES OF IMPRESSION MAKING

- Pressure theory/ mucocompressive theory
- Minimal pressure theory/ mucostatic theory
- Selective pressure theory.

### Pressure Theory/Mucocompressive Theory

- Proposes that tissues recorded under functional pressure (mastication) provided better support and retention for the denture.
- The peripheries of denture must be established during function.
- Tryde in 1965 advocated the use of closed mouth technique for making mucocompressive impression. Movements of oral cavity are recorded as they would in normal physiological activities such as swallowing, chewing, and talking.
- Preliminary impression is made with compound.
- Special tray is made with periphery short by 1/8th inch.
- Secondary impression is made in this tray with compound.
- Bite rims with uniform occlusal surface is made.
- Impression is softened and reinserted in mouth and held against biting pressure for 1-2 mins.
- Borders are molded by asking the patient to perform functional movements such as whistling, smiling, etc. PPS is recorded by swallowing movements under biting pressure.

#### *Advantages*

- Borders are recorded in their functional positions and not rest positions hence dentures will be better retained and not dislodged during functional movements of jaws.
- Positive posterior palatal seal is obtained.

#### *Disadvantages*

- Amount of pressure applied is too great.

- Pressure applied to tissues like incisive papilla, mid-palatine raphe, peripheral tissues, which is not suited for receiving maximum biting load, result in transient ischemia.

### Minimal Pressure/Mucostatic Theory

- Discovered by Harry L Page in 1938.
- Oral tissues are not distorted nor under stresses of any type but maintained in an undisplaced or normal relationship.
- The impression material used in this theory is softer than the softest denture bearing tissue placed in a custom made tray that does not impinge on tissues at any area and seated without pressure.
- The tray settles while the patients mouth is completely relaxed giving the most accurate reproduction of the bearing area at rest.

### Selective Pressure Theory

- Advocated by Carl O Boucher.
- Combines principles of pressure and minimal pressure.
- Importance is given to the tissue preservation combined with mechanical factors of achieving retention through minimum pressure which is within the physiologic limits of tissue tolerance.
- Certain areas of maxilla and mandible are by nature better adapted to withstand the masticatory loads.
- Equilibrium between resilient and non resilient tissue is created using spacer and reliefs.

#### *Advantage*

- The physiologic functions of basal seat tissues are considered.

#### *Disadvantages*

- Difficult to record areas with varying pressure.
- Some areas recorded under function, hence potential danger of tissue rebounding and subsequent loss of retention.

## 67. Functional impression technique.

### Material Used

Tissue conditioners.

### Advantages of Tissue Conditioners

- Good for refitting complete dentures with ease.
- Retaining compliance for many weeks.
- Good dimensional stability.
- Good bonding to the resin denture base.

### Indications for Relining

Lack of retention.

Hyperemic mucosa with sore spots in the denture-bearing mucosa (for tissue conditioning).

#### *Factors to be Checked Before Tissue Lining*

- Peripheral reduction or extension

- Posterior palatal seal extension
- Amount of ridge resorption
- Vertical dimension of occlusion.
- Centric relation, esthetic and artificial teeth for abrasion and wear.

### *Procedure*

The tissue surface of the denture is reduced uniformly at least 2 mm to create space for the liner material.

A treatment liner is placed inside the denture and allowed to flow while all the molding procedures as asking the patient to move the mandible to and fro and other steps are carried out. The lining material should flow evenly to cover the whole impression surface and the borders of the denture with a thin layer without voids. An excess of thick material in the border can go unsupported. Hence adequate border extensions are to be done before lining the denture.

The patient's mandible is guided into a retruded position, of maximum intercuspation, to help stabilize the denture while the lining material is setting.

Excess material is trimmed away with a hot scalpel.

The setting progress through plastic and then elastic stages before hardening, which takes several days.

The plastic stage permits movement of the denture base or bases so they are more compatible with the existing occlusion and also allows the displaced tissues to recover and assume their original position.

### *Instruction for Patient*

Simple rinsing and gentle brushing with a soft toothbrush minimize damage to the lining. No chemical agents should be used of cleaning the denture.

### *Clinical Reline*

After 10 to 14 days when the material is firm enough clinical reline can be done.

Before clinical reline the tissue surface is examined to evaluate the health of mucosa.

If the temporarily relined denture is well retained, with well-rounded peripheral borders and a healthy-appearing mucosa then clinical reline can be done.

If the surface or peripheral deterioration is slight after tissue conditioning then these areas can be trimmed with a carbide bur and the denture surface can be prepared for a wash, impression with a light-bodied material.

The stone cast must be poured immediately after removal of the relined denture base from the mouth.

Maxillary casts may have to be scored in the selected posterior palatal seal area, since the long period of plasticity of the material may not create sufficient displacement action in this area.

## Rerecording Centric Relation

A new CR record and remount procedure are needed.

### *Chairside Technique*

Both the static technique and the functional impression technique are good techniques in cases for simple situations and complicated situations as excessive tissue changes. Chairside technique was uncommon due to chemical burn on the mucosa; a bad odor; lack of color stability of the lined acrylic and if the denture was not positioned correctly, the material was difficult to remove.

Use of Visible Light-Cured (VLC) resin systems as substitutes to the liner was a better choice of material than acrylic cause of many of its advantages.

*Advantages* are good fit, strength, ability to polymerise without residual components, ease of fabrication and manipulation, patient acceptance, ability to bond with other denture base resins and low bacterial adherence.

## 68. Spacer designs in complete denture.

The selective pressure technique which was proposed by Carl O. Boucher combines the principles of both pressure and minimal pressure technique. Selective pressure can be achieved either by scraping of the primary impression in selected areas or by fabrication of a custom (special) tray with a proper spacer design and escape holes (relief).

***Various Spacer Designs***

1. **Design by Roy Mac Gregor:** Place a sheet of metal foil in the region of incisive papilla and mid palatine raphae. Other areas that may require relief are maxillary rugae, areas of mucosal damage, buccal surface of the prominent tuberosities.
2. **Design by Neill:** Recommends adaptation of 0.9 mm casing wax all over except PPS area.
3. **Design by Heartwell:** Two techniques:
    1. In the first technique, primary impression is made with impression compound in a non-perforated stock tray. The borders are refined and space is provided in selected areas by scraping the impression compound.
    2. In the second technique, a custom tray is fabricated (but did not mention about the wax spacer). Border molding is done with low fusing compound. Five relief holes are placed on the palatal region. Three holes in the rugae area and two in glandular region before making the secondary impression with ZOE paste.
4. **Design by Boucher:** 1 mm base plate wax is placed on the cast except posterior palatal seal (PPS) area as the PPS area will act as guiding stop to position the tray properly during the impression procedure. Escape holes are also made with No. 6 round bur in the palate.
5. **Design by Morrow, Rudd, Rhoads:** Undercut areas are blocked out with wax and a full wax spacer is adapted 2 mm short of the resin special tray border all over. Three tissue stops of 4×4 mm is placed equidistant from each other.
6. **Design by Sharry:** A layer of base plate wax is adapted over the whole area outlined for tray (even in PPS area). Four tissue stops of 2 mm width is located in molar and cuspid region which extended from palatal aspect of the ridge to the mucobuccal fold and one vent hole in the incisive papilla region before making the final impression with the metallic oxide impression material.
7. **Design by Bernard:** Layer of pink base plate wax of 2 mm thickness is attached to the areas of the cast that usually have the areas of the softer tissues. Wax spacer is placed all around except in the posterior part of the palate which are at right angles to the occlusal forces.
8. **Design by Sheldon:** Describes two techniques
    1. In the first technique, the primary impression is made with low fusing modeling compound. The borders are refined with green stick compound. Once the operator is satisfied with the retention, selective relief is accomplished by scraping in the region of incisive papilla, rugae and mid-palatal areas.

2. In the second technique, primary impression is made with an alginate primary impression. A primary cast is poured. After analysis of cast contours, undercuts are blocked out. Then placement of spacer or pressure control (but did not mention about the wax spacer design) is done. Border molding is done with green stick compound before making the secondary impression with ZOE paste.

9. **Design by Halperin:** Recommends the 'Philosophy of the custom impression tray with peripheral relief'. According to this, the slopes of the ridges are considered to be the primary stress bearing areas and therefore these areas are functionally loaded with compound during making of the final impression. In this technique, wash secondary impression is not made as the tray surface and the border-molded areas are considered as the final impression surface.

### An Alternative Custom Tray Design by Shetty Sanath et al

### (JIPS, Vol. 7, Issue 1, 2007)

A thin sheet of wax 0.4 mm major connector wax is placed in all the areas except the posterior palatal seal area. A 1.5 mm modeling wax is adapted on top of the already adapted wax sheet. Modeling wax is removed in the region of crest of the alveolar ridge and the horizontal plates of the palate, as these are the stress bearing areas. Tissue stops, which need to be four in number, are located in the canine and molar region.

### Considerations for the use of alternate design

- Can be used in patients with healthy basal seat areas.
- Clinical situations where the mucosa over the ridge or the palate is hyperplasic or flabby, severe undercuts, tori, etc.; an additional layer of wax can be added in these regions.
- In cases of inoperable severe hyperplasic tissues over the ridge an open tray technique is to be followed to obtain maximum relief.

## 69. Single complete denture.

The single complete maxillary denture opposing all or some of the mandibular natural dentition is the most common situation.

***Problems associated with this:*** Malposed, tipped, or supererupted teeth in the lower arch. Soreness, mucosal changes and ultimately ridge resorption in maxillary arch.

Abrasion of the artificial teeth if acrylic resin is used or the abrasion of natural teeth if porcelain is used.

### Diagnosis and Treatment Planning

The final maxillary impression is made and mounted on the articulator using a face-bow. The lower diagnostic cast is mounted using a provisional centric interocclusal record made at an acceptable vertical dimension. Eccentric records are made and the condylar elements of the articulator are set.

### Techniques for Tooth Modification (Swenson)

The maxillary and mandibular casts are mounted on the articulator, using a provisional centric relation record at an acceptable vertical dimension.

A maxillary base is made and denture teeth are set.

If the lower natural teeth interfere with the placement of the denture teeth, the area is marked with a pencil.

The natural teeth are then modified using the marked diagnostic cast as a guide.

After the occlusal modifications are completed, a new lower arch cast is made and mounted on the articulator.

The denture teeth are reset and prepared for the try-in.

## Other Techniques

By *Yurkstas*, involves the use of a metal U-shaped occlusal template that is slightly convex on the lower surface.

By *Bruce*: The inner surface of the template is coated with pressure-indicating paste. Interferences are noted through the template and removed by reshaping.

## Common Occlusal Disharmonies

Completely edentulous maxillary area opposing mandibular natural teeth with second molars present. These second molars are often severely inclined mesially and their distal halves supererupted.

### *Correction done by*

1. Grinding the distal half of the occlusal surface and the denture teeth set to occlude only with that area.
2. Crown prepared for second molars.
3. Onlay mesial rest.
4. Orthodontic repositioning of the tilted molars.

### *Methods Used to Achieve a Harmonious Balanced Occlusion*

1. Dynamically equilibrate the occlusion by the use of a functionally generated path.
2. Statistically equilibrate the occlusion using an articulator programmed to simulate the patient's jaw movement.

## Functional Chew-in Techniques

### *Technique by Stansbury, 1928*

- For an upper complete denture opposing lower natural teeth.
- A compound maxillary rim trimmed buccally and lingually for freedom in lateral excursions is used.
- Carding wax is added to the compound rim and patient is instructed to perform eccentric chewing movements.
- The carding wax is slowly molded to the functional movements, while the compound preserves the vertical dimension.
- Stone is vibrated into the wax paths of the cusps.
- The upper cast is mounted on the articulator with lower cast.
- One is a duplicate of the lower teeth and the other is a replica of the generated path.
- The denture teeth are first set to the lower cast of the patient's teeth.
- After the try-in is approved, the lower cast is removed and the lower chew-in cast record is secured to the articulator.
- All interfering spots are ground until the incisal guide pin prevents further closure.

### Technique by Vig

A fin of resin is placed into the central grooves of the lower posterior teeth. The resin fin maintains the vertical dimension and also helps diagnostically locate interfering mandibular cusps. In eccentric movements, the lower cusp tips are ground until equal contacts occur between the teeth and the resin. The fin is then built up using a soft wax and a functional path is generated.

### Technique by Sharry

Lateral and protrusive chewing movements are made so that the wax is abraded generating the functional paths of the lower cusps. This is continued until the correct vertical dimension has been established.

### Technique by Rudd

A thickness of recording matrix made up of 3 sheets of medium and pink base plate wax and two sheets of red counter, wax is added to the buccal and lingual surface of this compound rim.

### Articulator Equilibration Techniques

- The upper cast and lower cast is mounted on an articulator by a centric interocclusal record at an acceptable vertical dimension.
- If denture teeth placed too far to the buccal when articulated with the lower buccal cusps, they are reset to oppose the lower lingual cusps.
- If the denture teeth appear to be placed too far lingually when articulated with the lower lingual cusps, they are reset to oppose the lower buccal cusps.
- If the lower buccal cusps are selected for the holding cusps, the lingual cusps are reduced.
- If the lower lingual cusps are selected for the holding cusps, the buccal cusps are reduced. Thus a cusp-to-fossa relationship is achieved.
- If any of the natural teeth are supererupted or tipped, they are modified by selective grinding or by restoring with a crown or onlay to attain a proper occlusal plane.
- At the time of the wax try-in, eccentric records are made and the condylar inclinations are set on the articulator with the upper posterior teeth arranged in balance occlusion.
- After the denture has been processed, it is again related to the mounted lower cast with a new centric interocclusal record.
- Finally a denture that is in balanced occlusion that allows freedom in lateral excursions while maintaining maximum bilateral contacts in functional and parafunctional activities is made

### Occlusal Materials for the Single Denture

Occlusal materials are porcelain, acrylic resin, gold, acrylic resin with amalgam stops and interpenetrating polymer network resin.

### Subsequent Problems with Single Dentures against Natural Teeth

One of the major problems with dentures opposing natural teeth is abrasion.

When using maxillary porcelain teeth, will lead to rapid wear of the opposing natural teeth. Gold inlays or crowns and silver alloy restorations wear away more rapidly than tooth enamel when opposed by porcelain complete denture teeth.

The use of acrylic resin teeth is the best alternative.

## 70. Problems associated with single complete denture.

The major problems associated with single complete denture are associated with the following:

- Occlusal forces
- Occlusal form of the natural teeth
- Support for the denture base
- Intermaxillary relations.

### Occlusal Forces

These forces have been recorded as high as 198 lbs on a single molar natural tooth whereas the force with a complete denture is only 26 lbs. Hence natural tooth can impart a high force on the opposing complete denture.

Unfavorable force distribution can cause extensive morphological changes in denture foundation, extreme jaw relationships and excessively displaceable denture bearing tissue.

### Occlusal Form of the Natural Teeth

The occlusal form of the remaining natural teeth will dictate the occlusion of the denture. The natural teeth may be over-erupted or tilted and their cusps may be high and sharp. Denture will constantly be thrust or dragged horizontally on the ridge. Hence an occlusal plane correction will be required for eliminating the associated problem.

### Support for the Denture Base

Denture base should have the maximum extension within the functional anatomic limits. Lower complete denture opposing upper natural teeth should be normally avoided.

### Intermaxillary Relations

When upper complete denture is being made to occlude with lower natural teeth, an error may be made in recording the vertical dimension. The labiolingual thickness of the wax rim will usually not allow the lower incisor to close beyond the occlusal surface. Hence an increased vertical dimension may be recorded.

### Common Reasons for Fracture of Denture

- Occlusal stress on the maxillary denture and the underlying edentulous tissue from teeth and musculature of opposing natural dentition.
- The position of the mandibular teeth which may not be properly aligned for the achievement of bilateral balance for stability.
- Flexure of the denture base.

### Considerations to Overcome the Problems Associated with Single Complete Denture

- Acceptable interocclusal distance.
- Stable jaw relationship with bilateral tooth contact in retruded position.
- Stable tooth quadrant relationships with axially directed forces.
- Multidirectional freedom of tooth contact throughout a small range (within 2 mm) of mandibular movements.

## 71. Tissue conditioners

### Composition

The material is a three-component system
- Polyethyl-methacrylate (Polymer)
- Aromatic ester ethyl alcohol mixture the monomer (liquid)
- A liquid plasticizer.

These materials, when mixed, form a gel, the ethyl alcohol having a greater affinity for the polymer.

### Use of Tissue Conditioners

- Used as adjuncts in conditioning the denture-bearing tissues to a healthy state.
- For temporary obturation.
- Protection of surgical areas.
- Used as stabilizer of base plates or of surgical stents.
- In impression-making procedures.
- Used as adjuncts in the healing phase of tissue integrated implants.

#### *Adjuncts in Tissue Conditioning*

Tissue conditioners are used to condition selected oral structures to bear the stresses of denture prostheses, such as:
- In distorted tissues as hypertrophic, irritated, hyperemic and displaced oral mucosa associated with ill-fitting, poorly occluding dentures, bruxism, papillary hyperplasia, depressed areas associated with suction cups and patients with avitaminosis or general debilitating disease.
- For preservation of the residual ridge.
- To re-establish and maintain proper maxillomandibular jaw relationships.

#### *Temporary Obturators*

- Tissue conditioners may be added to an obturator on an existing complete or partial denture by direct or indirect method.
- Usually done seven to ten days after surgery.
- Tissue conditioners protects the tissues and enhances the healing process as in cases of resected maxillae.
- In obturator patients it can aid in improving masticatory function, deglutition and speech.

#### *Stabilizers of Base Plates*

- In an edentulous cast with undercuts, tissue conditioners can be used to stabilize recording bases and prevent breakage of the cast.
- Reduces the error in recording jaw relation records.
- Breakage and abrasion of the edentulous cast are prevented with a better finish for the final denture.

#### *Adjunct in the Impression-making*

- As a final impression material when it is difficult to determine the extent of the denture base due to movable oral structures.
- They will record the extension in a dynamic form which will help in making of an impression tray for the final impression.

## Technique in the Use of Tissue Conditioner

The dentures to be relined should have:

- Adequate coverage of the denture bearing area
- A good centric relation
- Adequate occlusal vertical dimension
- No occlusal interferences in eccentric jaw positions.

## Preparation of the Denture

The tissue surface of the denture is relieved of all undercuts and nearly 2 mm of denture material is relieved from all over the tissue surface sufficient to allow the displaced and traumatized tissue to recover to a normal state.

Retain the borders or flanges and the hard palatal area as vertical stops in seating.

If the denture base is short extend it by using activated acrylic resin to provide support for the soft material.

## Preparation and Placement of Tissue Conditioner in the Mouth

For conditioning tissues, a ratio of 1¼ parts of polymer to 1 part of monomer is used with the addition of 1/2 cc of the plasticizer.

Place the material on the denture base and seat without much pressure.

Allow the material to set. A new application of the material is needed every three to four days until the tissues have recovered.

Ideally eight to ten weeks is sufficient to determine the potential benefits from the use of a resilient liner.

After the denture base material has been removed and replaced with processed acrylic resin remount procedures are done as follows:

a. Eliminate undercuts to make an accurate remount cast of dental plaster of both arches.
b. Make a facebow transfer of the maxillary cast and mount the lower cast to upper in centric relation and eliminate all occlusal discrepancies in centric and eccentric relation by selective grinding procedures.

### 72. Neutral zone.

In the absence of all natural teeth, there exists a space called potential denture space bounded by maxilla and soft palate above, mandible and floor of the mouth below, tongue medially and lips and cheek laterally. Within the potential denture space is the area that is termed neutral zone.

## The Neutral Zone or the Neuromuscular Approach (Sir Wilfred Fish, 1933)

Objectives:

1. Maximum comfort
2. Maximum efficiency
3. Esthetic appearance.

## Factors Influencing Neutral Zone

*a. Cheeks*

1. *Masseter*

   It affects the distodental border.

2. *Buccinator*
   It helps to place food over the occlusal surface of the teeth in coordination with the tongue.

b. *Lips*
   1. *Orbicularis oris*
      It exerts force against teeth and alveolar process which is counteracted by the tongue.
   2. *Caninus*
      Pulls lower lip. Helps in sucking and swallowing.
   3. *Quadratus labii superioris*
   4. *Zygomaticus major*
   5. *Risorius*
   6. *Mentalis*
   7. *Triangularis*
   8. *Modiolus*

   If denture is not narrowed in the premolar area, it may unseat the lower denture.

c. *Tongue*
   Muscles of tongue.

d. *Denture surfaces*
   1. Impression surface
   2. Occlusal surface
   3. Polished surface

e. *Denture shape*
   It should be triangular in cross section in the molar area. This triangular shape stabilises the denture.

## Procedure

1. *Preliminary impression:*
   Modeling compound used.
2. *Construction of acrylic tray:*
   a. Modeling compound occlusal rims are made on the tray. Wire loops are made on the tray for the modeling compound to be attached as occlusal rims. Over extensions on the tray can be checked by disclosing wax.
   b. To serve as a tray for final impression.
3. *Location of neutral zone*:
   The modeling compound rims are placed in the patients mouth and the patient is instructed to do various movements as pursing of lips, swallowing, and tongue movements for lower arch and sucking fingers, swallowing for upper arch
   *Upper arch shape*: Palatal surface sloping buccally and downward and buccal surface sloping lingually and downward.
   *Lower arch*: Buccal surface inclined lingually with narrowing at the bicuspid area (modiolus function) and lingual surface inclined buccally.
4. *Final impression*:
   Zinc oxide eugenol with closed mouth technique, when patient does all the needed movements.
5. *Register* the retruded jaw relation while the patient moves the cheeks, lips and tongue through their full functional range for 5–10 min.

When recording the jaw relations in the patient's mouth, the occlusal surface of the upper rim is trimmed parallel to the nasoauricular line, and positioned at a height so that the incisal edges of the patient's artificial central incisors and the mesiopalatal cusps of the upper first molars will just touch it.

6. The resultant impression is poured with buccal and lingual registers or indices and after removing the acrylic base and impression material the resultant space is used to fabricate the denture.
7. *The position of the teeth:*
   In the horizontal plane, the position of the teeth and the alveolar ridges which support them is determined by the interaction of the forces of the muscles surrounding them.
   Lingually this force is provided by the tongue and buccally and labially by the cheeks and lips; thus the teeth is arranged in a zone of neutral muscular force.

## 73. Hanau's quint (Rudolph L. Hanau).

He proposed nine factors that govern the articulation of artificial teeth as (Fig. 9):

1. Horizontal condylar inclination
2. Compensating curve
3. Incisal guidance
4. Plane of orientation
5. Inclination of tooth
6. Sagittal condylar pathway
7. Sagittal incisal guidance
8. Tooth alignment
9. Relative cusp height.

These nine factors were called the laws of balanced articulation.

Later he condensed these nine factors and named *five factors, known as Hanau's Quint:*

1. Condylar guidance
2. Incisal guidance
3. Compensating curves
4. Relative cusp height
5. Plane of orientation of the occlusal plane.

### Modifications of Hanau's Quint

#### *Trapozzano's Triad of Occlusion*

His triad of occlusion included:

- Condylar guidance,
- Incisal guidance
- Cusp height.

He eliminated plane of occlusion as he considered that factor as a variant depending on the interarch distance. He also dismissed the need for setting compensating curves, as these curves are dependant on the cuspal inclination and not an individual factor.

#### *Boucher's concept gave importance to:*

- Orientation of the occlusal plane
- The incisal guidance
- Condylar guidance

- Angulation of the cusp
- Compensating curve.

Boucher compensating curve permits alteration of cusp height without changing the form of teeth. In zero degree teeth the equivalence of a cusp can be produced by a compensating curve. Others who modified Hanau's Quint were Lott and Levin.

## Factors Influencing Balanced Occlusion

The five basic factors that determine the balance of an occlusion are:

1. Inclination of the condylar path or condylar guidance.
2. Incisal guidance.
3. Orientation of the plane of occlusion or occlusal plane.
4. Cuspal angulation.
5. Compensating curves.

### *Condylar Guidance*

Condylar guidance can be defined as, "Mandibular guidance generated by the condyle and articular disc traversing the contour of the glenoid fossa."—GPT

The condylar path should be determined on the patient and set on the instrument so that the patient's temporomandibular joint is in harmony with the occlusion as programmed on the articulator. A steep condylar path needs a steep compensating curve for occlusal balance. If a lesser compensating curve is substituted for a steep condylar guidance it would result in a steep incisal guidance resulting in loss of molar balancing contacts.

### *Incisal Guidance*

It is defined as, "The influence of the contacting surfaces of the mandibular and maxillary anterior teeth during mandibular movements." –GPT

It is the effect the contact of the upper and lower anterior teeth have on the movement of the mandible. It is usually expressed in degrees of angulation from the horizontal by a line drawn in the sagittal plane between the incisal edges of the upper and lower incisor teeth when closed in centric occlusion.

If the incisal guidance is steep, it requires steep cusps, a steep occlusal plane, or a steep compensating curve to effect an occlusal balance. A steep inclined plane is detrimental to the stability and equilibrium of the denture base hence for complete dentures the incisal guidance should be as flat as esthetics and phonetics will permit. When the arrangement of the anterior teeth necessitates a vertical overlap, a compensating horizontal overlap should be set to prevent dominant incisal guidance (anterior interference) from upsetting the occlusal balance on the posterior teeth.

### *Plane of Occlusion*

It is defined as, "An imaginary surface which is related anatomically to the cranium and which theoretically touches the incisal edges of the incisors and the tips of the occluding surfaces of the posterior teeth. It is not a plane in the true sense of the word but represents the mean curvature of the surface." –GPT

It is established in the anterior by the height of the lower cuspid and in the posterior by the height of the retromolar pad. It is also related to the ala-tragus line, or Camper's line. Its position can be altered only slightly without creating serious functional problems.

### *Compensating Curve*

Compensating curve is defined as, "The anteroposterior and lateral curvatures in the alignment of the occluding surfaces and incisal edges of artificial teeth which are used to develop balanced occlusion." –GPT

## Types of Compensating Curves

- Anteroposterior curves
- Lateral curves.

### *Cusps on Teeth or the Inclination of Cuspless Teeth*

Cusp angle is defined as, "The angle made by the average slope of a cusp with the cusp plane measured mesiodistally or buccolingually."–GPT

The mesiodistal cusp heights that inter-digitate lock the occlusion so that reposition of the teeth due to settling of the base cannot take place. To prevent this problem, it is advocated that all mesiodistal cusp heights be eliminated, hence only the buccolingual inclines are considered as determinants of balanced occlusion in anatomic type teeth.

Once the vertical and horizontal overlaps of the anterior teeth have been established incisal guidance, the plane of occlusion, the compensating curve and the tooth form must harmonize with the three guiding elements, if balanced occlusion is to be achieved on the articulator. The incisal guidance and the plane of occlusion can be altered only a slight amount because of esthetic and physiologic factors. The compensating curve and the cuspal inclinations can be adjusted by the dentist.

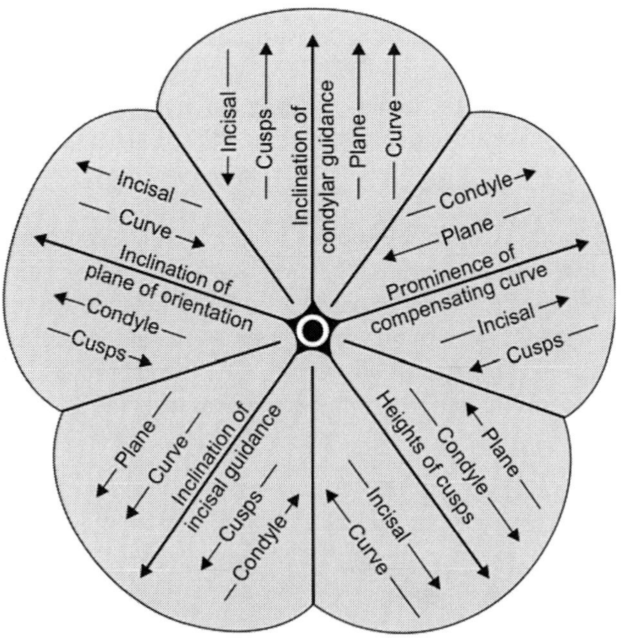


**Arrow pointing towards the center indicates Decrease**
**Arrow pointing away from the center indicates Increase**

**Fig. 9:** Hanau's quint

## 74. Balanced articulation.

Balanced articulation is the arrangement of the teeth done in any jaw relationship and when as many teeth as possible are in occlusion and when changing from one position to another they move with a smooth, sliding motion, free from cuspal interference and maintaining even contact.

Complete dentures made with balanced articulation will have only minor occlusal corrections.

### Factors in Balanced Articulation

These are the main four factors to achieve balanced articulation.

1. An adjustable articulator which can be adjusted to copy the movements and reproduce the relationships of the jaws of the patient.
2. A method by which the recorded movements and relationships can be measured and transferred to the articulator.
3. An understanding of the factors related to Balanced occlusion, which influence the arrangement of the anterior and posterior teeth.
4. Anatomic tooth form to be used for Balanced occlusion.
   According to Hanau Balanced articulation is the change from one balanced occlusion to another while the masticatory surfaces remain in balanced contact.

### Factors Affecting the Balanced Occlusion

1. Condylar guidance
2. Incisal guidance
3. Plane of occlusion
4. Compensating curve
5. Cuspal height.

## 75. Posterior Palatal Seal (Pps).

### Importance of PPS

1. A positive contact is established posteriorly thereby preventing the final impression material from sliding down the pharynx.
2. For positioning the impression tray, accurately.
3. To create slight displacement of the soft palate
4. To determine if adequate retention and seal can be achieved in the potential denture border.
5. Adequate border seal resist horizontal forces and lateral torquing of the maxillary denture.
6. The function of the posterior palatal seal in the completed maxillary prosthesis is to maintain contact with the anterior portion of the soft palate during functional movements as mastication, deglutition and phonation.
7. To aid the denture to achieve better retention.
8. The posterior palatal seal will reduce patient awareness of border of denture hence reducing gag reflex.

### Posterior Palatal Seal Area

The post-palatal seal extends medially from one tuberosity to the other. Laterally, the pterygomaxillary seal extends through the pterygomaxillary notch (hamular notch) continuing for 3 to 4 mm anterolaterally approximating the mucogingival junction.

The notch is covered by the pterygomandibular fold, which extends from the posterior aspect of the tuberosity posterior-inferiorly to insert into the retromolar pad which influences the posterior border seal, if the mouth is in a wide open position during the final impression procedure.

Exact position of the hamular process is to be located this will affect the length and direction of the pterygomaxillary seal. The hamular processes are covered by a thin layer of mucous membrane.

There are two glandular openings fovea palatini, into which the ducts of other palatal mucus glands drain. They are located, on average, 1.31 mm anterior to the anterior vibrating line. The median palatal raphe, overlies the medial palatal suture, contains little or no submucosa and will tolerate little compression.

#### *Anterior and Posterior Vibrating Lines*

*The anterior vibrating line* is an imaginary line located at the junction of the attached tissues overlying the hard palate and the movable tissues of the immediately adjacent soft palate. One way to locate the anterior vibrating line is to have the patient perform the Valsalva maneuver, which requires that both nostrils be held firmly while the patient blows gently through the nose. Another method is to the patient to say "ah" with short vigorous bursts. Due to the projection of the posterior nasal spine, the anterior vibrating line is not a straight line between both hamular processes. The anterior vibrating line is always on soft palatal tissues.

*The posterior vibrating line* is an imaginary line at the junction of the aponeurosis of the tensor veli palatini muscle and the muscular portion of the soft palate. It represents the demarcation between that part of the soft palate that has limited or shallow movement during function and the remainder of the soft palate that is displaced during functional movements. The posterior vibrating line is visualized by instructing the patient to say "ah" in short bursts in a normal, unexaggerated fashion. The posterior vibrating line marks the most distal extension of the denture base. The posterior palatal seal area lies between anterior and posterior vibrating line and is cupids bow shaped.

## 76. Impression of flat ridges: resorbed residual alveolar ridge.

## FLAT MANDIBULAR RIDGE IMPRESSION

### Material Used

- Tissue-conditioning materials.
- A preliminary impression with overextended registration is made.
- An activated resin tray is made with an occlusal wax rim which simulate the height and position of the anterior and posterior teeth.
- The borders of the tray are adjusted so that the lingual flange and sublingual crescent area are in harmony with the resting and active phases of the floor of the mouth.
- The buccal and labial extension of the acrylic tray is adjusted to be short of the reflections of the cheek and lip. The retromolar pad is covered by the tray.

## Technique

- Closed-mouth technique
- Open- mouth technique

### *Closed-mouth technique*

- Needs a well-fitting maxillary recording base
- An accurate occluding rims
- An acceptable vertical dimension.

### *Open-mouth Technique*

- Open-mouth technique in which the operator stabilizes the mandibular base, directs the patient's tongue to mold the lingual borders and digitally manipulates the cheek and lip tissues.

### *Technique*

- Three applications of Coe product is required.
- Two applications of the more viscous pink Coe-Soft are made, each application is allowed to remain in the mouth for eight to ten minutes, removed, rinsed and checked.
- Pressure areas corrected at the time of the first application.
- The third and final wash is made with the white Coe-Comfort which is a light-bodied material and is the final corrective wash.
- The impression that is made will be very thick with conforming buccal borders and a relatively thick lingual and sublingual crescent area.
- Some conditioning materials are not combatable with dental stone. If such a material is used, then the third and final wash can be made with a light-bodied polysulfide material, such as Kerr Class III Pennlastic.

## Maxillary Resorbed Ridge

In making an impression for the maxillary resorbed ridge, the difference from the mandibular is that the peripheral borders are thicker. Since much less surface area is being used to retain the denture, the tissue contact area via the peripheral border is important to maintain peripheral seal.

## 77. Denture adhesives.

The use of denture adhesives should be termed provisionally acceptable by the American Dental Association to be considered safe for use.

Woelfel states that, "all denture adhesives occupy space. Distribution of the adherent preparation into only the few limited regions where the denture does not fit alone is not possible to achieve."

## Disadvantages

- More viscous adhesive pastes, produce errors in vertical dimension and denture positioning.
- If the use of adhesive encroaches upon the interarch distance then clicking of teeth and other speech defects occur.
- The magnitude of this discrepancy is related to the amount applied and to the adherent itself.

### *Instruction to the Patient Regarding the use*

- If the dentist considers it necessary to temporarily enhance the retention of the denture, then an adhesive is recommended for a temporary period of time with instructions of how to use it.
- Adhesive powder is to be lightly sprinkled over the wetted tissue surface of the denture base. The excess powder should be shaken out of the denture before the patient inserts the prosthesis.
- Once properly seated, the patient should be instructed to close in the retruded jaw position to aid in final positioning of the denture.
- When the patient wants to renew the adherent, the denture should be removed, thoroughly cleansed of all remaining denture adhesive used and new adhesive reapplied as previously directed.

### *Available as:*

Powder form consisting of natural gums such as tragacanth or karaya with cellulose added.
Creams and liquids, containing the same substances as are in artificial saliva.

### *Uses*

a. To hold the upper record block in position when securing intraoral records.
b. To prolong the usefulness of an immediate upper denture for a short period of time.
c. To enable a patient to wear an old, ill-fitting upper denture, while the used denture is being repaired.
d. Public speakers, use adhesive to give them the assurance that the upper denture will not move while rendering speeches.

## 78. Effects of decreased vertical dimension.

## Definition

"It is distance between two selected points, one on a fixed and one on a movable member." – GPT—6

It is maintained either by occlusion of teeth or by the balanced tonic contraction of muscles of mandibular movements.

Vertical relations are classified as vertical dimensions of:

- Occlusion
- Rest and
- Other positions.

The *vertical dimension of occlusion* is established by the natural teeth when they are present and in occlusion. In case of edentulous patients vertical dimension is established by the vertical height of the two dentures when the teeth are in contact. Vertical dimension of occlusion must be established for edentulous people so that their denture teeth will be properly related to each other.

The *vertical dimension of rest* (or physiologic rest position of the mandible) is established by muscles and gravity. The interocclusal distance (formerly referred to as the "free-way space") is the distance or gap existing between the occluding surfaces of maxillary and mandibular teeth when the mandible is in the physiologic rest position.

The difference between the occlusal vertical dimension and the rest vertical dimension is the interocclusal distance. The interocclusal distance (formerly referred to as the "free-way space") usually is 2 to 4 mm when observed at the position of the first premolars. It was observed that clinically recorded rest position is not the same as the electromyographically determined one. A range of reduced muscle tension up to an interocclusal distance of about 10 mm has been noticed.

### Effects of Decreased Vertical Dimension

1. *Inefficiency:* The pressure that is exerted with teeth in contact decreases considerably in overclosure because attachment of muscles have been brought closer.
2. *Cheek biting:* When there is decreased vertical height the flabby cheek gets trapped between the teeth and gets bitten during mastication. Cheek biting often occurs because the buccal flange of denture is too narrow and cheek tends to fall.
3. *Esthetics:* Patients with decreased vertical height dentures look aged as the chin appears too close to the nose and forward. The lips lose their fullness and the vermilion borders are reduced to approximate a line. The corners of the mouth turn down as the orbicularis oris and its attachments are pushed too close to their origin.
4. *Muscular action:* The reduced vertical dimension of occlusion decreases the action of the muscles, with a resultant loss of muscle tone, giving the face an appearance of flabbiness instead of firmness.
5. *Angular cheilitis or Perliche:* Creases at corners of the mouth associated with Angular cheilitis.
6. *Pain in temporomandibular joint:* Loss of posterior occlusion subjects the joint to greater load damaging the meniscus resulting in clicking or crepitus which may be heard on movement. As the posterior teeth contacts are missing the temporalis and masseter muscles can lead to a source of pain and discomfort. The patients whose posterior tooth contact are absent tend to protrude mandible in order to occlude resulting in pain in lateral pterygoid muscle region which in turn is centered on or anterior to TMJ. In these patients vertical relation of occlusion should be gradually built up in successive dentures.
7. *Impaired hearing:* In case of decreased vertical dimension leading to less interarch space, the tongue will be pushed toward the throat region resulting in closure of eustachian tube opening leading to hearing problems.

### 79. Effects of increased vertical dimension

### Effects of Increased Vertical Dimension

1. *Appearance:* It will give the appearance of an elongated face with the expression of strain. There will be slight parting of lips.
2. *Discomfort:* An increased vertical height affects the patients talking, eating, tongue movements causing discomfort.
3. *Stability and retention:* Stability and retention of the denture is decreased due to premature contact of the teeth.
4. *Loss of freeway space:* Affects the overall function of the denture in all aspects
5. *Clicking teeth:* At increased vertical height opposing cusps frequently meet each other producing clicking sounds.
6. *Excessive bone resorption* due to loss of freeway space.

### 80. Burning mouth syndrome and "denture sore mouth".

Denture sore mouth is a vague burning sensation or pain under a well-fitting denture without any detectable lesions in some geriatric patients.

## Common Complaints

Burning tongue, burning sensation all over the mouth.
Always associated with prosthesis wear.

### *Causative Factors are:*

1. External
2. Internal
3. Psychologic
4. A combination of any two of these, or, in some cases, all three.

### *A. External Factors*

1. *Allergic response:*
   The high plasticizer content and the leaching of the plasticizer from soft denture liners to the tissue surface could be a causative factor. Free monomer present in incompletely cured denture bases or autopolymerized relines also result in allergy. This residual monomer usually disappears in a few hours when the denture is immersed in water or worn by the patient.
   Any of the above allergies can be confirmed by a patch test. If a positive result is obtained, the denture base has to be remade using another resin for the base, such as polystyrene, nylon, polycarbonate, a cast gold or chrome-cobalt base.
2. *Excessive pressure:*
   A burning sensation in the anterior portion of the palate may be due to excessive pressure from a denture base on the incisive papilla. Adequate relief in that region brings about disappearance of symptoms.
3. *Proper design and tooth arrangement:*
   An occlusal load beyond the capabilities of the denture-bearing tissues can cause a generalized burning sensation. The forces of mastication must be spread over as great an area as possible to minimize local stresses by proper design and tooth selection.
4. Smoking, tobacco chewing, mouth breathing, chronic alcoholism and tongue *habits*.
5. The continued ingestion of *excessively seasoned foods*.
6 The use of various *over-the-counter oral preparations*, such as mouth washes, denture adhesives and cleansers and tooth pastes and powders, can also cause allergy. If the cause is properly located avoiding the cause can bring relief to denture sore mouth.

### *B. Internal Factors*

1. Common causes are *nutritional or vitamin deficiencies* as, pernicious and iron-deficiency anemia, metabolic, circulatory disturbances, gastrointestinal disorders and hormonal imbalance. The tongue is often affected by a vitamin B-complex deficiency.
2. *Systemic disturbances* can account for a burning sensation of the oral structures, especially the tongue, palate and denture-bearing tissues. This can be followed by discernible oral lesions which can confirm the diagnosis.
3. *Metabolic, Hormonal imbalance*: A burning sensation of the tongue, palate and denture-bearing tissues is often associated with the climacteric, which is a period of transition from maturity to senility, as in menopause. A corresponding period occurs in men and is known as the male climacteric. The retrogressive changes of this period generally appear earlier in women.

Because of the endocrine, metabolic and structural changes associated with climacteric, oral symptoms can appear that may lead to the ultimate failure of prosthetic treatment. This is common in women after menopause.

### *C. Psychologic Factors*

When psychologic factors are involved it is difficult to diagnose and treat this group of patients as these patients consider the symptoms as real and expects an explanation whether reasonable or not. These patients are usually postmenopausal women, nervous, worried, tense and anxious, with a variety of actual or imagined systemic disorders. The psychologic and emotional response to the loss and replacement of teeth and age changes as wrinkling of the skin and greying or loss of hair, can also play a part. During menopause, women are often emotionally hypersensitive. These problems may not be discernible until the denture is inserted.

Patience, understanding and constant reassurance on the part of the dentist are important and only as a last resort and with the patient's permissiön should psychiatric consultation be sought as this can aggravate the present situation.

### *Treatment*

A thorough medical and nutritional history should be taken, any deviations from normal should be noted and if required referred to a physician. A complete physical examination with blood count and urinalysis or request of the results of recent examinations and laboratory tests can be asked for by the dentist. This can help to eliminate internal factors as a cause.

### *A treatment regimen followed by Payne and others*

- Vitamin C (ascorbic acid) 1500 mg per day, two tablets of 250 mg taken with each meal, for a four-week period.
- This dose is then reduces to 750 mg per day, one tablet of 250 mg with each meal, which is continued indefinitely.
- *Vitamin therapy is not a substitute for a well-balanced diet.* An adequate intake of protein with low carbohydrate should be recommended as diet regimen.

## 81. Camper's line.

It is a line projected from the ala of the nose to the superior edge of the tragus of the ear.

### Significance

After forming the rim with the above vertical heights, the plane of occlusion is modified until it is parallel with a line projected from the ala of the nose to the superior edge of the tragus of the ear (Camper's line) (Fig. 10).

When viewed from the front, the occlusal plane should be parallel to the interpupillary line. The cuspid eminences are marked on the occlusion rim by lines placed at the corners of the mouth. These lines represent the approximate location of the distal surface of the cuspid teeth.

From the cuspid line posteriorly the occlusion rim is sloped slightly inward This serves to create a buccal space, or corridor, between the teeth and the cheeks that can frequently be seen when a patient smiles.

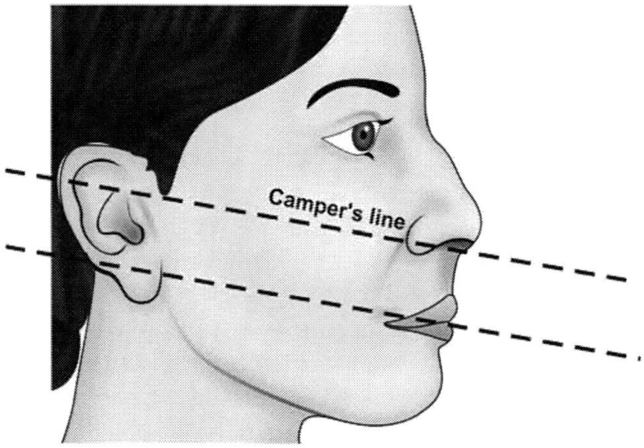


**Fig. 10:** Camper's line

## 82. Importance of balanced occlusion in complete denture

For balanced complete denture occlusion the following factors are important:

- The tooth size and position in relation to the ridge size and shape.
- The extent of denture base coverage.
- Occlusal balance with stable contacts at the retruded border position.
- Right and left eccentric occlusal balance by simultaneous contacts at the limit of functional and parafunctional activity.
- Intermediate occlusal balance for all positions between centric occlusion and all other functional or parafunctional excursions to the right, left and protrusive.
- It is important that both aspects of balance, one due to tooth position and one due to tooth contact, complement one another for total denture base stability.

### Advantages of Bilateral Balanced Occlusion

- It is important during activities such as swallowing saliva, closing to reseat the dentures and the bruxing of the teeth during times of stress.
- Patients with balanced occlusion do not upset the normal static, stable and retentive position of their dentures.
- If teeth are not arranged in balanced occlusion, the constant unseating of the denture bases create soreness and inflammation, which accelerates bone resorption.

### Factors Affecting Occlusal Balance

- Condylar guidance
- Incisal guidance
- Plane of occlusion
- Compensating curve
- Angulation of the teeth/Cuspal height

The incisal guidance and the plane of occlusion can be altered only a slight amount because of esthetic and physiologic factors.

The factors for the dentist to manipulate are the compensating curve and the inclinations, or cusps, on the occlusal surfaces of the teeth.

### Factors Affecting Protrusive Balance

1. Condylar inclination represents the path of the condyle in protrusion modified by the combined action of all of the tissues of the temporomandibular joint and the ridges covered by the recording bases.
2. The inclination of the incisal guidance is chosen for the patient.
3. The inclination of the plane of occlusion set to physiologic factors.
4. The compensating curve set to harmonize with 1 and 2.
5. Cusp heights and tooth inclination of the posterior teeth can be adjusted depending on other factors.

### Factors Affecting Lateral Balance

1. The inclination of the condylar path on the balancing side.
2. The inclination of the incisal guidance and cuspid end-to-end contact.
3. The inclination of the plane of occlusion on the balancing side and working side.
4. The compensating curve on the balancing side and working side.
5. The buccal cusp heights or inclination of the teeth on the balancing side.
6. The lingual cusp heights or inclination on the working side.
7. The Bennett side shift on the working side.

   The forces of occlusion should be balanced from right to left and anterior to posterior in complete dentures.

## 83. Classification of occlusion based on geometry.

In 1966 John P. Frush described occlusion in geometric terms as:

- Three-dimensional (cusped)
- Two-dimensional (flat plane)
- One-dimensional (linear).

### Three-dimensional (cusped)

In cusp occlusion, the contact between the opposing surfaces of any two teeth occurs in three dimensions such as:

- Width of the occluding surface
- Length of the occluding surface
- Depth of the occluding surface.

### Two-dimensional (flat plane)

The dimensions are:

- Width of the occluding surface
- Length of the occluding surface.

### One-dimensional (linear)

The contact occurs only in one dimension which is the length of the contacting blade (not surface).

This blade, being always in the form of a straight line, geometrically constitutes "length" in occlusal contact without either "width" or "depth" of occlusal contacts.

*Linear occlusion consists of the following basic parameters:*

- Zero degree teeth are opposed by bladed (line contact) teeth in which the blade is in a precisely straight line over the crest of the ridge
- Mandibular teeth set to a flat (monoplane) occlusal plane.There is no anterior tooth interference to protrusive or lateral movements.

### *Advantages*

- Reduction of needless problems due to complexities of occlusal contacts and resultant deflections
- Simplification of prosthodontic procedure
- Reduced post-insertion adjustments
- A general increase in chewing efficiency, comfort and stability of full dentures.

## 84. Organic concept of occlusion.

According to organic concept of occlusion, shapes of the teeth are altered to have cusps suitable for the patient. The movement of the condyle determines the direction of the ridges and grooves of the teeth and the mandibular movements determine other factors like cusp height, fossa, depth of the fissure, and concavity of the lingual surfaces.

### AIM

- To relate the occlusal surfaces of the teeth in harmony with the muscles and joints during function.
- Variations in the mesial-distal position of the cusps and fossae do occur. These variations require adjustments in the occlusal pattern of the teeth to maintain an organic occlusion.

### OCCLUSAL VARIATIONS

### Neutroclusion

The usual mesial-distal stamp-cusp position (class I occlusion) is known as neutroclusion.

i. The buccal stamp cusps of the mandibular premolars close into the mesial fossae of the maxillary premolars in centric occlusion.
ii. The buccal stamp cusps of the mandibular molars close into mesial, central and distal fossae of the maxillary molars.
iii. The lingual stamp cusps of the maxillary premolars close into the distal fossae of the mandibular premolars, and the lingual stamp cusps of the maxillary molars close into the central and distal fossae of the molars.
iv. The mesial fossae of the mandibular molars and the distal fossae of the maxillary premolars are vacant, since there are no available stamp cusps.
v. There is no cuspal interference during eccentric movements, as the working grooves are transverse and the idling grooves are oblique. The grooves are formed from developmental and supplemental occlusal grooves.

## Distoclusion

i. A variation to the normal mesial-distal stamp cusp position exists in centric relation when the mandibular premolar cusps are one half-tooth distal and the mandibular molars are one cusp distal to normal. This tooth position is called distoclusion.
ii. This causes the maxillary lingual premolar stamp cusps to be one half-tooth forward or to close into the mesial fossa of the mandibular premolars.
iii. The maxillary molar stamp cusps move one cusp forward so that they function in the mesial and central fossa of the mandibular molars respectively. This is also called a class II occlusion .
iv. This cusp position places the mandibular premolar stamp cusp posterior to the maxillary premolar stamp cusp.
v. As the mandible rotates around the vertical rotation center during function, the mandibular stamp cusp travel medially and forward and interfere with the maxillary stamp cusp.
vi. Because of the changed fossae in which the stamp cusps function, the maxillary premolars, the mandibular premolars, and the mandibular mesial fossae all have oblique paths that lead to a cusp tip which cause eccentric contact or interference.
vii. In restoring teeth in this mesiodistal position, the elimination of these eccentric interferences is done by moving the affected mandibular stamp cusps slightly distal and buccal and the affected maxillary stamp cusps slightly mesially and lingual.
viii. This allows further travel of the respective cusps in their idling grooves before coming to an opposing cusp tip position. As the advancing condyle travels further it also descends and further separates the idling teeth.
ix. Supplemental grooves along the idling cusp paths (oblique grooves) are placed to further enhance eccentric clearance.

## Mesioclusion

i. The mesial placement of the mandibular teeth by one-half tooth in the premolars and one cusp in the molars is called mesioclusion. This also places the maxillary lingual stamp cusps one-half tooth distally in the premolar area and one cusp distally in the molar relationship. This is a class iii occlusal relationship.
ii. In mesioclusion, the mandibular first premoiar buccal stamp cusp occludes with the maxillary canine, and the remaining buccal stamp cusps occlude with the indicated maxillary fossae in centric occlusion and centric relation.
iii. In mesioclusion the maxillary lingual stamp cusps occlude with the indicated mandibular fossae in centric occlusion and centric relation.
iv. The conflict in eccentric interference occurs when a mandibular stamp cusp is placed distal to its opposing maxillary stamp cusp.
v. Cuspal interference is corrected by moving the involved maxillary lingual stamp cusps slightly mesial and lingual.
vi. The involved mandibular buccal stamp cusps are moved slightly buccal and distal.
vii. Idling (oblique) grooves are also established to allow free travel to the border position for the cusps.

Variations of occlusion from neutroclusion which creates potential areas of conflict should be corrected so that the principles of organic occlusion would not be compromised even in these variations.

## 85. Posterior tooth forms.

## CLASSIFICATION

- Anatomic tooth forms (33° and more)
- Semi-anatomic tooth forms (20° modified anatomic)
- Other modified tooth forms.
- ***Anatomic Teeth of 33° or more (Trubyte)***
  Dr. Alfred Gysi of Switzerland was credited for designing the first anatomic porcelain tooth designed to function harmoniously with incisal and condylar guidances.
  After studying numerous natural dentitions he found that anatomic posterior tooth had a cusp angle of 33°. This tooth was marketed by The Dentists' Supply Company in 1914 and was called "Trubyte".
- ***Gysi*** recognized that his anatomic teeth would not satisfy all ridge relationships and in 1927 he designed a modified "cross-bite" posterior. In this tooth the maxillary buccal cusp was almost eliminated, resulting in one prominent lingual cusp that occluded into a lower anatomic tooth.
- ***Avery brothers*** in 1930 introduced modified form, the opposite of Sears, called the "scissor-bite" technique.

  ***Features of modified tooth form***
  - The posterior occlusal surfaces were locked anteroposteriorly by grinding steps on the surface of the teeth, with the angle determined by the inclination of the condylar path.
  - Sears teeth were modified to be free in lateral excursion.
  - The occlusion of these teeth was meant to shear food in lateral excursions.
  - These teeth were not marketed commercially.
- ***Curved cusp posterior tooth: (McGrane in 1936)***
  These too were designed to lock anteroposteriorly and be free laterally. The intent was to shear food in harmony with the lateral condyle guidance of the Bennett angle.
- ***French, 1935***
  The maxillary tooth had a central groove running mesiodistally but with very shallow buccolingual inclines to reduce lateral thrust.
  The mandibular teeth had a narrow mesiodistal food table moved to the lingual of the occlusal surface and a sloping buccal incline that was subocclusal. This design favored the stability of the lower denture.
- ***Max Pleasure's scheme, proposed in 1937***
  The reverse curve was set in the premolars, a flat occlusal surface on the first molar and a Monson curve (lingual tilt) at the second molar for balance. The reverse curve (buccal tilt of occlusal surfaces) is created to direct forces of occlusion lingually to favor the stability of the lower denture, while still retaining a balancing contact in the second molar.
- ***John Vincent in 1942***
  He used metal inserts in resin posteriors. Metal inserts of gold solder wire or stainless steel, protruded from the middle third of the maxillary posterior occlusal surfaces with shallow buccal and lingual cusps protruding beyond the metal inserts.

These teeth were set opposing French's mandibular self-adjusting quality of the resin teeth as they wear against the porcelain teeth.

- ***S. H. Payne, 1941***
  The lingualized occlusion concept was reported by Pound and Murrell. Ortman started using the term lingual cusp contact occlusion to describe the contact of the maxillary lingual cusp with the mandibular teeth.
- ***Sosin in 1961and Levin***
- Sosin replaced the maxillary second bicuspid and first and second molars with Vitalium forms, called "cross-blades", of slightly smaller size.
- During try-in stage, the lower posterior molars were removed and the case processed. At the time of insertion, wax was placed in this area, the dentures inserted and the patient "chewed" the occlusal form into the wax. This was then converted to gold and cured to the existing lower denture.
- Levin modified this scheme by reducing the size of the cross-blade to the maxillary lingual cusp (for esthetic reasons).

### *Advantage*

Increase in masticatory efficiency.

### *Evaluation of Occlusal forms*

Based on:

1. Masticatory efficiency
2. Forces directed to the ridges.
3 Tissue response
4. Denture wearer preference.

***Advantage*** of anatomic tooth form is that the masticatory efficiency is increased.

## 86. Classification of mandibular movements

1. ***Functional:***
   a. *Masticatory:*
      i. Mastication
      ii. Grasping of feed
      iii. Biting
      iv. Tearing
      v. Swallowing
   b. *Non-masticatory:*
      i. Smiling
      ii. Facial expression
      iii. Sneezing
      iv. Wetting of the lips (their own and others)
2. ***Parafunctional:***
   a. *Bruxism*
   b. *Clenching* (holding teeth intact under pressure)

### *Mandibular Movements are also Classified as (Fig. 11).*

1. ***Opening and closing:***
   a. Along the transverse axis

   b. Along the vertical axis
   c. Along the horizontal axis
2. ***Bennett movement*** (lateral shift of the mandible along lateral).

### *Mandibular Movements are also Classified as:*

1. Closing and opening
2. Protrusive
3. Retrusive
4. Left and right lateral
5. Border movements

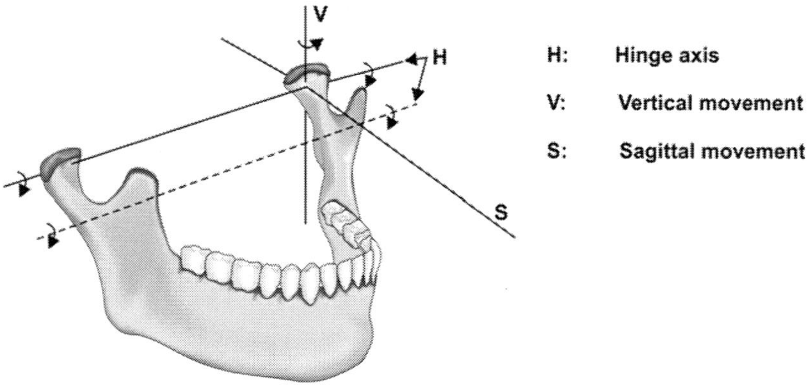


**Fig. 11:** Mandibular movement

### *Opening*

Condyles rotate and move. This brings incisors into vertical relationship.

### *Closing*

Food interposed between incisors and the condyle rotate upwards and backwards.

Teeth meet and lower incisors slide with shearing action on the palatal inclines of upper anteriors till heads of condyles are physiologically in glenoid fossa.

Factors that influence mandibular movements:

1. Muscles as force for the movement
2. Condylar path
3. Inclination of contacting surfaces of opposite teeth
4. Ligament
5. Occlusal surface of teeth
6. Mental well being of the patient
7. Bony structures.

## Structures that Limit Mandibular Movement

1. Bony structures
2. Soft tissues
   a. Muscles
   b. Ligaments

3. Neuromuscular control (proprioceptive mechanism)
4. Teeth.

### *Ligaments*

1. Sphenomandibular
2. Stylomandibular
3. Temporomandibular
4. Capsular.

In protrusion, a vertical drop of the mandible takes place by a distance which is equal to the depth of the anterior overbite. This was first noticed by Christensen and is called *Christensen's phenomenon.*

### *In Protrusion the Mandibular Movement is Guided by*

1. Condylar path posteriorly
2. Movement of lower anteriors against palatal inclines of maxillary anteriors in front.

### *In Lateral Movements, the Mandible is Guided by*

1. Path of moving condyle
2. Inclined planes of the teeth on the side of the movement of the mandible.

## 87. Envelope of motion.

When we combine the border movements of all the three planes, we get a three-dimensional space within which mandibular movement is possible. This three-dimensional limiting space is called the envelope of motion. It was first described by Posselt in 1952. The envelope of motion is longest and widest superiorly and narrows down to a point near the maximum mouth opening (MMO) position. Hence, as the jaw separation increases, space for movement decreases to a zero at the MMO position.

### *Border Movements*

- Border movement is defined as, "***mandibular movement at the limits dictated by anatomic structures, as viewed in a given plane.***" – GPT
- Border movements are recorded in three different planes. A pantograph is required to record all border movements.
- The pantograph is an extraoral tracing device, which has six sets of styli and flags (four posterior and two anterior). The styli is designed to draw tracings on their respective flags as the patient moves his mandible.

*Extreme movements in the horizontal plane*

- Border movements recorded in the horizontal plane produce a characteristic 'Diamond tracing'.
- While recording the tracing, the patient is instructed to move his mandible from the centric relation (CR) position to the maximum right lateral (MRL) position to the maximum protrusive (MP) position, to the maximum left lateral (MLL) position and return to centric.
- An arrow point tracing formed using Gothic arch tracers should and will coincide with this pattern.

*Extreme movements in the sagittal plane (Fig. 12)*

- A characteristic 'Beak tracing is formed while recording border movements in the sagittal plane.
- The patient is instructed to move the mandible from centric relation (CR) to centric occlusion (CO), then to the edge-to-edge relationship (ER) guided by the incisal guidance, progress further forward to the maximum protrusive (MP) position and then arc downward to the maximum mouth opening (MMO) position.
- Once this position is reached, the operator should guide the mandible backward and close the mouth.
- While closing the mouth the mandible arcs upward [RAT-rotation after translation] around a transverse axis passing through the mandibular foramen. Consecutively the condyle translates back to the centric relation position where the mandible continues to arc upwards around the true hinge axis passing through the condyle [true hinge axis (THA)].

*Extreme movements in the coronal plane (Fig. 13)*

- Border movements in this plane produce a characteristic 'shield tracing'.

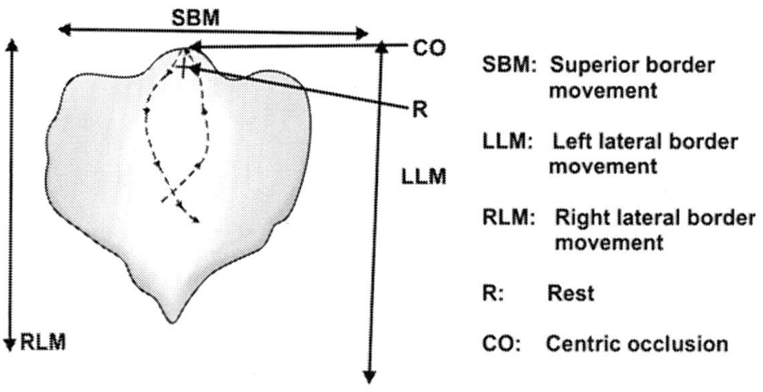


**Fig. 12:** Envelope of motion in frontal plane

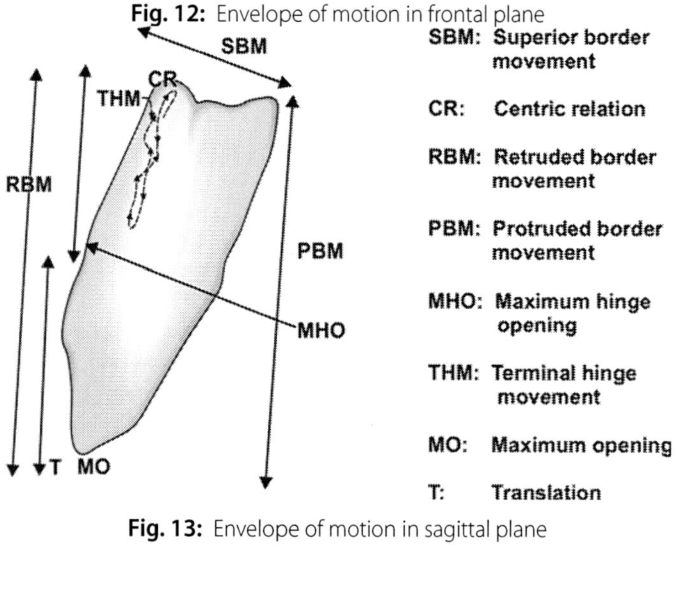


**Fig. 13:** Envelope of motion in sagittal plane

- The patient is instructed to move his mandible from centric occlusion (CO) to canine-guided disocclusion on the right side (RD) and then to the maximum right lateral (MRL) position then arc downwards to the maximum mouth opening (MMO) position. From this position, the patient is instructed to arc upward to the maximum left lateral (MLL) position, return medially to canine guided disocclusion on the left side (LD) and then return to centric occlusion (CO).

## 88. Denture stomatitis and epulis fissuratum.

Denture stomatitis is a chronic inflammation of the denture-bearing mucosa (the basal seat) that may be localized or generalized in nature.

### Etiologic Factors

a. Infection
b. Trauma from ill-fitting dentures
c. Parafunctional habit
d. Nocturnal denture wear
e. Hypersensitivity to some components of the denture material.

#### *Common Complaints and Findings*

a. Burning or itching sensation related to both the palatal and the glossal mucosa.
b. Inflammation which is localized or involving the entire basal seat.
c. Angular cheilitis and glossitis.
   Common in maxillary arch than in the mandibular arch.
d. Some times palatal inflammation—papillary hyperplasia, or papillomatosis—is seen.
   This can be due to the presence of relief chambers in dentures.
e. The presence of microbial plaque and yeasts on the fitting surface of the denture base.

### Treatment of Denture Stomatitis

1. Correct the factors that cause it.
2. Good oral and dental hygiene and rest for the tissues of the basal seat.
3. Construction of new well-fitting dentures.
4. Antifungal drugs: A therapeutic dose of one nystatin tablet taken three times a day for 10 to 14 days is usually sufficient to control the infection. Antifungal therapy may be required for up to 4 weeks in some patients.
5. 2% solution of chlorhexidine gluconate
6. Gingival massage with a toothbrush or fingers.
7. Surgical excision of papillomatosis: Excision is undertaken only after other methods of treatment have been used. Electrosurgery is frequently used to excise maxillary papillary hyperplasia. Cryosurgery also has been used, with good results.

## 89. Vertical dimension of rest and vertical dimension of occlusion

### Significance of Vertical Relations

- The value of the vertical dimension of rest in denture lies in its use as a guide to the lost vertical dimension of occlusion.
- The difference between the occlusal vertical dimension and the rest vertical dimension is the interocclusal distance.

- The interocclusal distance is the distance or gap existing between the upper and lower teeth when the mandible is in the physiologic rest position. It usually is 2 to 4 mm when observed at the position of the first premolars.
- The clinically recorded rest position and the electromyographically determined one have a range of about 10 mm.
- Failure to provide correct interocclusal distance will cause "clicking" of the dentures during speech, soreness of the tissues of the basal seat and rapid destruction of the residual alveolar ridges.

## Recording Rest Position

Following are the different methods.

### *Facial Measurements*

Instruct the patient to stand or sit comfortably upright with the eyes looking straight ahead. Insert the maxillary record base with the attached contoured occlusion rim. With either an indelible marker or a triangle of adhesive tape, place a point of reference on the end of the patient's nose and another on the point of the chin. Instruct the patient to wipe the lips with the tongue to swallow and to drop the shoulders. When mandible drops to rest position and then measure between the points with a millimetre ruler. Repeat the procedure until the measurements are consistent.

### *Tactile Sense*

Then ask them to close slowly until the jaws reach a comfortable, relaxed position, The distance Is measured between the points of reference and compared with the measurements made after swallowing.

### *Phonetics*

Have patients repeat "M" until they are aware of the contacting of the lips as "M" is pronounced. Repeat this procedure and ask that they stop all jaw movement when the lips touch. At this time measure between two points of reference.

## Occlusion Position Recording

### *Pre-extraction Records*

a. Profile photographs
   Measurements of anatomic landmarks on the photograph are compared with measurements using the same anatomic landmarks on the face.
b. Profile silhouettes
c. Facial measurements

### *Niswonger's Method*

The distance is measured and these measurements are compared with measurements made between these points when the occlusal rims are tried in.

### *Closest Speaking Space*

The closest-speaking space measures vertical dimension when the mandible and muscles involved are in physiologic function of speech. The 'F' or 'V' and 'S' syllables are used in locating closest-speaking space.

## Swallowing Followed by Relaxing

With denture in the mouth, instruct the patient to wipe the lips with the tip of the tongue, swallow and let the shoulders drop in a relaxed position. Watch the reference points and ask the patient to close the teeth together. If the teeth are together, it can indicate that no interocclusal distance exists.

***Another method*** is based on the theory that teeth make contact at or near centric occlusion. Two small cones of a soft wax are placed, one in each central sulcus of the mandibular first molars. Encourage the patient to swallow several times. If the vertical dimension of occlusion is correct, the wax will be penetrated and reduced to tooth contact.

### *Phonetics*

Have the patient repeat these words:

- "Three, thirty-three": There should be enough space for the tip of the tongue to protrude between the anterior teeth.
- "Fifty-five": Incisal edges of the maxillary central incisors should contact the vermilion border of the lower lip at the junction of the moist and dry mucosa.

### *Following are the Some of the tests:*

- Judgment of the overall facial support. When the patient closes jaw slowly until lips just touch, at this point mandible is at rest position. The lips are in constrained contact. Next ask the patient to close the jaw so that in closing through the interocclusal distance there is little or no movement of the lips. If patient has decreased vertical relation that is increased interocclusal distance, the lips close excessively, fold together and vermilion tend to disappear.
- Visual observation of the amount of space between the rims when the jaws are at rest.
- Measurements between dots on the face when the jaws are at rest and when occlusion rims are in contact.
- Observation made when sibilant - containing words are pronounced to ensure that occlusion rim come close together but do not contact.

## 90. Anterior teeth selection

## Size of Anterior Teeth

Seven anatomic factors are used as guides in the selection of anterior teeth for size:

1. *Size of the face:* The average width of the maxillary central incisor will be approximately one sixteenth of the width of the face measured between the zygoma.
2. *Size of the maxillary arch:* The mold selector can be used to make measurements of the maxillary cast. Measurements are made from the crest of the incisal papilla to the hamular notches and from one hamular notch to the opposite hamular notch. The combined length of the three legs of the triangle in millimeters is used on the selector. When there is a discrepancy between face size and arch size the selection of anterior teeth should be done by face size.
3. *Incisal papilla and the cuspid eminences or the buccal frenum:*
   Mark in the occlusion rim at each corner of the lips. The marker is passed on a line parallel to the pupils of the eyes. The distance between the marks following the contour of the arch measured in millimeters is the combined width of the six maxillary anterior teeth.

4. *Maxillomandibular relations:* Any disproportion in size between the maxillary and the mandibular arches influence the length, width and position of the teeth.
5. *The contour of the residual ridges:* The artificial teeth should be placed to follow the contour of the residual ridges that existed when the natural teeth were present.
6. *The vertical distance between the ridges:* The length of the teeth is determined by the available space between the existing ridges.
7. *The lips:* The labial surfaces of the maxillary anterior teeth support the upper lip.

## Form of Anterior Teeth

Three factors are used as guides in the selection of anterior teeth for form.

1. *The form and contour of the face:* The square, tapering, ovoid and combinations of face forms helps in selecting the tooth form. Profile is observed by checking forehead, the base of the nose and the point of the chin. If in line, the profile is straight.
2. *Sex:* Curved facial features are associated with femininity and square features are associated with masculinity.
3. *Age:* As age progress the lips lose their curves and the teeth wear at the incisal edges and interproximal surfaces. The labial surfaces seem flatter and the outline form appears squarer.

## Color or Shade of Anterior Teeth

Shade is the degree of darkness of a color with reference to its mixture with black. The yellow is more prominent in the gingival third and the gray is more prominent in the incisal third. To check the shade, the patient's mouth should not be opened too wide and white light after 10 o'clock in the morning and before two in the afternoon is preferred. The tooth and the shade guide should be viewed from a distance of six or eight feet and in different angles.

Harmony should exist between the color of the teeth and the color of the skin, hair and eyes.

To check the size, form and shades, the anterior and posterior teeth of both arches should be arranged in their anatomic positions on accurately adapted record or trial bases.

## 91. Buccal shelf.

It is primary stress bearing area of the mandible denture base (Fig. 14).

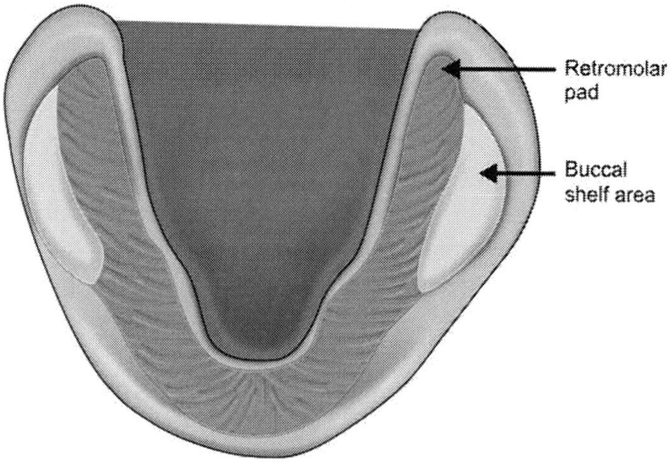


**Fig. 14:** Buccal shelf area

### Extension

Buccal shelf area extends from mandibular buccal frenum to the anterior edge of the masseter.

### Boundaries

- Medially by the crest of the residual ridge
- Anteriorly by the buccal frenum
- Laterally by the external oblique line
- Distally by the retromolar pad.

### Attachments

The inferior part of the buccinator is attached in the buccal shelf of the mandible and thus contraction of the muscle does not lift the lower denture.

### Bone quality

It is covered with good smooth cortical bone which is usually at right angles to the occlusal forces hence it can resist forces better than any other region.

## 92. Parts of a face-bow.

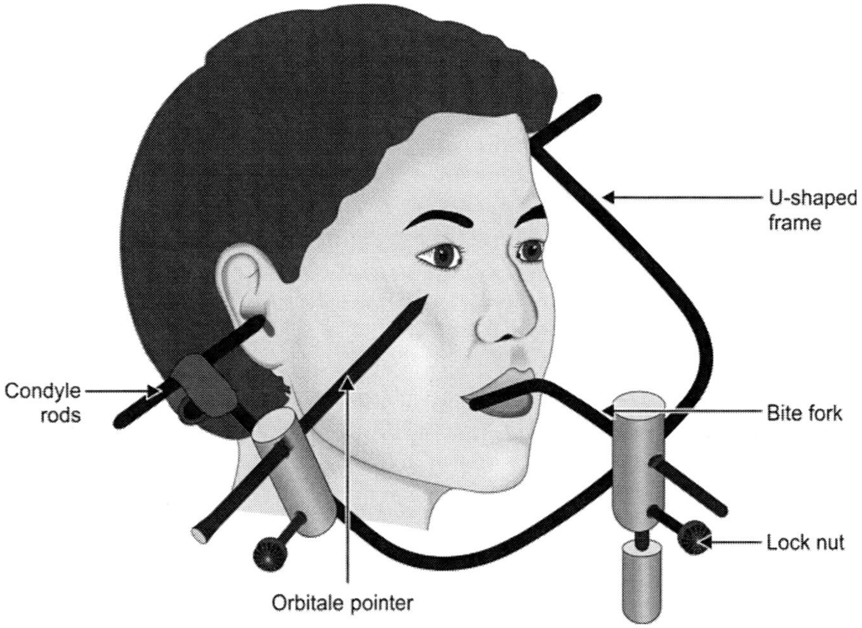


**Fig. 15:** Parts of a face-bow

## Parts of Face-bow (Fig. 15)

- U- shaped frame
- Condylar rods
- Bite fork with locking device
- Infraorbitale pointer.

### Procedure

- It consists of a U-shaped frame or assembly that is large enough to extend from the region of the TMJs to a position 2 to 3 inches (5 to 7. 5 cm) in front of the face and wide enough to avoid contact with the sides of the face.
- After recording a tentative jaw relation, the face-bow fork is heated and attached to the maxillary occlusal rim.
- The midline of the fork should correspond with the midline of the rim.
- The face-bow is then positioned so that the condylar styluses are on a point 13 mm in front of the line drawn from the outer canthus to the tip of the tragus.
- The bow is adjusted so that the stylus points are equidistant from the bow proper and have uniform readings on both sides.
- The U- shaped frame anteriorly should be parallel to the interpupillary line.
- After all adjustments are finalised the bow is locked firmly to the fork, ensuring that the styluses do not move from the recorded condylar positions.
- Then the infraorbitale pointer is directed at the infraorbital notch and is locked in place.
- The face-bow assemblage is removed from the patient and oriented to the articulator.
- The fork attached to the face-bow by means of a locking device, also serves to support the face-bow, the occlusion rims and the casts while the casts are being attached to the articulator.

### 93. Advantages of face-bow.

- Transverse hinge axis can be located with the aid of face-bow.
- Records the position of maxilla in three planes with reference to two points.
- To relate the maxillary casts to the transverse axis of the articulator.
- Mandibular hinge axis is coincided and related to the maxillary by centric relation record. The path of closure will be similar.
- It aids in securing the anteroposterior cast position in relation to the condyles of the mandible.
- It registers the horizontal relationship of the casts accurately and assists in incisal plane location.
- Helps in restoring vertical height in the articulator without change in the centric relation.
- Face-bow transfer allows more accurate arc of closure on the articulator when the interocclusal records are used.
- Helps in arbitrary mounting of the cast.

### 94. Reference points.

#### Anterior Reference Points

1. Orbitale
2. Orbitale minus 7 mm
3. Nasion minus 23 mm
4. Incisal edge plus articulator midpoint to articulator axis-horizontal plane distance.
5. Ala of the nose.

## Posterior Reference Point

1. Bergstrom point
2. Beyron point
3. Gysi point
4. Beck point
5. Luritzen and Bodner's point
6. Weinberg's point
7. Brandrup Wognsen point
8. Schlosser's point
9. Pothero point
10. Teteruck and Lundeens point
11. Swenson's point
12. Craddock and Symmon's point.

## Anterior Reference Points

- **Orbitale:** Is the lowest point of the infraorbital rim. One orbitale and the two posterior points that determine the horizontal axis of rotation will define the axis-orbital plane and can be transferred from the patient to the articulator with the face-bow.
- **Orbitale minus 7 mm:** The Frankfort horizontal plane passes through both poria and one orbital point. Because porion is a skull landmark, Sicher recommends using the midpoint of the upper border of the external auditory meatus as the posterior cranial landmark on a patient.
- Gonzalez pointed out that this posterior tissue landmark on the average lies 7 mm superior to the horizontal axis so position the orbital pointer 7 mm above the orbital indicator of the articulator.
- **Nasion minus 23 mm:** The nasion is located in the head as the deepest part of the midline depression just below the level of the eyebrows. The nasion guide or positioner of the face-bow fits into this depression. This guide can be moved in and out, but not up and down, from its attachment to the face-bow crossbar. The crossbar is located 23 mm below the midpoint of the nasion positioner.
- **Incisal edge plus articulator midpoint to articulator axis-horizontal plane distance:** In accordance with this concept, the distance from the articulator's mid-horizontal plane to the articulator's axis-horizontal plane is measured. This same distance is measured above the existing or planned incisal edges on the patient, and its uppermost point is marked as the anterior point of reference on the face. This point can be recorded for future use by measuring vertically downward to it from the inner canthus of the eye and recording this measurement. The inner canthus is used because it is an accessible, unchanging landmark on the head.
- **Ala of the nose:** The occlusal plane actually parallels the horizontal plane. Augsberger stated that the occlusal plane parallels the camper's line with minor variations. Knowing this, we can transfer Camper's line from the patient to the articulator by using either right or left Ala as the anterior reference point.

### Posterior Reference Points

- **Bergstrom point:** A point 10 mm anterior to the center of a spherical insert for the auditory meatus and 7 mm below the Frankfort horizontal plane.
- **Beyron point:** A point 13 mm anterior to the posterior margin of the tragus of the ear on a line from the center of the tragus to the corner of the eye.
- **Gysi point:** 10 mm in front of the tragus in the tragus-canthus line.
- **Beck point:** 10 mm anterior to center of EAM and 7 mm below FH plane.
- **Luritzen and Bodner' s point:** 13 mm in front of the tragus in the tragus-canthus line.
- **Weinberg 's point:** 11-13 mm anterior to the reference line drawn from the middle and the posterior border of the tragus of ear to the corner of eye.
- **Brandrup Wognsen point:** On line extending from the tragus to the lateral angle of eye, a point is marked at about 12 mm in front of posterior margin of the most prominent tragus.
- **Schlosser'point:** 13 mm in front of tensed anterior margin of EAM.
- **Pothero point:** A line drawn from top of richey condylar marker [placed in the external acoustic meatus] to the outer canthus of eye. A point 13 mm anterior to Richey condylar marker to this line is used as the arbitrary reference point.
- **Teteruck and Lundeens point:** 13 mm from the base of tragus to the canthus.
- **Swenson's point:** 11 mm anterior to the meatus of ear on reference line from top of the meatus to the corner of eye.
- **Craddock and Symmon's point:** 1 cm anterior along a line drawn from the upper margin of the tragus of ear to corner of eye.

#### *Importance of Selection of Third Point Reference*

1. The selection of the anterior point of the triangular spatial plane determines which plane in the head will become the plane of reference when the prosthesis is being fabricated.
2. The act of affixing a maxillary cast to an articulator relates the cast to the articulator's
   - Hinge axis
   - Vertical axes
   - Condylar determinants
   - Anterior guidance
   - Mean plane of the articulator.
3. It will allow the dentist and the auxiliaries to visualize the anterior teeth and the occlusion in the articulator in the same frame of reference that would be used when looking at the patient.
4. Reference points also eases the communication between dentists and laboratory personnels.

### 95. Graphic methods.

These methods use graphs or tracings to record the centric jaw relation.

Graphic methods are of two types:

a. Arrow point tracing
b. Pantograph.

   The arrow point tracing is a graphic record measured in a single plane whereas the pantograph is measured three-dimensionally.

## Factors Affecting Accuracy of Graphic Tracing

1. Stability of the denture base.
2. Resistance by the occlusal rims against occlusal forces.
3. Difficulty in placing the central-bearing device in certain clinical situations.
4. Presence of flabby tissue.
5. Height of the residual alveolar ridge.
6. Interference from the tongue.
7. Efficiency of the recording devices.
8. Obtaining a pointed apex in the tracing pattern.
9. Lack of coordinated movement can cause double tracing.
10. The graphic tracing should harmonize with the centric relation and centric occlusion.

### *Arrow-point Tracing*

It is a single plane graphic tracing using an arrow-point tracer. The characteristic pattern created is called a central arrow-point tracing.

It is defined as, "The pattern obtained on the horizontal plate used with a central-bearing tracing device." –GPT

### *Pantographic Tracing*

It is defined as, "A graphic record of mandibular movement in three planes as registered by the styli on the recording tables of a pantograph; tracings of mandibular movement recorded on plates in the horizontal and sagittal planes." –GPT

The instrument used to do a pantographic tracing is called a pantographic tracer. A pantographic tracer is defined as, "An instrument used to graphically record one or more planes paths of the mandibular movement and to provide information for the programming of the articulator." –GPT

### *Advantages*

- Most accurate method available to record centric jaw relation.
- Eccentric jaw relation can be recorded using these instruments.
- Used for full-mouth rehabilitation of dentulous patients.

## 96. Gothic arch tracers.

The apex of the arrow point tracing gives the centric relation.

### *Types of arrow point tracers (Based on the location of the tracer)*

- Intraoral tracers
- Extraoral tracers.

Intraoral arrow-point tracers: The central-bearing device is located intraorally and hence the name.

## Procedure

1. The central-bearing point and the central-bearing plate (coated with chalk) attached to record bases are inserted into the patient's mouth.
   The central-bearing point is adjusted to a predetermined vertical dimension such that it contacts the central-bearing plate when the patient closes his mouth.

2. When the patient is asked to make anteroposterior and lateral movements, the central-bearing point will draw the tracing pattern on the central-bearing plate.
3. After completing the movements, the tracing should resemble an arrow point with a sharp apex. If the apex is blunt, the record is repeated.

### Disadvantages

1. The tracer is not visible during the procedure.
2. The size of the tracing is very small, hence to determine the apex of the tracing is difficult.
3. It cannot be used in patients who cannot retract the tongue.

### In Cases of Macroglossia

1. A tentative vertical dimension is established.
2. The maxillary cast is mounted in the articulator using face-bow transfer and mandibular cast is positioned against the maxillary in a tentative centric relation and articulated.
3. The mandibular occlusal rim is reduced to obtain interocclusal distance.
4. The recording plate is attached to the mandibular occlusal rim coinciding with the midline of the rim.
5. The stylus or the central-bearing point is attached to the maxillary occlusal rim.
6. The record bases attached to the recording devices are inserted in the patient's mouth:
   - The Ney excursion guide can be used to train the patient for proper jaw movements.
   - The recording plate projecting extraorally (attached to the mandibular rim), is coated with precipitated chalk and denatured alcohol.
   - Intraorally, the central bearing point should touch central bearing plate at the predetermined vertical dimension.
   - The patient is asked to perform protrusive, lateral and anteroposterior movements.
   - It is an extra-oral tracing on the recording plate by the tracing pointer. The tracing should have a sharp apex.
   - After finalising the records, quick setting plaster is injected between the occlusal rims.
   - The assembly is removed and articulated and should be checked using an inter-occlusal check record.

#### *Advantages*

1. Extraoral tracing can be examined as it is made.
2. The size of the tracing pattern is easily seen.
3. The apex can be identified easily.

### 97. Pantographic tracing.

A pantograph is used clinically to measure mandibular movement. There are two types of pantographs:
1. Mechanical type developed by *McCollum and Stuart (1955)* and
2. Electronic type.

## MECHANICAL PANTOGRAPH

- Requires complex handling procedures in clinic and laboratory.
- It is heavy and difficult to use

- It is used to obtain information of the movement of TMJ in glenoid fossa.
- Face-bow is attached to the patient's lower teeth using a disposable plastic clutch tray.
- The side arms of the face-bow hold horizontal styli oriented to the patient's arbitrary or true hinge axis.
- Vertical parallel recording plates on the upper face-bow are located close to the face.
- Lead pencil marking tips of the styli draw the protrusive and lateral movement pathways on the vertical plates.

## ELECTRONIC PANTOGRAPH

Measures protrusive, right and left eccentric movements by means of a small optoelectronic sensor fixed to the maxilla. Since the condylar path data is computed, transferring the measurement apparatus is not necessary with the computer pantograph system.

***E.g. The Cyberhoby computer pantograph developed by Hobo and Takayama in 1983.***

### Parts of Electronic Pantograph

- Clutches
- Attitude meter
- Light source utilizing optical fibers and an opto-electronic sensors
- Computer
- Articulator that receive the data.

#### *Clutches*

Clutches are used to fix the pantograph sensor to maxillary and mandibular arches. The maxillary clutch has a central bearing plate and the mandibular clutch has a central bearing screw. With both clutches fixed intraorally, the screw tip contacts the plate at one point with all teeth disoccluded. Clutches are aligned vertically after guiding the mandible to centric relation position. The transverse horizontal axis is located and marked on the skin surface.

#### *Attitude Meter*

The attitude meter is similar to a face-bow but includes a gyroscope-like structure used for measuring clutch inclinations. The positions are determined in reference to the right and left posterior and anterior reference points. The attitude meter has seven color-coded scales. The attitude meter is attached to the maxillary clutch joint and the right and left styli is positioned toward posterior reference points and data is recorded based on the colors.

#### *Light Source*

A point light source utilizing optical fibers and an opto-electronic sensor are used as the sensing device for the computer pantograph. The point light source attached to the lower clutch is called the incisal satellite with lights emitted in three directions X, Y, and Z. The opto-electronic sensor is attached to the maxillary clutch joint. Mandibular movements are made in an order of protrusive movement three times, left and right lateral movement three times.

#### *Computer Operation*

Input data into the computer begins with the date of measurement. Next, input data is measured from the attitude meter; the data for <red>, <green>, and <blue> scales represent the angles of clutch inclination. The items and notations of the digital data including six items of measured data and four kinds of insert numbers will be displayed.

### *Digital Data*

Required for adjustment of the computer. Data recorded are:

- The distance between the rotational centers of the right and left condyles.
- The right and left lateral sagittal condylar inclinations.
- The lateral sagittal condylar inclination of the articulator.
- The sagittal protrusive condylar inclination.
- Immediate protrusive shift.
  - The distance between the intersection of the condyle path extension with the horizontal plane and the centric relation position.

## Selection of Analog Inserts

- Sixty possible combinations with analog inserts.
- The type of analog inserts used for a patient are indicated in the digital output of the computer pantograph.
- When data fits between two curve types on the gauge, select the greater analog number in order to make a prosthesis with less cuspal interferences.
- When the analog number for the horizontal condylar path is selected, read the sagittal inclination of lateral condylar path.
- When a sagittal inclination of lateral condylar path is less than 45 degrees, use the group A analog, and use the group B analog for an inclination greater than 45 degrees.
- The analogue inserts No.1, 2, and 3 are all convex-shaped in the superior direction with a curvature of 3/4 inch radius.
- For immediate protrusive shift use either Analogue insert No. 4 is linear-shaped and insert No. 5 is convex-shaped inferiorly with a curvature of 3/4 inch radius.

## Articulator Adjustment

- To maintain the centric relation position.
- The centric latch mechanism on the articulator insures a secure lock for centric relation position using lever arms inside the right and left ends of the maxillary fossa box that lock the condylar shaft to the mandibular frame.
- The centric latch mechanism is released by pushing the lock lever down on the rear-side of the maxillary frame.
- To help the operator, notches are incorporated into the undersurface to position the condyles by the levers.
- Adjustments in the articulator is done using the values in the obtained digital data.

### *Mounting the Casts*

The maxillary casts should be mounted using the axis jig and the face-bow record. With the centric relation record, position the mandibular cast against the maxillary cast. Set the incisal pole on "zero". Set the centric latch and mount the mandibular cast with dental stone. Mount the casts after all articulator adjustments have been completed. After this, do not change analogue inserts, center of rotation position, or sagittal inclination since changes may cause errors in the cast relation.

## 98. Hybrid dentures/overdentures

### *Advantages, Disadvantages and Indications*

A hybrid is a type of overdenture that looks like a complete denture but is retained and supported by natural teeth for which prefabricated or precision attachments have been made.

### Advantages

1. The retained natural tooth in overdenture aids in providing tensile stimulation to the residual alveolar ridge, hence preserving residual alveolar ridge.
2. Preservation of proprioceptive response.
3. The modified teeth provide a definite vertical stop for the denture base.
4. Horizontal and torquing forces are minimized.
5. Stability and support are increased.
6. The retention of only one tooth frequently makes for a more favorable prognosis.
7. Less post insertion problems.
8. Convertibility: Can be easily relined or rebased into a conventional complete denture.

### *Disadvantages of an Overdenture*

1. Caries susceptibility of the abutment teeth.
2. Periodontal disease can cause failure in overdenture functioning
3. Encroachment of the interocclusal distance when internal attachment is used.
4. Bony undercuts adjacent to the overlaid teeth (usually buccally), prevent close adaptation of the denture flange to the underlying tissue.
5. If undercuts are blocked it causes spacing between denture and tissue creating a food trap.
6. Esthetics, bony undercuts cause over contouring of denture resulting in improper lip fullness.
7. Under contouring leads to improper retention and stability.

### *Indications for Overdenture Treatment*

1. When few natural teeth remain and when patient has difficulty in adapting to complete dentures (Parkinson's disease).
2. Maxillofacial patients, e. g. congenital or acquired cleft palate, have a deficiency of tissue and retention of a few abutments increases the retention and stability of the overdenture and obturator.
3. When the remaining teeth are considered unsuitable as partial denture abutments because of position, angulation or state of the crowns.
4. Retaining a few teeth for overdenture treatment acts as a transition between partial dentures and complete dentures when eventually all teeth are extracted.
5. In cases of attrition, erosion or abrasion, where crown height is already diminished. Intentional reduction and preparation of the crowns for an overdenture is a logical form of treatment.

## 99. Non-anatomic or zero-degree cuspless teeth.

The presence of cusps on artificial teeth was felt by many dentists to present problems that were too difficult to control.

1. **Inverted cusp tooth (Hall, 1929)**
   - The tooth was flat with concentric cone-shaped depressions on the occlusal surface like inverted cusps.

- This design created a flat occlusal surface with sharp concentric ridges around the cup-like depressions, which provided an efficient shredding action on food as the upper and lower teeth sheared by one another.
- Disadvantages
- The depressions became clogged with food and lost their efficiency because no escape ways were provided in this design.

2. **True-Kusp (by Myerson in 1929)**
   It had a series of transverse buccal-lingual ridges with sluiceways between them Hall's and Myerson's teeth were the first teeth to be commercially produced that provided for complete free gliding contact in all horizontal directions. They were of anatomic width and breadth.
3. **Chopping block posteriors (1934, Nelson)**
   Were flat occlusal surfaces with numerous ridges. The ridges on the mandibular teeth ran transversely and on the maxillary they ran mesiodistally. Because they were perpendicular to one another in contact, an efficient shredding and cutting action was claimed.
4. **Non-lock (by Swenson 1939)**
   These were essentially flat teeth with sluiceways for shredding and allowing food to clear the occlusal table. They did provide balancing contacts, as a modest buccal and lingual incline was provided.
5. **Vitalium Occlusal (by Hardy in 1946)**
   Designed a metal insert upper and lower posterior. These were produced in resin blocks of three posterior teeth simulating a buccal facade of two bicuspids and one molar. A narrow zigzag of Vitalium ribbon was embedded on the occlusal surface and ran mesiodistally, establishing a narrow, flat, convoluted metal surface that was raised slightly above the encasing resin.
6. **Shear-cusp tooth by Myerson Tooth Corporation 1959**
   - First cross-linked acrylic tooth in a flat occlusal scheme
   - With the wear-resistant quality of the new tooth,
   - Sears and Myerson joined in proposing a combination porcelain and acrylic occlusal schemes. In this combination less horizontal forces were generated with porcelain against acrylic resin teeth as opposed to porcelain against porcelain.
   - Porcelain teeth opposing resin teeth causes faster wear on acrylic teeth than when acrylic teeth oppose acrylic teeth.
   - The IPN posterior tooth available now (Dentsply) are at least 30% more wear resistant.
7. **Coe Masticators (by Cook in 1952)**
   - Among the most unusual non-anatomic posterior teeth ever designed. The second pre-molar and the first molar were flat stainless steel castings with holes on the occlusal surfaces that exited diagonally to a port on the buccal surface.
   - These teeth occluded with flat upper porcelain teeth to push the food through the holes and, in a grinder-like fashion, break it into small particles.
   - Disadvantages
   - The ports clogged with fibrous food and it was difficult for the wearer to retrieve from the buccal pouch the chewed food that did pass through.

8. **Cutter-bar (Bader in 1957)**
   With an intent to increase the masticatory efficiency of flat teeth, scheme opposed upper porcelain cuspless teeth with a metal cutting bar replacing the second bicuspid, first molar and second molar.
   A similar approach was advocated by Frush in 1967, which he described as a "linear occlusal concept. "Maxillary and mandibular posteriors were flat, with a single mesiodistal ridge usually on the lower. The idea was not new, as many previous designs also intended to minimize the force of penetrating food by sharp linear contact.
   In 1954, DeVan formalized guidelines for using flat teeth in his *"neutrocentric concepts"*, which stated, *Flat occlusal surfaces should have*:
   1. Flat planes in all directions with no inclination at all in respect to the underlying denture foundation and
   2. Balance was considered unnecessary and undesirable, as the resulting inclines would create instability of the dentures. This concept was carried out by limiting the mesiodistal extent of the occlusal table to avoid setting the teeth over the lower molar slope inherent in the posterior portion of the residual ridge.

   Sears, in 1949, advocated a *balancing ramp* to obtain bilateral balance.

In 1961, Hughes and Regli used a modified chew-in technique to determine a functionally generated path to which flat teeth could be set in order to achieve bilateral balance and thereby improve the masticatory efficiency with control of both vertical and horizontal forces so that their function would be as innocuous as possible in the highly compromised edentulous mouth.

## 100. Arbitrary scraping of master cast.

This technique is the least accurate as it relies on the dentist's recollection of the palatal configuration and tissue compressibility to locate the anterior and posterior vibrating lines and the depth to which the cast should be scraped.

### *Disadvantages*

1. **Under extension**
   a. As a result of the practitioner's use of the fovea palatini as the landmark for terminating the denture base depriving 4 to 12 mm of tissue coverage, which otherwise can improve the retention of the denture.
   b. If the hard and soft palates and the accurate marking of the vibrating lines are not carried out, the proper posterior border extension cannot be determined.
   c. When the laboratory technician is asked to trim and polish the processed denture borders.
2. **Underpostdamming**
   When the mouth is in the wide-open position, the pterygomandibular fold becomes taut. When the patient assumes any position other than a wide-open position, a space will be present between the denture base and the tissue, since the fold is no longer activated. The diagnosis of this condition consists of placing the wet denture base into the mouth and slowly pressing in the midpalate region until it is firmly seated, all the while observing the distal denture border. If air bubbles can be seen escaping from beneath the distal border, then at that point the denture base is underpostdammed.

3. **Overpostdamming**
   If excessively overpostdammed upon denture insertion, the posterior border will be displaced inferiorly. If it is moderately overpostdammed, tissue irritation will be seen across the posterior palatal region.
4. **Overextension**
   If over extended, the patient complaints that swallowing is painful and difficult. Small ulcerated areas in the region of the soft palate will be seen. Mark these lesions and transfer it to the denture base, the precise position of the overextension can be removed with a bur and then carefully repolished.
   If the denture base covers the hamuli, the patient will experience sharp pain, especially during function.

## 101. Soft tissue hyperplasia/epulis fissuratum.

The hyperplasia occurring around the border of a denture may be a fibrous growth referred to as epulis fissuratum.

### Etiology

1. Changes in the alveolar sockets after extractions.
2. Trauma from denture wearing.
3. Gradual residual ridge reduction.
4. Changes in soft tissue profile and temporomandibular joint function.
5. Changes in the relative proportions of both jaws.
6. Habits and duration of wear.
7. Natural lower anterior teeth opposing a complete upper denture including parafunctional mandibular movements.
8. Excessive forces due to lack of balancing contacts in eccentric jaw positions.

### *Treatment*

Remove cause as chronic irritation from ill fitting denture, etc.

Surgical excision of epulis fissuratum is indicated, but only after a period of prescribed tissue rest to reduce the edema.

A program of regular and vigorous massage of the damaged site.

If attached mucosa is absent over the residual ridge, a graft is usually placed and a splint is then inserted to maintain the patency of the sulcus.

Sometimes the patient's old denture is modified to serve as a splint that is circumferentially wired into place with resin treatment liner.

The splint is worn postoperatively until adequate epithelialization has taken place, which usually takes about 6 to 8 weeks.

## 102. Significance of centric relation.

**Other names:** Retruded mandibular position, centric jaw relation, Hinge axis position and Ligamentous position.

### *Definition*

1. The most retruded relation of the mandible to the maxilla when the condyles are in the most posterior unstrained position in the glenoid fossa from which lateral movements can be made at any given degree of jaw separation.
   Or
2. The maxillomandibular relationship in which the condyles articulate with the thinnest avascular portion of their respective discs with the complex in the anterosuperior position against the shapes of the articular eminences.

### *Significance of Centric Relation*

a. This position is more constant and definite than vertical dimension, and is independent of the presence or absence of teeth.
b. It is a recordable and reproducible position.
c. It serves as a reference relation.
d. If the centric relation coincides with centric occlusion in the natural dentition the supporting structures are healthy.
e. If artificial teeth are not arranged and occluded in centric relation dentures will be unstable.
f. Errors in mounting casts on articulator can be detected when centric relation is used as the horizontal reference position.
g. An accurate centric relation orients the lower cast to the opening axis of the articulator and the mandible.
h. Accurately recorded centric relation aids in proper adjustments of condylar guidances for control of eccentric movements.
i. Helps in remounting procedures to correct occlusal discrepancies by selective grinding.
j. Dentist is able to verify the relationship of casts on articulator.
k. It is a position from which all other eccentric movements occur. It is an intersection of right and left border position.

## 103. Pre-extraction records

It's a mechanical means of recording the vertical dimension of an edentulous patient.

### Types of Pre-extraction Records

a. Profile photographs.
b. Profile radiographs.
c. Lead wire adaptation.
d. Swenson's method using acrylic face mask.
e. Willis gauge.
f. Dakometer.
g. Articulated models.

### *Profile Photographs*

Photographs are enlarged to life size and made with teeth in maximum occlusion. Measurements of anatomical landmarks in the photograph are compared with measurements of landmarks on the face. These measurements are compared when records are made and in selection of artificial teeth.

### *Profile Radiographs*

A lateral cephalograph is made with teeth in occlusion. After extraction a trial rims are made to an appropriate vertical dimension. This is placed in the patients mouth and another radiograph is taken. The first and second radiographs are compared to make needed adjustments in the trial rim.

### *Disadvantages*

1. Enlargement of radiographs can cause error.
2. Time consuming.
3. Exposure to radiation.

### *Lead Wire Adaptation*

Lead wires are adapted to pre-extraction profiles and this is transferred to a cardboard. This cut-out is stored until extraction. During the vertical dimension assessment this cut-out is placed against the patients profile to re-establish the original contour.
Swenson's method using acrylic face mask:
Same as for lead adaptation method. Instead of Lead wire acrylic mask is placed and checked for.

### *Disadvantages*

1. Time consuming
2. Requires good skill.
3. Face assumes different shape in different posture.

### *Willis Gauge*

A gauge is used to measure two points of reference.
1. On the base of nose
2. Lower border of chin.

The screw of the gauge is tightened after measuring the distance between these points before extraction and compared with the measurement after extraction.

### *Dakometer*

An instrument used to record the vertical dimension and position of upper central incisors. The readings are noted from the instrument. Later after extraction this instrument can be reassembled with the same readings.

### *Articulated Models*

Measurements between stable points as incisive papillae and the crest of lower ridge, height of lower and upper buccal freni or between two hamular notches, retromolar pads can aid in selection of size, shape and position of tooth.

## 104. Centric occlusion vs centric relation.

## Definition

The maxillomandibular relationship in which the condyles articulate with the thinnest avascular portion of their respective discs with the complex in the anterosuperior position against the shapes of the articular eminences.
Centric occlusion is the maximum intercuspation of natural teeth.

## Differences

1. Centric relation is a bone to bone relationship. Centric occlusion is the relationship of upper and lower teeth to each other.
2. Centric relation is established for denture occlusion where as centric occlusion is present in natural dentition.
3. Centric occlusion can be made to coincide with centric relation to provide a broad area of tooth contact (Freedom in centric) in dentures. In natural dentition it may not coincide because of habitual occlusion.
4. In natural dentition the centric occlusion is usually located anterior to centric relation (0.5 to 1 mm)
5. In natural tooth interferences in CR initiates impulses that direct mandible away from eflective contacts into CO. Once tooth is lost there are no proprioceptive impulses to guide the mandible away from deflective contacts and hence centric occlusion cannot be reproduced by the patient.
6. If in natural dentition the CR and CO coincides then it is called Centric relation occlusion.

## 105. Angular cheilitis/angular stomatitis

It is a painful inflammation of the corners of the mouth.

### Etiology

- Reduction of the vertical dimension of occlusion.
- Riboflavin and thiamine deficiency.
- Secondary to a denture stomatitis.
- Candida infection from contaminated saliva.

### Angular Cheilitis

1. The interface of skin and oral mucosa at the corner of the mouth, the angulus oris, is susceptible to inflammation (cheilitis).
2. The mucosal surface is unkeratinized and more vulnerable to microbial invasion than the keratinized skin region.
3. The constant exposure to saliva and a large and varied microbial flora increases the chance of angular cheilitis.
4. The incidence appears to be higher among women and denture wearers.
5. The inflammation can occur unilaterally or bilaterally and sometimes followed by an atrophic glossitis.
6. The presence of an angular fold of tissue delays the healing of angular cheilitis.
7. *Candida albicans* and *Staphylococcus aureus* have been isolated from lesions of angular cheilitis, they need not be the cause of Angular cheilitis.

### Treatment

Antimicrobial treatment.
The lesions recur frequently, even after antimicrobial treatment.

## 106. Fixed condylar articulators

An articulator may be defined as, "A mechanical device that represents the temporomandibular joints and jaw members to which maxillary and mandibular casts may be attached to simulate jaw movement."

### Types

1. Plane line or simple hinge
2. Mean value with fixed condylar path and incisal inclines
3. Adjustable: Again classified as semi-adjustable and fully adjustable. Semi-adjustable can be Arcon or Non-Arcon.
4. Fixed condylar articulators.

#### Fixed Condylar Articulators

- Are based on Bonwill's theory of occlusion/Theory of Equilateral triangle (WGA Bonwill):
- Proposed that the teeth move in relation to each other as guided by the condylar controls and the incisal point. In this theory there is a 4 inch distance between the condyles and between the condyles and incisor point.
- It permits lateral movements but as the condylar guidances are not adjustable they move in a horizontal plane.

### Different Names

Fixed condylar articulator, Mean value articulator, Non-adjustable articulator, Three point articulator.

### Features

1. It simulates mandibular movements but in a fixed condylar and incisal paths.
2. It is a non-adjustable articulator but is fixed to average values.
3. Does not accept a face-bow record.

## 107. Phonetics

Phonetics is the production of speech sounds. All speech sounds are made by controlled air. The controls are valves in pharynx, oral and nasal cavities.

### Importance

1. Aids in accurate recording of vertical dimension.
2. Helps in locating correct closest speaking space.
3. Helps in positioning anterior teeth properly.

### Types of Speech Sounds

Valves modifies the flow of air through them and produces speech sounds.

a. Labial
b. Labiodental
c. Dentoalveolar(Anterior)

d. Alveolar sounds
e. Palatal
f. Velar (Posterior)
Except velar all other sounds can be affected by the position of teeth.

A. **Labial Sounds (B, P, M)**
The above sounds are produced by air pressure build behind lips and released with or without sound.

***Affected by:***

a. Wrong anteroposterior position of anterior teeth.
b. Thickness of labial flange.

B. **Labiodental (F, V)**
When pronounced the upper incisors contact the posterior third of lower lips.

***Affected by:***

a. If upper central incisors are too short or long.
b. If placed in placed too forward or lingually.
c. The contact of upper central should be at the posterior third and not in any other position.

C. **Dentoalveolar ("th" in these, this, etc.)**
When pronounced the tip of tongue should contact between upper and lower anterior teeth close to the alveolus.

***Affected by:***

Labiolingual position of anterior tooth. Ideally 3 mm of the tip of the tongue should be visible when 'th' is pronounced. If not the anterior teeth positioning is wrong.

D. **Alveolar (T, N, D, S) and sibilants as sh, zh, ch and j**
When pronounced the tip of the tongue should contact the anterior most aspect of palate or the lingual side of anterior teeth.

***Affected by:***

a. Teeth placed too anteriorly.
b. Palate portion of denture base that is too thick in rugae area.

***Sibilants as sh, j, s:***

When spoken the upper and lower incisors should approach edge to edge but not contact.

***Affected by:***

a. Vertical and horizontal overlap
b. Positioning of anterior teeth.
c. Shape of lingual flange of lower denture.

E. **Palatal and Velar sounds (Year, she) and velar (k, g)**
Does not affect the dentures as the other sounds.
By asking the patient to pronounce these sounds the dentist should observe the relationships of the lips and tongue to the teeth and the denture bases instead to the clarity of sounds.

## 108. Transfer bases/recording bases

Defined as a temporary or permanent form representing the base of a denture.

The base plate is used for making jaw relation records, arranging artificial teeth, for try-in stage and to check the accuracy of previous records (Keyworth, 1929).

Stabilized baseplate is a baseplate lined with a plastic or other material, to improve adaptation and stability.

### Criteria for Recording Bases

1. Well adapted and accurate
2. Stable on the cast and in the mouth
3. Free of voids
4. 1 mm thickness over the crest and the facial slope of the ridge.
5. 2 mm in the hard-palate area of the maxillary base and the lingual flange of the mandibular base.
6. Ability to be removed with ease from the cast
7. Reproduce contours and the dimensions of the final cast
8. Made from materials that are dimensionally stable.

### Types

- Temporary recording bases.
- Permanent recording bases.

### For Temporary Bases four Materials are used

1. Shellac
2. Cold-curing acrylic resin
3. Vacuum formed vinyl or polystyrene
4. Baseplate wax.

### Four Basic Materials used for Permanent Bases

1. Processed acrylic resin
2. Gold
3. Chromium-cobalt alloy
4. Chromium-nickel alloy.

   Permanent bases become part of the actual base of the completed denture.

#### *Ideal base material should be:*

1. Readily adapted to the required shape and contours.
2. Rigid and strong.
3. Should be stable at mouth temperature
4. Should not warp or distort during procedures
5. A contrast color from tooth.

#### *Shellac Recording Base Material*

It is a brittle material, hence should be reinforced with wires of 12 to 14 gauge.

For the maxillary cast, the wire is placed across the posterior palatal seal area.

For the mandibular cast it is adapted within the lingual flange.

To adapt the shellac, a brush flame from a Bunsen burner is moved slowly over the surface of the shellac. The trimmed edges are readapted using a Hanau torch and folded onto themselves, and burnished with a No. 7 wax spatula.

### *Autopolymerizing Resin Recording Base Materials*

Three techniques are used:

1. Non-flasking.
2. Alternating applications of powder and liquid.
3. Flasking.

### *Non-flasking*

After applying petrolatum, acrylic is mixed when it reaches the doughy stage, it is rolled into a cigar shape, placed on a roller board and rolled to the desired thickness (2 to 3 mm).

### *Flasking Method*

A wax pattern of specific thickness is adapted on to cast and dewaxed after flasking.

Once dewaxing is over acrylic resin is mixed according to manufacturers instructions and cured after trial closure.

### *Sprinkle on Method*

Consists of coating cast with tin foil substitute, sifting polymer powder on the cast and saturating it with monomer (liquid).

### *Vacuum-Formed Bases*

The vacuum method provides a fast and efficient means of forming rigid, accurate-fitting recording bases.

The cast is prepared by blocking out the existing undercuts. A sheet of baseplate resin is inserted in the frame, and the heater is activated. Heating is continued until the resin sheet begins to sag. At this time, the softened resin is lowered onto the cast by means of the supporting frame, and the vacuum is turned on. The sheet of softened resin is adapted closely to the cast. The heater is then turned off and the base allowed to cool for one minute. After removal from the cast, the base is trimmed and finished.

## Cast Alloys

### *Advantages*

1. Rigid, accurate, and dimensionally stable.
2. More weight to mandibular dentures.
3. Thermal conductivity to maxillary dentures.

### *Disadvantage*

Expensive and time consuming.

## Stabilization of Recording Bases

Materials used are:

1. Zinc oxide and eugenol
2. Light-bodied rubber base impression
3. Soft denture-liner resin.

## 109. Classification of residual ridge resorption

1. Atwood classification (Fig. 16)
2. Neil classification
3. Branemark classification.

### Atwood Classification

- Order 1: pre-extraction
- Order 2: post-extraction
- Order 3: high, well-rounded
- Order 4: knife-edged
- Order 5: low, well rounded
- Order 6: depressed.

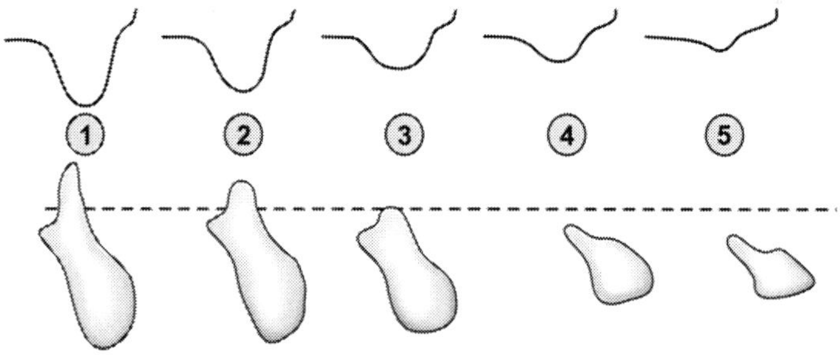


**Fig. 16:** At wood classification of residual ridge resorption

### Neil Classification

In relation with floor of the mouth and mylohyoid ridge:

- Class 1: 0.5 inch space exists between mylohyoid ridge and the floor of the mouth.
- Class 2: Less than 0.5 inch space exists between mylohyoid ridge and the floor of the mouth.
- Class 3: the mylohyoid muscle is at the same level as the mylohyoid ridge.

### Branemark Classification

Residual ridge resorption depending on bone quality and quantity.

### Bone Quantity

- Class A- Most of the alveolar bone is present.
- Class B- Moderate residual ridge resorption occurs.
- Class C- Advanced residual ridge resorption occurs.
- Class D- Moderate resorption of the basal bone occurs.
- Class E- Extreme resorption of the basal bone occurs.

### Bone Quality

- Class 1- Almost the entire jaw is composed of homogenous compact bone.
- Class 2- A thick layer of compact bone surrounds a core of dense trabecular bone.
- Class 3- A thin layer of compact bone surrounds a core of dense trabecular bone.
- Class 4- A thin layer of compact bone surrounds a core of low-density trabecular bone.

## 110. Residual ridge resorption

Residual ridge resorption is a chronic, progressive, irreversible and cumulative disease.

### Pathology

Porosity of medullary bone on the crest of the ridge, osteoclastic activity, smooth lamellar bone on all aspect except on the crest of ridge.

*Bone loss can be classified as :*

a. Pre-extraction
b. Post-extraction
c. High well rounded
d. Knife edge
e. Low well rounded
f. Depressed.
   The amount of bone loss can be determined by cephalometric radiograph.

### Pathophysiology

Mechanism of disordered functioning of bone. It is a localised process of bone loss with no bone deposition, and hence the bone loss is not reversible.

### Etiology

1. Anatomic
2. Metabolic
3. Mechanical
   a. Functional
   b. Prosthetic.

### Anatomic Factors

1. Size and shape of ridge
2. Type of bone
3. Type of mucoperiosteum.

### Metabolic Factors

1. Age
2. Sex
3. Hormonal balance
4. Vitamins
5. Diet
6. Osteoporosis.

#### *Age*

Old persons more resorption than young patients.

#### *Systemic Factors*

Diabetic mellitus, Tuberculosis increase resorption.

### *Local Factors*

Osteoclast activating factor, Prostaglandins, Human gingival - bone resorption stimulating factor increase resorption.

### *Sex*

Female patients after menopause are prone to osteoporosis which increases bone resorption.

### *Hormonal*

If high values of parathyroid hormone is present it increases bone resorption.

### *Vitamins*

Vitamin A, D and C are important. Excess of vitamin D can cause resorption. Vitamin A and C deficiency affects bone growth.

## Mechanical Factors

### *Functional Factors*

The frequency, direction and amount of force applied on the mucoperiosteum affects the rate of bone resorption.

Cancellous bone can withstand compressive forces better than any other type of bone.

### *Prosthetic Factors*

As the form and type of teeth, arrangement of teeth, interocclusal distance, etc.

## Management of Residual Ridge Resorption

1. *Preventive methods*
   a. Overdentures
   b. Submerged roots to preserve alveolar ridge structure
   c. Implants.
2. *Surgical methods*
   a. Removal of high frenal attachments
   b. Extension procedures (Vestibuloplasty)
   c. Ridge augmentation procedures
   d. Implants.
3. *Prosthetic management*
   a. Minimum pressure impressions.
   b. Use of tissue conditioners.
   c. Teeth arranged in bilateral balanced occlusion with acrylic material as ideal choice.
   d. Teeth arranged in neutral zone.
   e. Well contoured flanges and denture base.

## 111. Lasers in complete denture.

Laser is an acronym, which stands for Light Amplification by Stimulated Emission of Radiation. Lasers are an alternative to conventional surgical systems.

### Advantages

- Easy access to the anatomic site
- Possess inherent hemostatic properties.
- Capable of ablation of lesions in proximity to normal structures, with minimal damage to normal structures.
- Reduced pain during surgical procedures and less postoperative pain.
- Enhanced healing.
- Bactericidal and virucidal effects of laser result in decreased rates of wound infection.

### Uses of Lasers

1. Frenectomy
   Maxillary midline
   Lingual (Tongue tie).
2. Incisional and excisional biopsies.
3. Removal of benign fibrous lesions as:
   - Papillous
   - Pyogenic granuloma
   - Lichen planus
   - Erosive lichen planus
   - Nicotinic stomatitis
   - Verruca vulgaris
   - Inflammatory papillary hyperplasia
   - Epulis.
4. Soft tissue tuberosity reduction.
5. Soft tissue distal wedge procedure.
6. Aphthous ulcer.
7. Removal of hyperkeratotic lesions.
8. Removal of malignant lesions.
9. Coagulation
   - Graft donor sites
   - Vestibuloplasty.
10. Removal of vascular lesions
    - Hemangiom
    - Pyogenic granuloma.
11. Removal of lesion in patients with hemorrhagic disorders.
12. Implants – pilot drill and stage II – at the time of recovery.

## 112. Implant biomaterials.

The common biomaterials used are:

- Pure Titanium (In compromised bone beds CP titanium is the safest alternative)
- Titanium - 6Aluminum - 4Vanadium (Ti-6Al-4V) alloy
- Niobium

- Hydroxyapatite(calcium phosphate ceramic material)
- Hydroxyapatite coated titanium implants
- Plasma sprayed Ti implants
- Cobalt- chromium-Molybdenum alloy
- Iron- Chromium-Nickel based alloy
- Ceramics and carbon
- Aluminum, Titanium and Zirconium oxides
- Calcium phosphate ceramic biomaterials
- Bioglass or Ceravital (Sodium lithium invert glasses with calcium phosphate)
- Glass ceramics.

### *Advantages of Ceramic Biomaterials Over the Other Materials*

1. Pure chemical composition and constituents similar to biological tissue.
2. Biocompatible
3. Minimal thermal and electrical conductivity
4. Moduli of elasticity similar to bone
5. Color similar to bone, dentin and enamel.

### *Disadvantages*

1. Relatively low tensile and shear strength
2. Limited information regarding stability of coatings
3. Low fatigue strength
4. Variable solubility for different materials.

Ideally any biomaterial that does not corrode, abrade, biocompatible with good strength and osseointegration properties, with minimum thermal conductivity are good implant materials.

## 113. Geriatric age changes.

### *Gerodontology*

Gerodontology is dentistry for patients above 75 years of age.

### Epidemiology

1. Increase in proportion of the elderly.
2. Improved dental health.

### Problems

1. Age changes, physiological and pathological
2. Disease and drug therapy
3. Delivery of care.

### General Aspects of Aging

1. Decreased microcirculation
2. Decreased cellular production
3. Decreased tissue repair
4. Increased fibrosis.

Overall there is reduced function of body systems.

## Oral Aspects of Aging

1. Loss of teeth: Mainly due to degeneration of periodontal structures.
2. Attrition: Increases due to diet and masticatory habits.
3. Oral mucosa: Loss of elasticity, dryness, atrophy and hyperkeratosis.
4. Gingiva: Edematous, thin keratinized layer, friable tissue and loss of stippling.
5. Saliva: Xerostomia due to atrophy of cells lining the intermediate ducts. Abnormal taste sensations.
6. Tongue: Atrophic glossitis due to vitamin deficiency.
7. Lips: Angular cheilitis due to decreased vertical dimension or vitamin B deficiency.
8. Bone: Osteoporosis, excessive alveolar ridge resorption (Knife edge ridge) due to senile atrophy.

### *Prosthetic Problems*

1. Reduced adaptive capacity
2. Age changes in denture bearing areas as resorption and atrophy.

## Complete Denture Construction

### *Impression*

If the patient was wearing a ill fitting denture and the tissues are abused, then tissue conditioning should be done.

An impression with maximum tissue coverage with no peripheral displacement during functional movement is to be made.

Preliminary impression are to be made in stock trays with final impression in custom trays.

### *Vertical Dimension*

In geriatric patients more time is needed for accurate recording of all jaw relations. An adequate interocclusal distance is required for proper mastication, phonetics and patient comfort.

Geriatric patients need more than 3 mm of interocclusal space. In some situations a 5 to 10 mm of space is needed.

In cases of difficulty in recording vertical dimension, other methods as old dentures or pre-extraction records have to be used.

Vertical dimension should not be opened more than 5 mm at one time.

### *Centric Relation*

Centric relation must be recorded at the established vertical dimension.

In case of a patient with habitual forward position of mandible, sufficient time should be given for the accurate jaw relation record to be registered.

For patients with muscular incoordination muscle relaxants can be used.

In geriatric patients interocclusal wax records are favored as patient might find the gothic arch tracing difficult due to many reasons.

### *Posterior Tooth Selection*

Zero degree tooth is highly recommended as:

1. Can adapt to unusual jaw positions.
2. Eliminates horizontal forces
3. They adapt to negative changes in ridge height better.

### *Adjustments*

Geriatric patients should be seen the day after insertion. No border or tooth should be reduced until sure of the problem. Home care, cleaning procedure and oral hygiene instructions should be reinforced.

## 114. Bennett movement and Bennett angle (Norman G. Bennett, 1908)

### Bennett Movement

It is defined as the bodily lateral movement or lateral shift of the mandible resulting from the movements of the condyles along the lateral inclines along the mandibular fossae in lateral jaw movements.

- Recorded in the region of the translating condyle of non-working side.
- The mandible shifts 1 to 4 mm towards working side in lateral movement called Bennett movement.
- If major part of Bennett movement occurs in first 4 mm, it is called distributed side shift.

#### *Factors Affecting Bennett Movement*

1. Shape of fossa
2. Looseness of capsular ligament
3. Contraction of medial pterygoids.

#### *Types of Bennett movement in relation to the forward movement of nonworking condyle*

a. Immediate side shift: Occurs in lateral movement before the nonworking condyles move forward (Average 0.75 mm).
b. Precurrent side shift: Is the initial 2 to 3 mm of forward movement of non-working condyles.
c. Progressive side shift: Lateral translation occurring beyond 2 to 3 mm of forward movement.

### Effects of Bennett Movement on Cusp Paths

1. Depending on the value of side shifts cusp path vary in mandibular and maxillary teeth.
2. The balancing and working cusp paths in maxillary and mandibular vary with the different types of side shifts.
3. Greater the side shifts, shorter the cusps and shallower the fossa.
4. Lesser the side shift, longer the cusp and deeper the fossa.

#### *Methods of Recording Bennett Movement*

1. Electronic pantograph
2. Polyether interocclusal records
3. Mechanical pantography (Denar, Panadent)
4. Simplified mandibular motion analyser.

### Bennett Angle

It is defined as the angle formed by the sagittal plane and the path of the advancing condyle during lateral mandibular movements as viewed in the horizontal plane.

- This angle is formed between the path of the non-working condyle and the sagittal plane.
- Average Bennett Angle is 7.5 to 12.8 degree.
- In Hanau articulator it is calculated as $L = H/8 + 12$.

### 115. Overjet and overbite.

**Overjet** is the distance between upper and lower incisors and Overbite denotes horizontal overlap of upper and lower incisors (Fig. 17).

**Incisal guidance:** is defined as, "The influence of the contacting surfaces of the mandibular and maxillary anterior teeth during mandibular movement." –GPT

It is usually expressed in degrees of angulation from the horizontal by a line drawn in the sagittal plane between the incisal edges of the upper and lower incisor teeth when closed in centric occlusion.

Increase in overjet and overbite will alter the incisal guidance of occlusion.

With a given vertical overlap incisal guide angle can be made flatter by increasing the horizontal overlap.

It can be made less steep by reducing vertical overlap.

If the incisal guidance is steep, it needs steep cusps, a steep occlusal plane and a steep compensating curve to produce occlusal balance.

Ideally the incisal guidance should be as flat as esthetic and phonetics will permit.

If the anterior teeth necessitates a vertical overlap, a compensating horizontal overlap should be set to prevent anterior interference from upsetting the occlusal balance on the posterior teeth.

Increased horizontal overlap will provide freedom of the anterior teeth during normal functional and parafunctional activities.

Repeated anterior interference of the teeth during mastication unstabilizes the denture bases and causes damaging effects to the anterior region of the supporting structures.

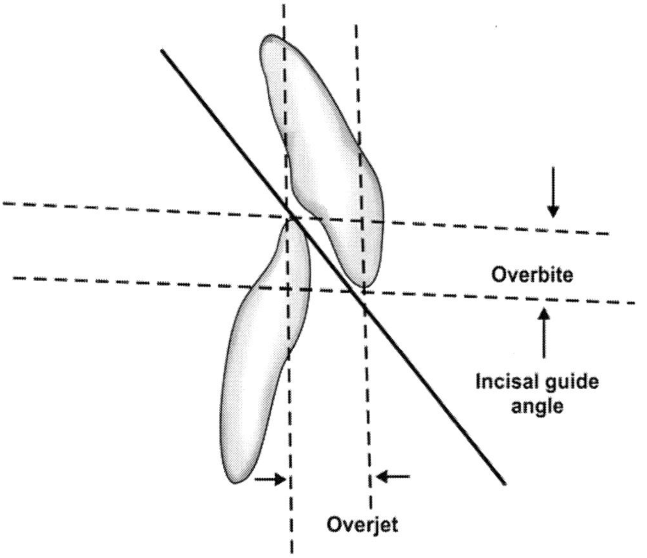


**Fig. 17:** Overjet and overbite

#### *Values*

- Normal overjet and overbite values should not exceed 2 mm in class 1 situation.
- In class 2 the overjet is more than 2 mm .
- In class 3 the overjet is less than 2 mm.

## 116. Biofunctional prosthetic system (BPS)

BPS is an idea of denture prosthetics developed by Ivoclar Vivadent.

This treatment concept is used for treating edentulous and partially edentulous patients.

### *Steps Involved in the BPS Denture Fabrication*

- Anatomic impression
- Provisional jaw relation (recording vertical jaw relation and tentative centric relation using centric trays)
- Facebow transfer with centric trays in position
- Articulation
- Functional impression
- Determining definite jaw relation
- Definite facebow transfer
- Selection and arrangement of teeth
- Try-in
- Denture insertion.

### *Anatomic Impression*

**Materials used:** Impression trays – Accu- trays ( 5 differently sized maxillary and mandibular trays).

Impression material – System 1 Accu-gel material available as syringe gel and tray gel to be mixed with water.

### Procedure

- Appropriate size tray is selected for maxilla and mandible based on ridge size and shape
- Accu-gel tray material is mixed and loaded on the tray
- Accu- gel syringe material is mixed, loaded in a syringe and dispensed in patient's mouth
- Tray material is inserted over the syringe material
- Accu- dent cast with markings of anatomic landmarks is prepared from the impression for the fabrication of special tray and occlusal rim.

### *Provisional Jaw Relation: Materials Used*

Centric tray

Accu gel tray material

### *Procedure for Jaw Relation*

- Centric tray helps to determine the occlusal position, centric relation and also helps in mounting the models in proper relation
- Vertical dimension is measured at rest
- Load the centric tray with Accu-gel and ask the patient to close the mouth until desired VD is obtained.
- A facebow transfer is done with the centric tray in position
- Cast is seated in the impression on the centric tray and it is mounted.

## Definitive Jaw Relaton and Functional Impression

- Serrated light cure resin rim is placed on maxillary custom tray and a normal wax rim on the mandibular custom tray
- Correct vertical dimension is obtained by adjusting the lower wax rim
- Border molding is done with this tray and maxillary and mandibular functional impression is made
- For centric relation, gothic arch tracing is done.
- For this, a Gnathometer M (metal trays) is attached on the occlusal surface of the rims with a white spacer in between to maintain the vertical dimension
- After recording the functional impression, white spacer is removed and intraoral needle point tracing is done
- Interocclusal centric and protrusive bite registration is done for programming the articulator
- The entire assembly is transfered to the Stratos articulator after making the master cast
- Articulation and model orientation is done according to average values with the help of a 'horizontal guide' based on the Bonwill triangle of the articulator.

## Teeth Selection and Arrangement

Teeth selection and arrangement is done based on anatomical landmarks like:

- Mid-palatine raphe
- Incisive papilla
- First large pair of rugae
- Maxillary tuberosity
- Ridge line in the posterior region of the mandible
- The retromolar pad
- Teeth arrangement is also based with standard parameters like Curve of Spee and Curve of Wilson. Arrangement of teeth is done using the special teeth set for BPS dentures with the help of a setting up template which follows these landmarks.

### *Denture Processing*

- Done using injection molding technique.

## Advantages of BPS Dentures

- Improved stability and retention
- Posterior teeth will be correctly positioned allowing sufficient tongue space
- Reduced food trapping adjacent to the molar teeth
- Good esthetics.

# VIVA FINAL

## CHAPTER-1 INTRODUCTION

1. **Define prosthodontics.**
   Prosthodontics is a dental specialty pertaining to the diagnosis, treatment planning, rehabilitation and maintenance of the oral function, comfort, appearance, and health of the patient with clinical conditions associated with missing or deficient teeth and/or maxillofacial tissues using biocompatible tissues.
2. **What are various branches in prosthodontics?**
   Removable prosthodontics, fixed prosthodontics, maxillofacial prosthodontics and implant prosthodontics.
3. **What are the surfaces of a complete denture prosthesis?**
   Polished surface, tissue surface and occlusal surface.
4. **What are the various types of teeth based on materials?**
   Acrylic resin teeth, porcelain teeth, IPN resin teeth.
5. **Define complete denture prosthesis?**
   A removable dental prosthesis that replaces the entire dentition and associated structures of the maxillae or mandible are called a complete removable dental prosthesis.
6. **What is the differences between a prosthesis and an appliance?**
   A prosthesis replaces the missing structure and is passive in nature while an appliance actively moves the tooth and its associated structures.

## CHAPTER -2 DIAGNOSIS AND TREATMENT PLANNING

1. **Define case history?**
   Case history is defined as the collected data about an individual, family, environmental factors and any other information that may be useful in analyzing and diagnosing conditions or for instructional purpose, best termed the patient history.
2. **Define diagnosis?**
   Diagnosis is the examination of physical state, evaluation of mental or psychological make up and understanding the needs of each patient to ensure predictable results.
3. **Define treatment plan.**
   Treatment plan is developing a course of action that encompasses the ramification and sequelae of treatment to serve the patient's needs.
4. **What is the relevance of occupation in case history?**
   Public speakers and singers require perfect seal for good retention, wind instrument players need special modification of the teeth and professional people need good esthetics as well as retention.
5. **Which type of mental attitude is the best and why?**
   Philosophical is the best mental attitude as these patients are calm, sensible, organized and have better acceptance of complete denture.
6. **What are the causes for variation in the color of mucosa in an edentulous patients?**
   The common causes for variation in color of mucosa are over extension of periphery of denture, ill-fitting denture, dirty denture, continuous wearing of denture, faulty articulation of teeth, use of suction disc, traumatic injury, bony spicules, allergy, manifestation of systemic diseases and other infective oral lesions.

7. **Why is a 'V' shaped palate not preferred?**
   A high 'V' shaped palate is usually associated with thick bulky ridges. The force of adhesion and cohesion are not at right angles to surface when counteracting the normal displacing forces of gravity. Hence retention is compromised in these cases.
8. **What are the functions of rugae?**
   Rugae aids in speech as well as enables tongue to make seal when it is pressed against the palate while making linguopalatal consonants. They are associated with sense of taste and also aids tongue to absorb fluid containing flavors.
9. **Classify soft palate.**
   According to Milsap soft palate is classified into:
   Class I : it is horizontal and forms 10 degree
   Class II : soft palate makes 45 degree angle to hard palate
   Class III : soft palate makes 75 degree angle to hard palate.
10. **Classify cosmetic index.**
    Class I- high cosmetic index patients
    Class II- average cosmetic index patients
    Class III-medium cosmetic index patients.
11. **How will you manage a mandibular tori?**
    The mandibular tori should be surgically removed as the mucosa over it is very thin.
12. **What is the approximate force applied by the muscles of mastication during contraction and which muscle attachments are seen superiror in a highly resorped ridges?**
    400 lb is the appropriate force of muscles of mastication. Attachements of mylohyoid, genioglossus and buccinator muscles are seen superior in highly resorbed ridges.

## CHAPTER -3 ANATOMIC LANDMARKS

1. **What is the mean denture bearing area of maxillary and mandibular arch?**
   The mean denture bearing area of maxillary arch is 22.96 $cm^2$ and of mandibular arch is 12.25 $cm^2$.
2. **What are the limiting structures of maxillary and mandibular arch?**
   The limiting structures of maxillary arch is labial frenum, labial sulcus, buccal frenum, buccal sulcus, hamular notch and PPS.
   The limiting structures of mandibular arch is labial frenum, labial sulcus, buccal frenum, buccal sulcus, distobuccal region, retromolar pad, lingual frenum and alveolingual sulcus.
3. **What are the supporting structures of maxillary and mandibular arch?**
   The supporting structures of maxillary arch are the crests and slopes of maxillary arch, rugae, anterior palate and posteriolateral slopes of hard palate.
   The supporting structures of mandibular arch are the crest and slopes of residual alveolar ridge, retromolar pad and the buccal shelf area.
4. **What is the primary and secondary stress bearing areas of maxillary and mandibular arch?**
   The primary stress bearing areas of maxillary arch is crest of residual alveolar ridge and posteriolateral aspect of hard palate. The primary stress bearing areas of mandibular arch is buccal shelf area.

5. **What are the relief areas of maxillary and mandibular arch?**
The relief areas of the maxillary arch are incisive papillae and midpalatine raphe. The relief areas of the mandibular arch is the crest of residual alveolar ridge, mental foramen and mylohyoid ridge.
6. **What are the contents of retromolar pad and what is its relevance in complete denture construction?**
Retromolar pad is a pear-shaped pad which forms the posterior seal of the mandibular denture. It consists of glandular tissue and fibers of temporalis posteriorly, buccinator laterally and medially by the pterygomandibular raphe and superior constrictor. The muscles determine the denture extension as well as prevent the application of excessive pressure during impression making. Hence the denture base should be extended only to two-third of the retromolar pad. It also helps in determining the height of occlusal plane and also provide retention of lower denture.
7. **What is pterygomandibular raphe?**
Pterygomandibular raphe is a tendon arising from hamular process of medial pterygoid and attached to mylohyoid ridge. Superior constrictor and buccinator is inserted to the pterygomandibular raphe. Overextension causes inflammation of tissues, soreness of throat and falling of denture.
8. **What is masseteric notch?**
Masseteric notch is a notch or depression seen on the distobuccal region of mandibular arch which is due to the influence of masseter over buccinator.
9. **What is retromylohyoid curtain?**
Retromylohyoid curtain forms the posterior extension of the retromylohyoid fossa. It is formed posteriolaterally by superior constrictor, posteriomedially by palatoglossal muscle and lateral surface of tongue and inferiorly by submandibular gland and mylohyoid muscle.

## CHAPTER -4 TMJ MANDIBULAR MOVEMENTS

1. **Classify mandibular movements?**
Based on type it is classified into hinge movement, protrusive movement, retrusive movement and lateral movements.
2. **What is border movement?**
The extreme movements of mandible are called the border movements.
3. **What is Bennett movement?**
Bennett movement is defined as the condylar movement on the working side in horizontal plane. Introduced by *Norman Godfrey Bennett*, British Dental Surgeon.
4. **What is immediate side shift?**
During lateral movement of mandible, the condyle on the non-working side condyle moves forward by 0.75 mm and this is called immediate side shift.
5. **What is Bennett angle?**
Bennett angle is defined as the angle formed between the sagittal plane and the average path of advancing condyle as viewed in horizontal plane during lateral mandibular movements.

6. **When do you get shield pattern?**
   The border movement of mandible recorded in the frontal plane.
7. **When do you get diamond tracing?**
   The border movement of mandible recorded in the horizontal plane.
8. **What pattern do you get during chewing?**
   Tear drop pattern.
9. **What is Posselt's envelope?**
   The border movements of mandible in all three planes were put together by Posselt. Hence, it is called as Posselt's envelope.

## CHAPTER -5 COMPLETE DENTURE OCCLUSION

1. **What are the various occlusal schemes?**
   - Balanced occlusion
   - Neutrocentric concept of occlusion
   - Lingualized occlusion.
2. **What is Bonwill's triangle?**
   Bonwill's triangle is an eponym for a 4 inch equilateral triangle bounded by lines connecting the contact points of mandibular central incisors incisal edge or midline of the mandibular residual ridge to each condyle and from one condyle to other, first described by Bonwill in 1858 while introducing his anatomic articulator.
3. **Define and classify compensatory curve. What is its function?**
   Compensatory curve is defined as the anteroposterior curving and mediolateral curving within the alignment of occluding surface and incisal edges of artificial teeth that is used to develop balanced occlusion. They are classified into anterior posterior curves and mediolateral curves. Curve of Spee is the anterior posterior curve while curve of Monson and curve of anti-Monson are the mediolateral curves incorporated in complete denture construction. It is used to provide balanced occlusion in complete denture when mandible is protruded.
4. **What is lingualized occlusion?**
   Lingualised occlusion is a form of denture occlusion articulates with the maxillary lingual cusps with the mandibular occlusal surfaces in centric working and non-working mandibular positions. It was put forward by Payne.
5. **What is monoplane occlusion?**
   Monoplane occlusion is an occlusal arrangement wherein the posterior teeth have masticatory surfaces that lack any cusp height.
6. **What is the length of each sides in Bonwill's equilateral theory of occlusion?**
   Four inches
7. **What is the amount of discrepancy allowed between centric relation and centric occlusion?**
   0.5–1 mm.
8. **In Monson theory of occlusion, what should be the diameter of the sphere?**
   Eight inches.

## CHAPTER -6 RESIDUAL RIDGE RESORPTION AND PRE-PROSTHETIC SURGERY

1. **What is residual ridge?**
   Residual ridge is that the portion of the residual bone and its soft tissue covering that remains after the removal of teeth.
2. **Define RRR.**
   Residual ridge resorption (RRR) is the term used for the diminishing quantity and quality of the residual ridge after teeth are removed.
3. **What is the pattern of resorption of edentulous mandible?**
   In mandible the resorption pattern is on lingual aspect in posterior region and labial aspect in anterior region.
4. **What are the various factors responsible for RRR?**
   1. Anatomic Factors: Quantity and quality of bone, type of bone and density of bone
   2. Metabolic Factors: Local resorption factors-endotoxins from plaque, osteoclast activating factor,prostaglandins. Heparin is a cofactor in causing resorption.
   3. Mechanical Factor: Force distribution and damping effect of underlying tissues.
5. **Which radiographic technique is used to determine the amount of RRR?**
   Wical and Swoope's panoramic radiographic technique.
6. **What is the mean ratio of anterior maxillary RRR to anterior mandibular RRR?**
   1:4
7. **What is the difference between alveoloplasty and alveolectomy?**
   Alveoloplasty is the surgical reshaping of the excess bone and alveolectomy is the surgical reduction of excess bone.
8. **Classify various ridge augmentation procedures.**
   Ridge augmentation procedures are Visor osteotomy, Onlay border grafting, Inter-positional bone grafting and Inferior border grafting of mandible.
9. **What are the various ridge extension procedures?**
   Ridge extension procedures are Vestibuloplasty, Transpositional vestibuloplasty, Maxillary submucosal vestibuloplasty and Vestibuloplasty with skin grafting.
10. **What are the impression procedures for highly resorbed ridges?**
    Lingual flange and sublingual flange techniques.

## CHAPTER -7 GAGGING

1. **What are the various factors causing gag?**
   Systemic disorders, psychologic factors, physiologic factors and intraoral stimuli.
2. **What are the pharmacologic techniques to reduce gag?**
   Topical local anesthetic, alcohol injection, centrally acting drugs like antihistamine, sedatives, tranqulizers and antidepressants are used to reduce gag.
3. **Name few general techniques to reduce gag?**
   Two milliliter anesthetic solution can be injected to lower labial frenum or sprinkle table salt at tip of tongue for 5 seconds before impression making.

## CHAPTER -8 IMPRESSION

1. **Define impression.**
   Impression is defined as a negative likeness or copy in reverse of the surface of an object; an imprint of teeth and adjacent structures for use in dentistry.
2. **Define impression tray.**
   Impression tray is defined as a device that is used to carry, confine and control impression material while making an impression.
3. **What are the theories of impression making?**
   The mucocompressive theory, mucostatic theory and selective pressure theory are the various theories of impression making.
4. **What are the various materials used for making primary impression?**
   Impression compound, alginate, silicone impression material.
5. **Define secondary impression.**
   Secondary impression is the negative likeness made for the purpose of fabrication of prosthesis.
6. **Define border molding and what are the various techniques to perform border molding?**
   The shaping of border areas of an impression material by functional or manual manipulation of the soft tissue adjacent to the borders to duplicate the contour and size of vestibule.
7. **Name the muscles influencing buccal frenum?**
   Caninus, depressor anguli oris.
8. **What are the various materials used for fabrication of special tray?**
   Shellac, autopolymerization acrylic resin, vacuum formed trays.
9. **What are the various materials used for making spacer?**
   Base plate wax, tin foil, non-asbestos ring liner.
10. **What is the purpose of a spacer?**
    Spacer provides space for impression material.
11. **What should be the thickness of a spacer?**
    The ideal thickness of a spacer should be 2 mm.
12. **What are the various materials used for making secondary impression?**
    Metallic oxide paste, addition silicon impression material.
13. **Why is zinc oxide eugenol used in making master impression?**
    Zinc oxide eugenol records the palatal tissues more accurately as it does not absorb the mucus secretion. It can also record the border accuarately as the material is more plastic in nature.
14. **Name an impression procedure for flabby ridge.**
    Open window technique.
15. **Which among the factors of retention is considered as the emergency retentive force?**
    Atmospheric pressure is considered as the emergency retentive force or temporary retaining force and is about 14.7 lb/inch$^2$.

16. **Which impression is made first, mandibular or maxillary impression?**
There will be excessive accumulation of saliva in the floor of the mouth during impression making procedure. Hence mandibular impression is made first. In case of maxillary impression, there will be gagging sensation for the patient, hence it is preferred to do mandibular impression first.

## CHAPTER -9 POSTERIOR PALATAL SEAL

1. **Define PPS.**
Posterior palatal seal (PPs) area is defined as the soft tissue area at or beyond the junction of the hard and soft palates on which pressure within physiologic limits can be applied by a complete removable dental prosthesis to aid in retention.
2. **What are the parts of PPS?**
PPS area is divided into two parts—the pterygomaxillary region and the post-palatal seal area. The post-palatal seal area is that part of PPS that extends between two maxillary tuberosity.
3. **Describe the boundaries of PPS.**
PPS is bounded anteriorly by anterior vibrating line (AVL), posteriorly by posterior vibrating line (PVL) and laterally by hamular notches.
4. **What is the ideal dimensions of posterior palatal seal area?**
PPS is 1-1.5 mm high and 1.5 mm broad.
5. **What are the type of mouth temperature waxes used to record PPS?**
Korecta wax No. 4, IOWA. HL Physiologic paste, Adaptol.
6. **What are the various methods to record PPS?**
Conventional method, fluid wax method and extended palatal technique.
7. **Why is the patient asked to bend the head at 30 degree while recoding PPS?**
The depression of the PPS is maximum when the Frankfort horizontal plane is 30 degree below the horizontal plane and the tongue is firmly positioned against the mandibular anterior teeth.Hence patient is asked to bent the head at 30 degree while recording PPS.
8. **What is post-damming?**
Post-damming is method to record depressibility of PPS.
9. **What is the common cause of failure of seal?**
Under extension of posterior border.

## CHAPTER -10 ARTICULATORS

1. **Define articulators.**
A mechanical instrument that represents the temporomandibular joints and jaws, to which maxillary and mandibular casts are attached to simulate some or all mandibular movements.
2. **What is the differences between arcon and non-arcon articulators?**
ARCON ARTICULATOR is an articulator that applies the arcon design; this instrument maintains anatomic guidelines by the use of condylar analogs in the mandibular element

and fossa assemblies within the maxillary elements while a non-arcon articulator has the condylar analogs in the upper member and fossa in lower member.

3. **Who coined the word "ARCON"?**
   Bergstrom coined the word "ARCON" which stands for articulator condyle.
4. **Define fully adjustable articulator with example?**
   Fully adjustable articulator is an articulator that allows replication of three-dimensional movement of recorded mandibular motion.
   E.g.: Denar D5A, TMJ stereographs.
5. **Which Hanau's principle is applied in Hanau articulators?**
   Bennett angle (L) = H/8 +12, where H is the horizontal condylar guidance.
6. **Define condylar guidance.**
   The mechanical form located in upper posterior region of an articulator that controls movement of its mobile member is called condylar guidance.
7. **Define incisal guidance.**
   Incisal guidance is defined as the influence of the contacting surfaces of the guide pin and guide table on articular movements OR the influence on mandibular movements caused by the contacting surfaces of the mandibular and maxillary anterior teeth during eccentric excursions.
8. **Why three point articulator is called mean value articulator?**
   A three point articulator is based on Bonwills theory of occlusion. Here the distance between two condylar analogs and, the distance between the condylar analogs and incisal pin is considered to be a mean value of four inches. Since three points are used in fabrication, it is also called three point articulator.
9. **Name few semi-adjustable articulators.**
   Hanau wide vue, Whipmix articulator, Denar Mark II.

## CHAPTER -11 PHONETICS

1. **Define speech.**
   Speech is a sophisticated, autonomous and unconscious activity of producing sound.
2. **Classify sounds.**
   Bilabial, labiodental sounds, lingua-alvoeslar sound, linguopalatal sounds and velar sounds
3. **Name some labiodental sounds?**
   F,V, and p are the labiodental sounds.
4. **If the thickness of the denture base is more in anterior region pronunciation of which syllables are affected?**
   S, t, d, n and z.
5. **Which sound is affected if there is change in the length of the upper anterior teeth?**
   F and v.
6. **Which is called the pounds syllable?**
   "s"

## CHAPTER -12 JAW RELATION

1. **Define jaw relation.**
   Jaw relation or maxillo mandibular relation is defined as any spatial relationship of the maxillae to the mandible.
2. **Define denture base.**
   Denture base is defined as the portion of a denture that supports the artificial dentition and replaces the alveolar structures and gingival tissues.
3. **What are the modifications to be done to an occlusal rim prior to jaw relation?**
   Adjust fullness, visibility or low lip line, high lip line, anterior and posterior plane of occlusion.
4. **What is high lip line?**
   High lip line is the greatest height to which the inferior border of the upper lip is capable of being raised by muscle function.
5. **Define occlusal plane.**
   Occlusal plane is the average plane established by incisal and occlusal surfaces of the teeth.
6. **Define occlusal rim.**
   Occlusal rim is the occluding surfaces fabricated on interim or final denture bases for the purpose of making maxillomandibular relation records and arranging teeth.
7. **What are the various mechanical methods of determining vertical dimension?**
   1. Ridge relation
      - Distance from the incisive papilla to mandibular incisors
      - Parallelism of ridges
   2. Pre-extraction method
      - Profile photographs
      - Profile silhouettes
      - Radiographs
      - Articulated casts
      - Facial measurements.
   3. Mesurement of former denture.
8. **What is closest speaking space?**
   Closest speaking space is the space between the anterior teeth that, according to Dr. Earl Pound, should not be more or less that 1 to 2 mm of clearance between the incisal edges of the teeth when the patient is unconsciously repeating the letter "S".
9. **Define centric relation.**
   Centric relation is defined as the maxillomandibular relationship in which the condyles articulates with the thinnest avascular portion of their respective discs with the complex in the anterior-superior against the shapes of the articular eminencies. This position is independent of tooth contact. This position is clinically discernible when the mandible is directed superior and anteriorly. It is restricted to a purely rotatory movement about the transverse horizontal axis.

10. **What is Christensens phenomenon?**
Christensens phenomenon is the space between opposing occlusal surface during mandibular protrusion.
11. **What are the two concepts of recording centric relation?**
Concept of minimal closing pressure and heavy closing pressure.
12. **What are the methods to record centric relation (CR)?**
Static method and functional method.
13. **Name few functional methods.**
Needle house and Patterson's technique.
14. **Which is one of the most accurate method of determining CR?**
Graphic method.
15. **What are the various types of tracers for recording centric relation?**
*Extraoral tracers:* Height extraoral tracers, Sears extraoral tracers.
*Intraoral tracers:* Microtracers, Cobble tracer.

## CHAPTER -13 NEUTRAL ZONE

1. **Define neutral zone.**
NEUTRAL ZONE is the potential space between the lips and the cheek on one side and the tongue on the other; that area or portion where the forces between the tongue and cheeks or lips are equal.
2. **What are the various methods to record neutral zone?**
Phonetics and physiologic method.
3. **What are the various materials used to record neutral zone?**
Impression compound and tissue conditioners.

## CHAPTER -14 FACE-BOW

1. **Define face-bow.**
A caliper like instrument used to record the spatial relationship of the maxillary arch to some anatomic reference point or points and then transfer this relationship to an articulator, it orients the dental cast in the same relationship to the opening axis of the articulator.
2. **What is the purpose of doing face-bow transfer?**
Face-bow is used to record the axis-orbital plane. It also records the arc of closure of mandible against the maxillae or base of cranium. It also determines the orientation of maxillae to base of skull.
3. **Define hinge axis?**
Hinge axis is an imaginary line around which the mandible may rotate within the sagittal plane.
4. **How is hinge axis located in an edentulous patients?**
Hinge axis is located accurately using a kinematic face-bow or a hinge-axis locator. It can be recorded approximately using an arbitrary type facebow. In completely edentulous patients, hinge axis is recorded using arbitrary face-bow. The kinematic face-bow cannot be used in edentulous patients as this bow is attached to mandibular rim. This results

in movement of denture bases causing instability which further leads to inaccurate recording of hinge axis.

5. **How is occlusal plane determined?**
   Posterior occlusal plane is determined by the ala tragal line or relation with Stensen duct and anterior plane using lower lip as a reference plane.
6. **What is Frankfort horizontal plane?**
   It is a plane established by the lowest point on the margin of the right or left bony orbit and the highest point on the margin of right or left auditory meatus.
7. **Name some anterior reference points.**
   Nasion, infraorbital notch.
8. **Name some posterior reference points.**
   Beyron's point, Bergstrom's point, Gysi point, Teteruck-Lundeen's point, Prothero's point.
9. **What is Beyron's point?**
   Beyron's point is a posterior reference point, which is 13 mm anterior to posterior margin of tragus on a line from the center of tragus to outer canthus.
10. **What is Bergstrom's point?**
    Bergstrom's point is a posterior reference point which is 10 mm anterior to the center of spherical insert of the face-bow and 7 mm below FH plane.
11. **What is the difference between arbitrary and kinematic face-bows?**
    Kinematic facebow is used in full mouth rehabilitation procedure or in-fixed partial denture procedure whereas arbitrary bow is used in complete denture procedures. Kinematic facebow is fixed to clutches attached to mandible while arbitrary facebow is fixed to maxillary arch.

## CHAPTER -15 TEETH SELECTION AND TRY-IN

1. **What is Berry biometric index?**
   - The width of the maxillary central incisor = Bizygomatic width/16
   - The width of the maxillary central incisor = Length of the face/ 20.
2. **What is Pounds formula?**
   - The width of the maxillary central incisor = Bizygomatic width/16
   - The length of the maxillary central incisor = Length of the face /16
4. **What is Leon Williams theory?**
   Leon Williams in 1917 formulated the "Typal form theory" which states that, "the shape of the teeth should be like the shape of face."
5. **What are the factors which determine the posterior teeth selection?**
   Posterior teeth selection is based on: (1) size of teeth which depends on the capacity of ridges to receive and resist forces of mastication, space available for teeth and esthetic requirements. Space available for posterior teeth depends on the mesiodistal teeth and the interridge space, (2) shade of teeth and (3) tooth material.
6. **Classify posterior teeth form.**
   - Posterior teeth is classified based on cusp angle into:
   - Anatomic- teeth with cusp angle of 33 degree
   - Semianatomic- teeth with cusp angle of 20 degree
   - Non-anatomc form- teeth with cusp angle of 0 degree.

7. **What should be the buccolingual width of the posterior teeth?**
   The buccolingual width of the posterior teeth should be less than the width of the natural teeth that they replace. This reduces the width of the occlusal table, thereby helps in developing a proper polished surface of the denture which reduces the stress on the supporting tissues.
8. **What are the indications of non-anatomic teeth?**
   Non-anatomic teeth is indicated in highly resorbed ridges, knife edge ridges, if inter- ridge distance is more, in bruxers, in patients with neuromuscular disorders and in debilitated patients.

## CHAPTER -16 DENTURE INSERTION AND POST-INSERTION INSTRUCTIONS

1. **Why is the patient asked not to wear the previous denture for at least 24 hours before impression making?**
   This is to avoid the distortion of the tissues by the old denture which will result in occlusal errors and fit.
2. **If there is defective contact in centric relation, then how will you perform selective grinding?**
   Reduce fossa or marginal ridge.
3. **What is BULL's law?**
   Upper buccal cusp and lower lingual cusp can be selectively trimmed in case of occlusal correction as these cusps are nonfunctional cusps.
4. **When will you do selective grinding based on BULL's law?**
   BULL's law is followed if there is deflective contact on working side.
5. **After denture insertion if the patient complains of difficulty in swallowing, what would be the cause?**
   Difficulty in swallowing can be due to increased VD, over extension of the lingual flange in the lateral throat form and overextension in the PPS.
6. **What is the cause of generalized soreness in the crest of the ridge?**
   Increased vertical dimension.
7. **What is the reason for burning sensation in the anterior third of palate?**
   This is due to inadequate relief of incisive papillae.
8. **What type of denture cleansers are preferred for acrylic dentures?**
   Soak the denture in alkaline hypochlorite solution for 2 minutes in the evening.
9. **What is the composition of denture adhesives?**
   Karaya Gum, Tragacanth or Sodium Carboxymethyl cellulose, antimicrobial agents, the additives, the plasticizing agent, the wetting agent and the flavoring agents.

## CHAPTER -17 POST-INSERTION COMPLETE DENTURE PROBLEMS AND THEIR MANAGEMENT

1. **Classify the factors causing problems after denture insertion.**
   - Adverse intraoral anatomical factors, e.g. atrophic mucosa.
   - Clinical factors, e.g. poor denture stability.
   - Technical factors, e.g. failure to preserve the peripheral roll on a master cast.
   - Patient adaptional factors.

2. **What are the two common problems associated with basal seat mucosa after complete denture insertion?**
   - Hypertrophy—associated with midpalatal suture area (papilloma-like hypertrophy) and incisive papilla area.
   - Inflammation—as a result of constant wear of the denture, insufficient interocclusal distance, loosely attached or detached submucosa in the mandibular lingual side, a complete denture opposed by natural teeth, an unbalanced diet, endocrine disturbances, systemic debilitating diseases and allergic reactions.
3. **What are the causes of abrasions appearing on the mucosa of cheeks and lips?**
   - Cheek biting
   - Rough margins on the teeth
   - Unpolished denture bases.
4. **Causes of ulcerations and other lesions appearing on the margins and apex of tongue.**
   - Tongue biting caused by improper placement of teeth either in vertical or horizontal position (lack of lingual overjet).
   - An unpolished denture base or a too pronounced rugae area.
   - Rough margins on the teeth.
5. **What is bone sore mouth?**
   - This is a rare condition seen in senile patients following denture use and is characterized by normal appearing mucosa, but a feeling of constant soreness and urge to remove the denture whenever possible. They also possess the desire to remove glasses from nose as well as shoe from the foot.
6. **What are the causes of dislodgement of maxillary denture when the jaws are at rest?**
   - Underfilled buccal vestibule
   - Inadequate border seal
   - Excessive saliva
   - Xerostomia.
7. **Causes for clicking with complete dentures.**
   - Insufficient interocclusal distance.
   - A dropping of maxillary denture.
   - Vertical displacement of mandibular denture.
8. **Commonest cause of epulis fissuratum.**
   Over extended denture borders.
9. **Causes for commissural cheilitis.**
   - Excessive interocclusal distance.
   - Maxillary posterior teeth set closer to cheeks, saliva collects at the neck of the teeth and makes its escape at the canines.
   - Too high an occlusal plane preventing the regular action of cheek in eliminating the saliva from the lower buccal vestibule, causing saliva to exit through the corners of the mouth, i.e. drooling results.
10. **Causes for gagging.**
   - Loose dentures, poor occlusion,
   - Incorrect extension or contour in the posterior area of the palate and the retromylohyoid space, underextended denture borders,

- Incorrect positioning of teeth causing dorsum of the tongue to be forced into the pharynx during swallowing,
- Increased vertical dimension of occlusion
- Psychogenic factors.

11. **Classification of burning mouth syndrome (Lamey and Lewis, 1989).**
    Type I–There are no symptoms on waking. A burning sensation then commences and becomes worse as the day progresses. This pattern occurs every day (33%).
    Type II–Burning is present on waking and persists throughout the day. This pattern occurs everyday (55%).
    Type III–Patients have symptom free days. Burning occurs in less usual sites such as the floor of the mouth, the throat and the buccal mucosa (12%).
12. **Causes for generalized pain over denture supporting area.**
    Under extended denture
    Increased vertical dimension.
13. **Pain about the periphery of the denture with the pain increasing as the day progresses with associated pain in the masseter and temporalis muscle is classically seen in relation to———.**
    Increased vertical dimension.
14. **Pain in the posterior aspect of the upper denture upon opening.**
    Too thick flange on the buccal aspect of tuberosity limiting the mobility of coronoid process.
15. **Causes of midline fractures of dentures.**
    **Denture factors**
    - Stress concentrators (scratches, median diastema and a deep frenal notch)
    - Absence of a labial flange
    - Incomplete polymerization of acrylic resin
    - Previous repair
    - Shape of the teeth on the denture
    - Poor fit
    - Lack of adequate relief.

    **Patient factors**
    - Anatomical factors
    - High occlusal loads.

## CHAPTER –18 SEQUELAE CAUSED BY WEARING COMPLETE DENTURES

1. **What are the direct sequelae caused by wearing removable prosthesis?**
    - Mucosal reactions
    - Oral galvanic currents
    - Altered taste perception
    - Burning mouth syndrome
    - Gagging
    - Residual ridge reduction
    - Periodontal disease (abutments)
    - Caries (abutments).

**2. What are the indirect sequelae of wearing complete dentures?**

- Atrophy of masticatory muscles
- Nutritional deficiencies.

**3. Synonyms for denture stomatitis.**

- Denture induced stomatitis
- Denture sore mouth
- Inflammatory papillary hyperplasia.
- Chronic atrophic candidiasis.

**4. Newton's classification of denture stomatitis.**

- Type I—A localized simple inflammation or pinpoint hyperemia.
- Type II—An erythematous or generalized simple type seen as more diffuse erythema involving a part or the entire denture covered mucosa.
- Type III—A granular type (inflammatory papillary hyperplasia) commonly involving the central part of the hard palate and the alveolar ridges. Type III is often seen in association with Type I or Type II.

Type I is often trauma induced. Type II and Type III due to microbial plaque accumulation.

**5. How will you diagnose *Candida*-associated denture stomatitis?**

Presence of mycelia or pseudohyphae in a direct smear or the isolation of *Candida* species in high numbers from the lesions ( ≥ 50 colonies).

**6. What are the factors predisposing to *Candida*-associated denture stomatitis?**

| **Systemic Factors** | **Local Factors** |
|---|---|
| Old age | Dentures (changes in environmental conditions, trauma, denture usage, denture cleanliness) |
| Diabetes mellitus | Xerostomia (Sjogren's syndrome, irradiation, drug therapy) |
| Nutritional deficiencies (iron, folate or Vit $B_{12}$) | High carbohydrate diet |
| Malignancies (acute leukemia, agranulocytosis) | Broad spectrum antibiotics |
| Immune defects | Smoking tobacco |
| Corticosteroids, immunosuppressive drugs | |

**7. How will you manage a case diagnosed as Candida-associated denture stomatitis?**

- Institution of efficient oral and denture hygiene.
- Correction of denture wearing habits.
- Antifungal drugs (especially local therapy with nystatin, amphotericin B, miconazole or clotrimazole).
- Surgical elimination of deep crypts formed by Type III denture stomatitis.
- Correction of ill-fitting dentures.
- Efficient plaque control.

**8. Differentiate between burning mouth sensations and burning mouth syndrome (BMS).**

**In burning mouth sensation,** the patients mucosae are often inflamed due to mechanical irritation, infection or allergic reaction. Whereas in burning mouth syndrome (BMS) patients the oral mucosa appears clinically healthy.

**9. Symptoms associated with BMS.**

- Symptoms have a gradual onset. Pain present in the morning and tends to become aggravated during the day.
- Quality of pain is a burning sensation associated with a feeling of dry mouth and persistent altered taste sensation.
- Other associated symptoms include headache, insomnia, decreased libido, irritability or depression.

**10. Etiological factors associated with BMS**

| Local Factors | Systemic Factors | Psychogenic Factors |
|---|---|---|
| Mechanical irritation | Vitamin deficiency | Depression |
| Allergy | Iron deficiency anemia | Anxiety |
| Infection | Xerostomia | Psychosocial stresses |
| Oral habits and parafunction | Menopause | |
| Myofascial pain | Diabetes | |
| | Parkinson's disease | |
| | Medication | |

**11. Trigger centers for gagging.**

Soft palate, uvula, the posterior dorsal part of the tongue and the fauces or posterior pharyngeal wall.

**12. What are the causes of persistent gagging in complete denture wearers ?**

- Overextended borders, especially in the posterior part of the maxillary denture and the distolingual part of the mandibular denture.
- Poor retention of the maxillary denture.
- Unstable occlusal conditions.
- Increased vertical dimension.

**13. Etiological factors for reduction of residual ridges.**

- Anatomical Factors
  - › More important in the mandible versus the maxilla
  - › Short and square face associated with elevated masticatory forces
  - › Alveoloplasty
- Prosthodontic Factors
  - › Intensive denture wearing
  - › Unstable occlusal conditions
  - › Immediate denture treatment
- Metaboloic and Systemic Factors
  - › Osteoporosis
  - › Calcium and Vitamin D supplements for possible bone preservation.

**14. What are the consequences of residual ridge reduction?**

- Loss of sulcus width and depth
- Displacement of muscle attachment closer to the crest
- Loss of vertical dimension of occlusion
- Reduction of lower face height

- Anterior rotation of mandible and increase in relative prognathia
- Changes in interalveolar ridge relationship (which is essentially centripetal in the maxilla and centrifugal in the mandible)
- Morphological changes of the alveolar bone such as sharp, spiny uneven residual ridges and location of the mental foramina close to the top of the residual ridge.

## CHAPTER – 19 RELINING AND REBASING

1. **Define relining.**
   The procedures used to resurface the tissue side of a removable dental prosthesis with new base material, thus producing an accurate adaptation to the denture foundation area (GPT 8).
2. **Define rebasing.**
   The laboratory process of replacing the entire denture base material on an existing prosthesis (GPT 8).
3. **What are the clinical changes manifested in the supporting tissues that warrant a reline, rebase or a remake?**
   - Loss of retention and stability
   - Loss of VDO
   - Loss of support for facial tissues
   - Horizontal shift of dentures : incorrect occlusal relationship
   - Reorientation of occlusal plane
   - Minimal to moderate changes warrant a reline , whereas moderate to maximal changes need a rebase. If the vertical dimension is reduced by 2-3 mm and the centric relation is incorrect to a large degree, then denture should be remade.
4. **Why there is a forward displacement of the mandible with loss of vertical dimension?**
   Closure of the mandible is a rotary movement around an imaginary axis passing through the condyles. As the mandible rotates to a closed position without translation of the condyles, it frequently moves forwards as the space between the maxillae and the mandible is reduced. As a result centric relation position of the condyle may be retained but the occlusion may not be correct in the patients mouth.
5. **What is the main problem associated with relining and rebasing?**
   Alteration of jaw relationships.
6. **Classify relining techniques.**
   A. Clinical Procedures
      1. Static impression technique
         › Open mouth
         › Closed mouth
      2. Functional impression technique
      3. Chair side impression technique
   B. Laboratory Procedures
      1. Articulator method
      2. Jig method.
         Jectron jig, Hooper duplicator
      3. Flask method

7. **What are the various static impression techniques?**
   - Open mouth technique or Technique F (Boucher, 1973)
   - Closed mouth techniques
     - › Maxillary
       - » Technique A (Shaffer FW, Filler WH, 1971)
       - » Technique B (Hansen NJ, 1964)
       - » Technique C (Christensen FT, 1971)
       - » Technique D (Jordan LG, 1972)
     - › Mandibular
       - » Technique E (Gillis RR, 1960)
8. **Minimum acceptable thickness of tissue conditioner.**
   1-1.5 mm
9. **Uses of tissue conditioner material.**
   - Tissue treatment
   - For lining surgical splints
   - For stabilizing a record base
   - Functional impression material.
10. **Impression materials used for relining and rebasing.**
    - Zinc oxide eugenol paste
    - Wouth temperature waxes
    - Plaster of Paris
    - Elastomers
    - Tissue conditioner or fluid resin (functional impression technique, Hydrocast)
    - Visible light cured resin.
11. **What special preparation is done for the denture in Technique A and why?**
    A large part of the middle of the palatal portion of the maxillary denture is removed during impression making. This allows better seating of the maxillary denture and alleviate the increase in vertical dimension.
12. **Classify soft denture liners.**
    - Short term liner – Used intraorally for up to 30 days (ISO 10139-1:1991)
      E.g., Coe-Comfort (GC America), Softone (Bosworth)
    - Intermediate liners – Used for 1-6 months
    - Long term liners – Used for more than one year (ISO 10139-2:1991)
      E.g., Molloplast-B (Buffalo).
13. **What are the commonly used soft denture lining materials?**
    a. Plasticized acrylic resins—They may be heat cured or chemically cured.
    b. Silicones—Heat cured liners (Molloplast-B, Silastic 390, 616) and those vulcanized at room temperature.
    c. Vinyl resins (polyvinyl chloride and polyvinyl acetate).
    d. Polyurethane, Polyphosphazine.
14. **What are tissue conditioners?**
    Chemically-activated plasticized acrylic resin liners are known as short term soft liners or tissue conditioners. They may be comprised of poly(ethylmethacrylate) mixture of phthalate plasticizer and upto 25% ethanol. Powder—PEMA, Liquid—Ethyl alcohol solvent and Butylphthalylbutylglycolate. Liquid component contains no monomer and

the powder no initiator. When powder and liquid are mixed together a purely physical process occurs. The final set material is gel-like. With swollen plasticized spheres being cemented together with a matrix which is a saturated solution of polymer in a solvent/ plasticizer mixture. The large size of the plasticizer minimises entanglement of polymer chains allowing individual chains to slip past each other resulting in rapid changes in shape of soft liner. The plasticizer lowers the glass transition temperature (Tg) of resin below that of mouth temperature rendering it rubbery and resilient. If poly(methyl methacrylate) is replaced with higher methacrylates (e.g., ethyl, n-propyl and n-butyl), the Tg becomes progressively lower. Hence the amount of plasticizer can be reduced. Lowering of Tg temperature results in increased dimensional instability in the relined denture.

**15. What are the disadvantages of tissue conditioners?**

- Plasticized acrylics results in loss of plasticizers due to flushing action of saliva and hardens over a period of time.
- Surface becomes rough and irritating to mucosa.
- There will be food entrapment and absorption of cleanser component resulting in discoloration.

**16. What are the disadvantages of silicone liners?**

- Lack of bonding between the silicone liner and the acrylic resin base material. High incidence of fungal growth on and within processed soft liners.
- It is difficult to adjust or alter cured silicone.
- Patient abuse of the liner from poor home care habits and the use of improper cleansers.
- The use of hypochlorite solutions that are too strong produced a bleaching and wrinkling of the silicone material. Associated with this there will be swelling of the material placing undue stress on the supporting mucosa.
- If the hard soft junction is irregular or insecure, there may be accumulation of calculus, especially in the mandibular anterior lingual region.

**17. What are the physical stages of tissue conditioner material that make them useful as a reline material?**

- A tissue conditioner material passes through plastic and elastic stages before it sets into a hardened phase. In the initial stage, i.e. in the plastic stage, which lasts for few hours to few days, the denture base responds to functional and parafunctional stresses because the tissue conditioner permits movement of denture base in response to existing occlusion. Fit is also improved.
- In the elastic stage, lasting for 1–2 weeks, the stress is cushioned and recovery of the tissues takes place.
- In the firm stage which serves as the reline impression, the surface is similar to polymerized resin surface, except that it is vulnerable to deterioration.

**18. Why a new mix of tissue conditioner material is not being used as a final impression material for relining in functional impression technique?**

In the freshly mixed state, the material will be in the plastic or "self flow" stage, where the materials own weight may deform the impression. Moreover the weight of the stone poured can also cause distortion of the impression. Hence when there is minor surface deterioration of the impression, the areas should be trimmed with a carbide bur and secondary impression obtained with a light bodied material.

## CHAPTER - 20 GERIATRIC DENTISTRY

1. **What is the average life expectancy of females?**
   80 years.
2. **Average life expectancy of males.**
   73 years.
3. **Average energy consumption for 65-74 years old women.**
   1300 kcal.
4. **Factors affecting acceptability of food for denture wearers.**
   Texture and hardness of food.
5. **Saliva substitute that serves as a nutrient source and has excellent buffering capacity.**
   Milk.
6. **Residual ridge resorption is a manifestation of which type of osteoporosis?**
   Type I or post-menopausal osteoporosis.
7. **What are the effects of aging on the edentulous mouth?**

| | |
|---|---|
| Mucosa | • Stomatitis and mild inflammation<br>• Increased incidence of oral cancer due to increased atrophy, Increased mitosis with slow turnover of cells and increased number of elastic fibers. |
| Bone | • Bone quality decreases because osteoblasts are less efficient, estrogen production decreases and calcium absorption decreases.<br>• Resorption surpasses formation<br>• Osteoporosis |
| Saliva | • Hyposalivation of minor salivary gland of palate, food may have a metallic or salty taste, unpleasant sensitivity to bitter and sour foods and reduced sensitivity to sweet taste generate an unhealthy craving for food |
| Jaw movements | Chewing strokes are shortened and chewing time prolonged |
| Taste and smell | • Preferred taste in old age is sugar and salt<br>• Sensitivity to taste declines in disease conditions such as Alzheimer's<br>• Sense of taste is impaired in upper respiratory infection or neurological disorder |
| Skin | • Skin reveals wrinkles, puffiness and pigmentations<br>• Undesirable immunological responses are prevented due to fewer Langerhan's cells<br>• There will be mottling of skin which protects against sun<br>• Epidermis thickens, dermis thins, enzymes dissolves collagen and elastin and wrinkles appear when layers of fat are lost<br>• Concavity and pout of upper lip decreases and philtrum flattens<br>• Nasolabial groove deepens producing sagging to middle third of the face<br>• Atrophy of subcutaneous and buccal pad of fat hollows the cheeks<br>• Presymphyseal pad of fat disappears and upper lip droops |
| Teeth | • Jagged brownish appearance<br>• Incisal edges break and exposed dentin gathers extrinsic stains |

8. **How does protein loss manifest in the elderly?**
   As a decrease in skeletal muscle mass.

9. **Daily calcium requirement in elderly.**
   1000 mg per day.
10. **Daily protein requirement in elderly.**
    0.8 gm per kilogram body weight.
11. **Deficiencies in denture bearing tissues that account for prosthetic failures.**
    - Tissue dehydration caused by negative water balance in the elderly.
    - Calcium deficiency and excessive bone resorption (osteoporosis) especially in post-menopausal women.
    - Epithelial thinning and fragility of oral mucosa.
    - Muscle weakness resulting from inadequate intake of high quality protein and/or poor preparation of protein foods with poor digestion and absorption.

## CHAPTER -21 IMMEDIATE DENTURE

1. **Define immediate denture.**
   A complete or removable partial denture constructed for insertion immediately following the removal of natural teeth (GPT 8) .
2. **Classify immediate dentures.**
   - Conventional (or classic) immediate denture (CID)
   - After this immediate denture is placed and after healing is completed, the denture is refitted or relined to serve as the long term prosthesis
   - Interim (or transitional or nontraditional) immediate dentures (IID)
   - After this immediate denture is placed and after healing is completed, a second, new complete denture is fabricated as the long term prosthesis.
3. **Define interim prosthesis.**
   A prosthesis designed to enhance esthetics, stabilization and/or function for a limited period of time, after which it is replaced by a definitive prosthesis (Academy of Prosthodontics, 1999).
4. **What is a "jiffy" denture?**
   It is an abbreviated type of IID (described by Raczka and Esposito, 1995) which is fabricated in emergency situations. In this type of denture, "teeth" are usually made with tooth colored autopolymerising resin or from portions of patients preexisting partial removable or fixed prosthesis. This will later be replaced by a second complete denture after healing.
5. **Advantages of immediate denture.**
   - Prevent patient embarrassment, i.e. his/her psychological and social well being is preserved.
   - The digestive function is uninterrupted.
   - Minimal change in muscle tone and the occlusal vertical dimension can be maintained.
   - No development of unfavorable speech and chewing habits and tongue is not given a chance to enlarge.
   - Centric relation is easier to record.
   - Because the ridges are subjected to early function, less resorption

- Promote patient adaptation to dentures
- Provide protection to surgical site and less postoperative pain.
- Better duplication of the size and position of natural teeth.

6. **Disadvantages of immediate denture.**
   - Need for later reline or remake, usually within 6 months to a year.
   - The presence of anterior ridge undercut and remaining teeth in various locations may complicate the impression procedures and jaw relations of the posterior segment.
   - Increased treatment costs due to increased chair time, more appointments, post-operative adjustments and need to reline or remake.
   - Limit evaluation of anterior try in.
   - Increased patient discomfort.
7. **Compare and contrast CID and IID.**

| CID | IID |
|---|---|
| Better initial retention and stability | Retention and stability less at insertion (tissue conditioner proves useful) |
| Overall cost is less | More costly, because needs fabrication of new denture |
| Results in only one denture | Results in two dentures |
| 2 Surgical visits | Only one surgical visit |
| Period of posterior partial edentulism | All teeth or existing RPD retained until the day of extraction and insertion of denture |
| Takes longer to fabricate | Overall time is less |
| Easier surgical session on the second surgical visit | The single surgical visit for IID takes more chair time than that for a CID |
| Not useful for converting an existing RPD | Useful in converting an existing prosthesis to complete denture |

8. **Contraindications for immediate dentures.**
   - Patients with poor surgical risk or in poor health
   - Post-irradiation of head and neck region.
   - Systemic conditions that affect healing or blood clotting.
   - Cardiac disturbances.
   - Endocrine disorders.
   - Psychological disorders.
   - Uncooperative patients
   - When surgical correction of malrelated jaws is anticipated.
   - Excessively mobile teeth or teeth related to large abcess or cysts.
9. **Indications for immediate dentures.**

| CID | IID |
|---|---|
| Only anterior teeth are present or few posterior teeth remain that do not support an existing RPD | Multiple anterior and posterior teeth remaining |
| Indicated when patient can function without posterior teeth for approximately 3 months (3-4 weeks healing time and two months for fabrication) | These teeth support a RPD which the patient deserves to retain until insertion |

**10. Impression techniques for immediate denture.**

- **Single step technique using custom impression trays:**
- The undercuts and remaining teeth are blocked out and a custom tray covering teeth and edentulous ridge is fabricated. The tray is border molded and final impression made with an elastomeric impression material.
- **Double step technique using a combination of custom and stock trays:**
- Custom tray fabricated covering the residual ridge, palate and lingual surfaces of anterior teeth. Border molding done and final impression made using impression paste or light bodied elastomeric impression material. A second impression made over it with alginate in a stock tray.
- **Campagna impression technique (1968):**
  It utilizes a full arch tray with a hole cut where there are remaining anterior teeth. A stock tray is used over the full arch tray to capture the anterior teeth in the impression.

**11. How will you arrange anterior teeth in immediate dentures?**

Alternative or every other tooth set up – Remove one tooth at a time from the cast, allowing adjoining tooth to act as a guide.

Or

Remove the cuspid, lateral and central incisor from one side of the cast. The teeth on the opposite side will serve as a guide.

**12. Name guidelines that can be used for trimming the socket of anterior teeth.**

- Pocket depth, free gingival margins, a line marking the interproximal of each tooth and a drawing of where the new tooth position should be.
- Pocket depth (Jebri, 1966) can be used as a guide for trimming anterior socket. Facially the extraction site can be further trimmed conservatively to the pocket depth line. The lingual or palatal tissues should not be trimmed because they will not collapse to the pocket depth after extraction.

**13. What results in a knuckle-shaped residual ridge?**

Knuckle-shaped residual ridge results when the tissue conditioner used underneath the denture projects into the extraction sockets and interfere with the proper healing of the socket. The ridge will heal with small concavities overlying the extraction sites resulting in a knuckle-shaped ridge.

## CHAPTER – 22 TOOTH SUPPORTED OVERDENTURE

**1. Define overdenture.**

A removable partial or complete denture that covers and rests on one or more remaining natural teeth, the roots of natural teeth and/or dental implants; a prosthesis that covers and is partially supported by natural teeth, natural tooth roots, and /or dental implants (GPT 8).

**2. Synonyms for overdenture.**

Tooth supported complete denture, overlay denture, overlay prosthesis, superimposed prosthesis, telescopic denture, hybrid denture, biologic denture.

**3. Classification of overdenture.**

- According to Heartwell based on abutment preparation:
  - Noncoping
  - Coping – short and long
  - Attachments
- According to Morrow and Brewer:
  - Immediate
  - Transitional
  - Remote
- According to Prieskel
  - Transitional overdentures
  - Training overdentures
  - Immediate overdentures
  - Definitive overdenture.

**4. Goals of overdenture therapy.**

- It maintains teeth as part of residual ridge. This gives the patient a denture that has far more support than any conventional prosthesis
- Decrease in the rate of bone resorption
- An increase in the manipulative skills in handling the denture.

**5. Requirements of overdenture.**

- Maintenance of health of the underlying tooth structure
- A reduction in crown-root ratio
- A well fitting base to distribute the load over as wide an area as possible.
- Simplicity of construction
- Ease of manipulation.

**6. Advantages of overdenture.**

- Preservation of alveolar bone.
- Preservation of proprioceptive response.
- Extra support and retention.
- Patients with congenital defects such as cleft palate, partial anodontia, amelogenesis imperfecta, etc. can be treated.
- Periodontal maintenance possible easily if not splinted.
- Patient acceptance, cost effectiveness and convertibility are excellent.

**7. Disadvantages of overdenture.**

- Caries susceptibility
- Bony undercuts can pose a problem as close adaptation of denture flange is not possible.
- Poor esthetics: at times due to undercuts especially in the canine region one may have to excessively block out the region and this can lead to an overcontoured flange. If one prefers to underextend this area then peripheral seal may be compromised. To avoid this proper case selection is vital and also proper preparation of the underlying teeth.

- Encroachment of vertical space.
- Periodontal breakdown of abutment teeth.
- Increased cost of treatment.
- Increased bulk of prosthesis.

**8. Indications for overdenture therapy.**

- Patients who face the loss of remaining natural adult dentition.
- Complete denture opposed by retained mandibular anterior teeth.
- Attachments are particularly indicated when retention is difficult to obtain such as xerostomia or sialorrhea, absence of residul ridge in edentulous areas, loss of maxilla or partial loss of a mandible, congenital deformity, especially the cleft palate.

**9. Contraindications for using periodontally involved teeth as support for overdenture.**

- Class III mobility
- Soft tissue and osseous defects that are not correctable by surgery
- Poor oral hygiene maintenance by the patient
- Lack of attached gingival
- Excessive reduction of adjacent residual alveolar ridge.

**10. Contraindications for using endodontically treated teeth as support for overdenture.**

- Vertical fracture of the root or roots
- Mechanical preparation of the root
- Internal resorption that has perforated through the side of the root
- Broken instrument in the root canal
- Horizontal fracture of the root below the bony crest.

**11. Advantages of treating the abutment teeth endodontically**

- Crown-root ratio can be made more favorable
- Reduction of clinical crown provides more interocclusal distance.

**12. Which is the most favorable location and number of abutments?**

Two teeth in each quadrant, i.e. canine or first premolar and a second molar, is the ideal situation. This provides for distribution of stress over a rectangular area. The tripod is the next most favorable form for support and stability.

**13. Application of overdenture therapy in other areas**

- Congenital and acquired defects such as cleft palate, microdontia, amelogenesis imperfecta, dentinogenesis imperfecta, partial anodontia and traumatic loss of many teeth.
- Partial overdenture.
- Use of overlaid teeth in immediate and interim dentures.
- Implants.

**14. Various techniques for preparation of teeth to serve as abutments for overdenture.**

- Simple tooth modification and reduction
- Tooth reduction and cast coping
- Endodontic therapy and amalgam plug
- Endodontic therapy and cast coping
- Endodontic therapy with cast coping utilizing some form of attachments.

**15. What are the two types of stud attachments?**
- Extraradicular in which the male element projects from the root surface of the preparation or implant.
- Intraradicular in which the male element forms part of the denture base and engages a specially produced depression within the root contour of the implant.

**16. Name a few stud attachments.**
Gerber units, Dalbo series, Ceka, Zest anchor system, Rothermann, Introfix, Schubiger, Quinlavan, etc.

**17. Two types of bar attachments**
- Bar units (rigid fixation)—tooth borne
- Bar joints (permit rotational movement)—utilizes more of residual ridge for support.
- Single sleeve, e.g. Dolder bar
- Multiple sleeve, e.g. Ackermann system, CM clips, Hader bar.

## CHAPTER – 23 SINGLE COMPLETE DENTURE

**1. Define single complete denture.**
A single complete denture is a complete denture that occludes against some or all of the natural teeth, a fixed restoration, or a previously constructed removable partial denture or a complete denture.

**2. Rehabilitation of a patient with single complete denture is difficult, why?**
- Supraerupted, tipped or malposed teeth in lower arch making it difficult to achieve a harmonious balance occlusion
- The fixed positions of the mandibular anterior teeth make the phonetic and esthetic placement of maxillary anterior teeth difficult
- Abrasion of artificial teeth if made of acrylic resin and abrasion of natural teeth if opposed by porcelain teeth
- Decreased ability of the complete denture to resist a static load when compared to natural teeth (198 lb for natural teeth, whereas it is only 26 lb for a denture). Hence when the natural teeth occlude with them the denture is the loser
- Occlusal form of the natural teeth will dictate the occlusal form of the denture.

**3. What are the various techniques used to determine the necessary tooth modifications?**
- Swenson technique (1964)
- Yurkstas technique (1968)
- Bruce technique (1971)
- Boucher et al technique (1975).

**4. Which technique makes use of a preformed "U" shaped convex occlusal template to identify cuspal inclines?**
Yurkstas technique.

**5. Which is the commonly found occlusal disharmony?**
Completely edentulous maxilla opposed by mandibular partially edentulous situation with missing first molars or second premolars. The remaining molars will be severely

inclined mesially with their distal halves supraerupted. If maxillary molars are set in maximum intercuspation with these molars, the result would be horizontal movement of the denture base on closure.

6. **What are the adverse treatment outcomes with single complete maxillary denture?**
   - Natural tooth wear
   - Denture fracture due to heavy anterior occlusal contact
   - Deep labial frenum notches
   - High occlusal forces due to strong mandibular elevator musculature.
7. **Why endosseous implants are preferred over single complete dentures in mandible?**
   - Limited quality of mucosa
   - Amount of denture border adjacent to movable mucosa
   - Impact of occlusal forces from the moving mandible contacting the static dentate maxillary arch.
8. **In which situattlions a lower complete denture opposing upper natural teeth is indicated?**
   - Patients with class III jaw relationship where the mandible is larger
   - Cleft palate patient
9. **What are the methods to achieve a harmonious balanced occlusion?**

   **Dynamic method**—Functionally generated chew-in techniques
   - Stansbury (1928) using compound maxillary rim and carding wax as recording medium.
   - Vig (1964) using a fin of resin placed into the central grooves of lower posterior teeth to maintain vertical dimension.
   - Sharry (1968) using a maxillary rim of softened wax.
   - Rudd (1973) using compound maxillary rim and a recording medium made of a combination of medium hard pink baseplate wax and red contour wax.

   **Static technique**—Articulator equilibration technique.
10. **Which is the most accurately used method to achieve a harmonious balanced occlusion?**

    Functionally generated chew-in technique.
11. **Which is the commonly used method to achieve a harmonious balanced occlusion?**

    Articulator equilibration method because it can be used in cases of poor denture base stability and patients with poor neuromuscular control.
12. **Occlusal materials used for single complete dentures.**
    - Porcelain
    - Acrylic
    - Gold occlusals
    - Acrylic resin with amalgam stops
    - IPN resin.
13. **Another term for combination syndrome.**
    - Anterior hyperfunction syndrome.
14. **Who coined the term combination syndrome?**

    Ellsworth Kelly (1972).

**15. What are the signs and symptoms of combination syndrome?**

- According to Kelly
  - › Loss of bone from the anterior part of maxillary ridge.
  - › Overgrowth of the tuberosities.
  - › Papillary hyperplasia in the hard palate.
  - › Extrusion of lower anterior teeth.
  - › The loss of bone under partial denture bases.
- According to Saunders et al the six additional signs include:
  - › Loss of vertical dimension of occlusion
  - › Occlusal plane discrepancy
  - › Anterior spatial repositioning of mandible
  - › Poor adaptation of the prosthesis
  - › Epulis fissuratum
  - › Periodontal changes.

**16. How can combination syndrome be prevented?**

- Avoid combination of complete maxillary dentures opposing Class I mandibular RPD.
- Retain weak posterior teeth as abutments by means of endodontic and periodontic techniques.
- An overdenture on the lower teeth.
- Mandibular implant supported fixed prosthesis (Wennerberg et al, 2001) opposing maxillary complete dentures.
- Develop an occlusal scheme that minimizes pressure on the maxillary anterior region.
- The mandibular RPD should have maximum coverage and provide positive occlusal support from remaining natural teeth.
- Posterior teeth should be in balanced occlusion.
- Anterior teeth should be used for phonetic and cosmetic purposes only (Saunders et al, 1979).

## CHAPTER – 24 MAXILLOFACIAL PROSTHETICS

**1. Classification of maxillofacial patients based on the etiology of their defects.**

- Acquired defects – Due to cancer surgery or severe trauma.
- Congenital defects – Cleft lip and palate
- Developmental defects.

**2. Stages of grief process in a maxillofacial patient.**

- Shock and denial
- Guilt, anger and a search to find ways to discharge the emotional pain
- Adjustment, acceptance and growth.

**3. Healing period required after tooth extraction before initiation of radiation treatment.**

- 10 days to 3 weeks.

4. **Oral manifestations of radiation treatment.**
   - Mucositis
   - Loss of taste
   - Xerostomia and dental caries
   - Trismus and fibrosis.
5. **Name two sialogogues.**
   - Pilocarpine
   - Antholetrithione.
6. **Waiting period for denture construction following irradiation.**
   6 months to one year.
7. **The type of tooth preferred in complete denture for an irradiated patient.**
   Plastic monoplane teeth.
8. **Advantages of providing a skin graft in the cheek flap for a maxillectomy patient.**
   - Forms a sound prosthetic bearing surface that will not abrade easily and does not secrete mucus
   - Allows for vigorous cleaning of the defect
   - Aid in retention by forming a scar band.
9. **Methods for retention of maxillofacial prosthesis.**
   Intraoral
   - Anatomic retention
   - Mechanical retention
     › Temporary mechanical Retention
     › Stainless steel wrought wire of 18-gauge size
     › Preformed stainless steel bands or crowns
     › Extra soldered lugs or bands
     › Permanent mechanical retention
     › Cast clasps
     › Prefabricated precision attachments
     › Semiprecision attachments
     › Snap-on attachment
     › Overlay (Telescoping) crown and Thimble crown
     › Magnets
     › Gate type or swing lock device
     › Intermaxillary "George Washington" springs
     › Auxiliary retentive devices, e.g. buccolingual continuous clasps, valve seal, Fourchard wing device
     › Screws
     › Implants
     › Suction cups
     › Adhesives
     › Occlusion
   - Extraoral
     › Anatomic retention
     › Mechanical retention

- Eyeglasses
- Magnets
- Snap buttons and straps
  - › Adhesive retention
  - › Combination of anatomic, mechanical and adhesive retention.

**10. Classify cleft lip and palatal defect.**

Veau's classification

- Class I – Involves only soft palate
- Class II - Involves soft and hard palate but not alveolus
- Class III - Complete unilateral clefts involving soft and hard palate, lip, alveolar ridge.
- Class IV - Complete bilateral clefts involving soft and hard palate, lip and alveolar ridge.

**11. Functions of an obturator.**

- Aids in feeding purposes
- Keeps the wound or defective area clean
- Enhances the healing of post-surgical defect.
- Helps to reshape and reconstruct the palatal contour and/or soft palate
- Improves speech
- Can be used to correct lip and cheek position
- Improves deglutition and mastication
- Can be used as a stent to hold post-surgical dressing.

**12. Define an obturator.**

A maxillofacial prosthesis used to close a congenital or acquired tissue opening, primarily of the hard palate and/or contiguous alveolar/soft tissue structures (GPT7).

**13. Aramany's classification for partially edentulous maxillectomy dental arches.**

- Class I – Midline resection
- Class II – Unilateral resection
- Class III – Central resection
- Class IV – Bilateral anteroposterior resection
- Class V – Posterior resection
- Class VI – Anterior resection.

**14. Classify obturators for acquired defects or based on intervention time.**

- Surgical (immediate temporary obturator)
- Interim (treatment or transitional obturator)
- Definitive.

**15. Types of obturators for congenital defects of the palate.**

- A simple base plate type to correct an opening of the palate
- An obturator with a tail consisting of a speech appliance
- An overlay or superimposed denture.

**16. A definitive obturator prosthesis may be placed how long after the surgical phase?**

- After 6-12 months.

**17. Trouble shooting with an obturator prosthesis.**

- Leakage into the nose
- Hypernasal speech.

## 18. Name a few splints and stents used in maxillofacial rehabilitation.

| **Splints** | |
|---|---|
| Gunning splint | To hold together the fractured segments of mandibular or maxillary bones of an edentulous patient and to immobilise the jaws in occlusion |
| Modified gunning splint | Existing denture can be modified by removing the incisors and used as a splint |
| Labiolingual splint | For reduction of fractures in dentulous or partially edentulous arches. Divided into labial and lingual sections |
| Fenestrated splint | One-piece prosthetic device contoured to fit a dentulous maxilla and mandible through fenestrations created for the occlusal surfaces of the teeth |
| Kingsley splint | Used for raising a fractured maxilla in dentulous or edentulous patients. It is immobilized by means of an extraoral plaster headgear |
| Cast metal splints | Used to immobilize displaced fragments, used in mandibular resection cases, for periodontal stabilization. Indicated for long-term immobilization |
| **Stents** | |
| Anti-hemorrhagic stent | For control of post-extraction bleeding, as in hemophiliac patients |
| Occlusal stent | In temporomandibular dysfunction cases to temporarily disengage the occlusion. |
| Dynamic bite opener (Trismus stent, TMJ exerciser) | It is a modified Kingsley's splint with a combination of maxillary and mandibular occlusal stents with rod bows coming out from the commissures of the mouth to exercise the temporomandibular joint or to open and close the mouth |
| Drainage stent | Purpose is to allow the escape of blood or other fluids with the aid of a polyethylene tube inserted into the stent |
| Pedodontic stents | To prevent the healing of uncovered tissue and to facilitate the eruption of the impacted teeth |
| Labial periodontal stent | Used as a false gingival after extensive periodontal surgery |
| Mouth protector | Recommended in – contact sports, bruxism, for general anesthesia when anterior fixed bridge works or crowns are present, mouth breather, periodontal dressing |
| Radiation stents | To position diseased tissues in a repeatable position, shielding the undiseased tissue, to carry radioactive material or dosimetric devices to a site, recontour certain sites so that therapy can be simplified. |

## 19. Classify soft palate defects

- Based on etiology
  - Congenital, acquired, developmental
- Based on anatomy and physiology of involved structures
  - Palatopharyngeal insufficiency
  - Palatopharyngeal incompetence
  - Palatopharyngeal inadequacy.

**20. Types of soft palate prosthesis.**

- Pharyngeal obturator prosthesis (replaces missing portions of soft palate)
- Meatus obturator (projects vertically at the posterior aspect of the prosthesis to obturate the posterior nasal choanae)
- Palatal lift prosthesis (for patients with speech disorders due to palatopharyngeal incompetence).

**21. What is a palatal augmentation prosthesis?**

Indicated in cases of tongue mobility limitations, where the contour of the palate can be augmented by a prosthesis to modify the Donder's space to allow food manipulation to be more easily transferred posteriorly into the oropharynx.

**22. Classification of mandibular resection defects by Cantor and Curtis (1974).**

- Type I resection – The inferior border is intact.
- Type II resection – Mandible resected in the region of second premolar and first molar.
- Type III resection – Produces a defect to the midline or farther toward the intact side, leaving half or less of the mandible remaining.
- Type IV resection – Resection of almost half of mandible and the tempormandibular joint of that side.
- Type V resection – Anterior or posterior denture bearing area of the mandible has been surgically reconstructed.

**23. What is the function of mandibular guide flange prosthesis?**

It is used as an interim training device in mandibular discontinuity defect. It is used in dentulous patients with nonreconstructed lateral discontinuity defects with severe deviation of mandible towards the surgical side and are unable to achieve unassisted intercuspation on the non-surgical side.

**24. Classify maxillofacial materials.**

M.F. prosthetic devices were divided into 3 categories by National Institute of Health (1970).

- Extrinsic cosmetic
- Insertive removable
- Permanent implants.

**25. What are the various types of MFP materials?**

- Acrylic resin
- Acrylic copolymers
- Polyvinyl chloride
- Chlorinated polyethylene
- Polyurethane elastomers
- Isophorone elastomers
- Silicone elastomers - Heat temp vulcanizing (HTV)<br>- Room temp vulcanizing (RTV)
- Visible light-Cured resins
- Ceramics
- Newer materials - Silicone block copolymers<br>- Polyphosphazenes

**26. Classify silicone elastomers.**

According to their applications, silicones are classified into 4 groups:

- Implant Grade (requires the material to undergo extensive testing and must meet or exceed FDA requirements)
- Medical Grade (for external use only, most commonly used for fabrication of MFP)
- Clean Grade
- Industrial Grade (used for industrial applications).

**27. Name a few RTV silicone elastomers.**

- Silastic 382,399
- MDX 4-4210
- Silastic 891 (Silastic Medical Adhesive Silicone Type A)
- Cosmesil.

**28. Name a few HTV silicones**

- Silastic 370, 372, 373, 4-4514, 4-4515
- Q7-4635, Q7-4735, SE-4524U

**29. Classify adhesives.**

Adhesives are classified by the method in which they are dispensed:

- Pastes
- Liquid emulsions
- Spray-on
- Double-sided tapes.

# SYNOPSIS

1. Functions of a complete denture are to restore mastication, phonetics and esthetics.
2. Primary stress-bearing area in the maxilla is the horizontal slopes of the maxilla.
3. Primary stress-bearing area in the mandible is the buccal shelf.
4. The mean denture bearing area in the edentulous maxilla is 22.96 sq cm and mandible is 12.25 sq cm.
5. Residual ridge resorption is the continuous loss of bone after tooth extraction and even after placement of complete denture.
6. The rugae is the secondary stress bearing area in the maxilla.
7. Slopes of the residual ridges are the secondary stress bearing area in the mandible.
8. Mid-palatine raphe and incisive papilla are the relief areas in the maxilla.
9. The greater palatine foramen is positioned in such a way that it does not need a relief.
10. Mid-palatine raphe needs relief as there is very minimal thickness of mucosa coverage.
11. Incisive papilla covers the incisive foramen.
12. Nasopalatine nerves and vessels are transmitted through the incisive foramen.
13. Crest of the residual ridge is the relief area in the mandible.
14. A torus needs to be relieved if present in either of the denture-bearing areas.
15. The retromolar pad area resists resorption as it has insertion of temporalis, buccinator and fibers of superior pharyngeal constrictor.
16. The sublingual cresent area is also called the premylohyoid region.
17. Posterior palatal seal (PPS) is the seal achieved in the posterior aspect of the maxillary denture, which prevents air and fluid entry.
18. The posterior palatal seal area lies between the anterior and posterior vibrating lines.
19. Over extended PPS can lead to gagging and loss of denture retention.
20. The massetric notch is seen in the buccal flange of the mandibular denture.
21. Maxillary torus is seen commonly in the midpalatal area.
22. Objectives of impression making are preservation of the residual ridge, retention, esthetics, stability, and support. [PRESS]
23. Different theories of impression making are mucostatic, mucocompressive, and selective pressure.
24. Mucostatic impression technique is proposed by Harry L Page.
25. Mucostatic or minimal pressure technique was first proposed by Richardson and later popularized by Henry Page in 1946.
26. Mucocompressive or definite pressure theory was put forward by Greene brothers.
27. Selective pressure technique was put forward by Boucher.
28. Contents of the retromolar pad are loose connective tissue, glandular tissue, fibers of temporalis tendon, buccinator, superior constrictor and pterygomandibular raphe.
29. The temperature of water used for manipulating impression compound is 60 to 70° C.
30. A mucocompressive impression can cause ischemia of the tissues leading to excessive basal bone resorption.
31. Mucocompressive technique exerts excessive pressure continuously over the denture bearing area leading to increased bone resorption and loose denture.

32. Materials used for mucostatic technique are impression plaster and thin mix of alginate.
33. Lack of peripheral seal in mucostatic technique can lead to poor retention.
34. The mucostatic impression technique utilizes adhesion, cohesion, and interfacial surface tension for retention.
35. A mucostatic impression is indicated when there is loss of resiliency of the mucosa, e.g. Submucus fibrosis.
36. Ortho-ethoxybenzoic acid is used to replace eugenol in eugenol free impression pastes.
37. The spacer thickness needed for zinc oxide eugenol impression paste is 0.5 mm.
38. Elastomeric impression materials require a spacer thickness of 0.5 to 1.5 mm depending on viscosity of the impression material.
39. A full spacer is used for minimal pressure technique in diabetic patients and submucus fibrosis patients.
40. An I shaped spacer is indicated in shallow vault.
41. A dumbbell shaped spacer is indicated in deep palatal vault.
42. In anterior flabby tissue ridges a T spacer is the choice.
43. Tissue stops in the impression trays are used to obtain uniform thickness of the impression material and for correct positioning (reorienting) of the trays after the removal of spacers.
44. During impression procedure the patient should be seated up right with the occiput resting firmly on the headrest.
45. Under extended stock trays can be corrected by using impression compound or modeling wax.
46. The temperature of the water bath for softening impression compound is 55° to 70°C.
47. Border molding is done by incremental method using green stick or one step method with rubber base material.
48. Tempering is the procedure of immersing in warm water before insertion of impression compound or low fusing green stick compound.
49. Try adhesives has to be applied over the acrylic tray before doing border molding and secondary impression using rubber base impression materials.
50. Alpha butyl styrene is used as tray adhesive for rubber base impression material.
51. Tray exposures seen on the fitting surface of the impression after making the secondary impression shows the impression is made with too much pressure and these areas can become pressure spots in the denture.
52. The shapes of the occlusal rims can be square, tapering or ovoid.
53. The maxillary denture is primarily retained by the negative atmospheric pressure complemented by the intact peripheral seal.
54. Posterior palatal seal compensates for the volumetric shrinkage of the denture during curing.
55. Boundaries of PPS are anterior vibrating line, Posterior vibrating line, and pterygomaxillary notch.

56. The anterior vibrating line is cupids bow shaped due to the presence of the posterior nasal spine.
57. Anterior vibrating line is always located on the soft palate.
58. Posterior vibrating line marks the most distal extension of the denture base.
59. Jaw relation recording is considered as the most important step in complete denture fabrication.
60. Orientation jaw relation orients the mandible to the cranium.
61. A face bow records the axis of rotation of the mandible and transfers this axis to the articulator.
62. The axis around which the mandible rotates is known as the transverse axis or hinge axis.
63. The face bows can supports the maxillary cast during mounting in the articulator.
64. Face bows are of two types : arbitrary and kinematic.
65. Arbitrary face bows can be either fascia type or earpiece type.
66. During face bow transfer three reference points are considered in the skull. Two points are located posterior to the maxilla and one located anteriorly.
67. Plane of orientation is the spatial plane obtained by joining the anterior and posterior reference points.
68. The posterior reference points represent the terminal hinge axis position.
69. An arbitrary face bow is used for the fabrication of complete denture.
70. An arbitrary face bow is attached to the maxillary occlusal rim whereas the kinematic face bow is attached to the mandibular occlusal rim or clutches.
71. When the external auditory meatus is used as the posterior reference point, it is considered to be positioned with in 5 mm of the true center of the opening axis of the jaws.
72. Kinematic face bow locates the true terminal hinge axis.
73. Kinematic face bows are generally indicated for FPDs and full mouth rehabilitation.
74. Fascia type face bows have condylar rods instead of earpiece.
75. Intercondylar scale is a part of whip-mix quick mount face bow.
76. Face bow transfer avoids errors in occlusion of finished prosthesis.
77. Freeway space = vertical dimension at rest – vertical dimension at occlusion.
78. A freeway space of 2 to 4 mm at the premolar region is recommended in complete denture.
79. Silverman's closest speaking method is a technique to verify the freeway space.
80. Philp Paff was the first person to describe the technique of recording jaw relation.
81. Centric relation is the most posterior relation of the maxilla to the mandible at the established VD.
82. Centric relation is a reliable, repeatable, and recordable position (3R).
83. In CD patients the proprioceptive impulses from the TMJ guide the mandible to centric relation.
84. The centric relation and centric occlusion in CD patients should coincide.
85. Any relationship of the mandible to maxilla other than the centric relation is eccentric jaw relation.

86. Eccentric jaw relation records are used to programme adjustable articulators, i.e. to adjust the lateral and horizontal condylar inclinations in the articulator.
87. As the mandible protrudes the condyles moves downward and forward to create a triangular space between the posterior teeth called as the Christensen phenomenon.
88. As the mandible moves to one side, the condyle on the opposite side moves downward, forward and inward. This movement of the balancing side condyle is known as Bennett movement.
89. In Hanau articulators lateral condylar angles are set by the formula L=H/8+12.
90. In Hanaus formula H is horizontal condylar angle.
91. The posterior reference points are marked 13 mm anterior to the tragus on the tragus-canthus line.
92. Earpiece face bows are positioned directly in the external auditory meatus.
93. The graphic methods of recording centric relation are arrow point tracing (gothic arch tracing) and pantographic tracing.
94. In intraoral tracing, the central bearing plate is attached to maxillary rim and central bearing point or stylus is attached to mandibular rim.
95. In intraoral tracing the arrow points posteriorly.
96. It is difficult to see the intraoral tracing hence guiding the patient is difficult.
97. In extraoral tracing the central bearing plate is attached to the lower occlusal rim and the central bearing pin is attached to the upper occlusal rim.
98. Pantographic tracing records the mandibular movements in three planes.
99. Pantographic tracing is the most accurate method of recording centric jaw relation.
100. A fully adjustable articulator is needed to accept pantographic tracing.
101. Typal form theory for the shape of the teeth is proposed by Leon Williams.
102. Anatomic teeth are having a cuspal inclination of 33° or 30°.
103. Pilkington-Turner teeth are having a cuspal inclination of 30°.
104. Semianatomic teeth have a cuspal inclination of 10 or 20°.
105. Balanced occlusion is obtained easily with semi-anatomic teeth.
106. Non-anatomic teeth are 0° teeth also called as monoplane teeth.
107. Non-anatomic teeth are indicated in patients with flat and severely resorbed ridges, poor neuromuscular control and bruxism.
108. Anthropometric measurements are used to determine the mesiodistal width of the anterior teeth.
109. Buccal corridor is the space present between the buccal teeth and buccal mucosa.
110. The natural teeth occupy a zone of equilibrium between the buccal musculature and lingual musculature. This zone is known as neutral zone.
111. Artificial teeth are arranged in the neutral zone for better stability.
112. Squint test is used to select the shade of the tooth. It is used to compare the colour of the tooth with the color of the face.
113. Frush and Fisher proposed the dentogenic concept for the arrangement of anterior teeth based on the patient's age, sex and personality.

114. Interpenetrating polymer network (IPN) teeth are preferred over conventional acrylic teeth.
115. Different types of occlusal concepts in complete denture are:
    a. Balanced occlusion
    b. Non-balanced occlusion
        i. Spherical concept of occlusion
        ii. Organic concept of occlusion
        iii. Neutrocentric concept of occlusion
    c. Lingualized occlusion.
116. Who introduced the cusp to fossa occlusion --S.H. Payne (1941).
117. Sheppard stated that, "Enter bolus, Exit balance" according to this statement, the balancing contact is absent when food enters the oral cavity
118. Alfred Gysi 1927 introduced the concept of lingualized occlusion.
119. Hardy's concept proposed a flat occlusal plane with non-anatomic teeth.
120. Types of balanced occlusion are unilateral bilateral and protrusive.
121. Balanced occlusion is absent in natural dentition.
122. The factors which affect balanced occlusion are known as Hanau's Quint.
123. Hanau's quint
    a. Condylar guidance
    b. Incisal guidance
    c. Compensating curves
    d. Relative cusp height
    e. Plane of orientation of occlusal plane.
124. The condylar path is only factor which is not under the control of the dentist.
125. Teeth with a high cuspal height are required for patients with steep condylar guidance.
126. The compensating curves compensate Christensens phenomenon during excursive movements of the mandible.
127. Anatomic curves which are present in the natural dentition are:
    a. Curve of Spee
    b. Curve of Monson
    c. Curve of Wilson
128. Anteroposterior curvature is the counterpart of curve of Spee.
129. Lateral curvature is the counterpart of Monson's curve.
130. Arcon articulators have the condylar elements as part of the lower member.
131. The anterior teeth should be arranged with the incisal edge visible by 1 to 2 mm.
132. Central incisor should be positioned 8 to 10 mm anterior to the midpoint of incisive papilla.
133. Bi-labial sounds are b, p and m.
134. Labiodental sounds are f and v.
135. Lingo-alveolar sounds are t, d, n, s and z.
136. Lingo-dental sound is th.

137. Valar sounds are k, g and kg.
138. The more closer the teeth are arranged to the ridge the better the stability.
139. Wax surface around the teeth are called the art portion.
140. The mandibular denture has to be inserted before the maxillary denture.
141. Occlusal harmony of the denture is checked using interocclusal check records and articulating paper.
142. First appointment should be made 24 hours after insertion to correct occlusal disharmony and immediate tissue reaction.
143. Relining is adding new material to the fitting surface of the existing denture.
144. Relining techniques are:
    a. Static
    b. Functional
    c. Chairside
145. Functional reline technique utilizes tissue conditioners as impression material.
146. An immediate denture is one that is fabricated before all the remaining teeth have been extracted and is inserted immediately after the removal of the teeth.
147. An intrim immediate denture is to be used for a short period of time for reasons of esthetics, mastication, etc. until a more definitive prosthetic therapy can be provided.
148. Porosity is a processing error in acrylic denture which may compromise physical, aesthetic, and hygienic properties of the processed denture.
149. The longevity of tissue conditioners is limited due to leaching out of plasticizer and alcohol within 4-8 weeks of time.
150. Tissue conditioners are composed of Polymethyl methacrylate and a mixture of aromatic esters and ethyl alcohol.
151. Selective grinding is the procedure used for the final correction of any occlusal disharmony of the complete denture.
152. If the incisal guide pin rises from the incisal table of the articulator during lateral movements, the buccal cusps of the upper and the lingual cusps of the lower on the working side are to be reduced (BULL grinding).
153. Combination syndrome is the most common problem seen in patients wearing maxillary single complete denture opposing distal extension mandibular partial denture.
154. Over extended borders of the complete denture can lead to epulis fissuratum.

## SUGGESTED READING

1. Rahn O, Heartwell CM. Textbook of Complete Dentures, 5th edn. Pennsylvania, USA: Lea and Febiger; 1993.
2. Morrow RM, Rudd KD, Rhoads JE. Dental Laboratory Procedures Complete Dentures, 2nd edn. St Louis, Toronto, Princeton: Mosby; 1986.
3. Sheldon Winkler. Essentials of Complete Denture Prosthodontics, 2nd edn. Ishiyaku Euro America, Inc: USA; 1996.
4. Zarb GA, Bolender CL. Prosthodontic Treatment for Edentulous Patients: Complete Dentures and Implant-Supported Prostheses, 12th edn. St Louis, MO: Mosby; 2004.

# RECENT ADVANCES IN COMPLETE DENTURE PROSTHODONTICS

## INTRODUCTION

The scientific and technological basis of dentistry are expanding rapidly in the world where alternative changes in the managements and financing of health care have raised the public expectations of better "quality of life". Dentistry has come a long way from just replacing missing teeth to replacing lost alveolus supporting facial structures, recreating esthetics, reestablishing phonetics and many other major developments. Most of all we can say that in prosthetics by using all the artificial materials as well as technologies we can give a natural appearance to an individual at its best. Improvements in material science form just one aspect of complete denture prosthodontics. These are driven by the change in theoretical concepts, perceptions of the dentists and a need to fulfill the above.

Advancements in complete denture prosthodontics can be classified into two broad categories.

1. Advancements in theoretical concepts
2. Advancements in material science.

History of dentistry is strewn with examples of new materials or techniques developed for entirely different purposes triggering a revolution in the way things were done in an entirely different field. Similarly the need for specific purpose in one field has accelerated the field of research in a different field. For example, the need for accurate replication of terminal hinge axis and jaw positions in relation to base of cranium has spurred an interest in biomechanical engineering thereby combining the two entirely different fields of science. Necessity has indeed proved to be the mother of invention.

## RECENT ADVANCEMENTS IN THEORETICAL CONCEPTS

Theoretical concepts form the basis of perfection in several instances, since a concept has to be developed prior to its application in a patient. There have been numerous advancements in theoretical concepts pertaining to different stages in complete denture fabrication. These can be enumerated as follows:

1. Advancements in diagnostic aids
2. Advancements in impression procedures
3. Advancements in jaw relation records
4. Esthetic guides
5. Advancements in fabrication techniques
6. Miscellaneous

### Advancements in Diagnostic Aids

Graphoanalysis method for evaluating complete denture patient psychology is a relatively new concept for predicting the prognosis.[1] It is proved that Graphoanalysis in addition with properly structured interview and questionnaire is useful in evaluation of behavior of an individual especially for recognizing difficult patients.

A new classification of psychology of complete denture patients has been proposed, which provides a theoretical approach, a step-by-step guide to clinicians to better understand the thoughts, aspirations and expectations of complete denture patients and their effects and consequences in different patients, when not met with. This approach attempts to overcome the disadvantages of House classification of patient psychology which over simplifies the behavior of patients into just 4 categories.

Recent advances in computer-aided design/computer-aided manufacturing (CAD/CAM) technology, medical imaging and rapid prototyping have added to the armamentarium of implant dentistry in terms of efficiency, accuracy and predictability. Rapid prototyping and CAD/CAM technology are used to fabricate stereolithographic surgical templates for flapless implant placement.

A photogrammetric technique for analysis of jaws positioning and hidden surfaces attitude analysis is proposed recently. It uses original photogrammetric system for noncontact 3D measurements and surface 3D reconstruction. Two techniques are proposed for jaws 3D models mutual arrangement according to their original position in a mouth. The first one is point-based and it allows in determining jaw displacement concerning a set of reference points. The second technique is surface-based and it uses a scan of teeth occlusion for jaws positioning. Both methods provide adequate accuracy for dentistry. It is of huge diagnostic value in complete dentures.

## Advancements in Impression Procedures

Apart from the basic principles of complete denture impression making which were introduced in the middle of nineteenth century as listed below, many changes happened in the concept of impression.

1. Concepts of atmospheric pressure.
2. Maximum extension of denture bearing area.
3. Equal distribution of pressure.
4. Adaptation of denture bearing tissues.

To this were added the principles of retention, stability, comfort, biocompatibility, accuracy, etc. Some of the new techniques added to the already existing techniques for complete denture impressions in the last 10 years are as follows:

*Management of flabby tissue:* Flabby tissues are common clinical finding which poses no problem of pain and discomfort but adversely affect the support, retention and stability of complete dentures. Several techniques have been proposed as nonsurgical alternatives to such cases focusing on a modified impression technique to record the flabby tissue in its undisplaced form. For example, one technique[1] describes the custom tray to be made in two parts, the first part of which contains a "lattice-work", which strengthens the tray followed by a second tray, which adequately supports the final impression. A standard neutral zone technique was additionally employed for the mandibular ridge as it was severely resorbed. lynch et al[2] describes the use of polyvinyl siloxane material that is used very commonly in dental practice in a judicial manner, instead of using complicated techniques and materials to manage flabby ridges.

Onur et al[7] describes a modified impression procedure and a method of fabricating a 2-piece collapsible denture for a patient with limited oral opening as a result of the resection of a precancerous lesion on the maxillary lip. Fabricating the denture in 2 pieces (a smaller anterior piece and a larger, hinged, collapsible posterior piece) enabled the patient to place and remove the denture.

In 2005, a modified functional impression technique described by Alexander et al used a removable functional acrylic resin handle that was attached to custom impression trays allowing an excellent peripheral sealing zone got by patient conducted muscular and jaw motion.[8]

In 2008, Dr. Joseph Massad described an impression technique which involves the layering method of impression making that maintains the integrity between layers of the impression materials of varying viscosities and controls the path of insertion, thus minimizing the incidence of overextension.[9]

*Digital impression systems:* In the case of digital impressions, the creators of the impression-taking devices have introduced scientific developments in the fields of optics, digitization and CAD/CAM into the art of capturing impressions of prepared teeth and surrounding structures to develop 3D digital and even physical representations from which dental restorations can be made. They include the CAD/CAM products CEREC® (Sirona Dental Systems,www.sirona.com) and E4D Dentist (D4D Technologies, www.d4dtech.com) and the dedicated impressioning products Cadent iTero™ (Cadent, www.cadent.com) and Lava™ Chairside Oral Scanner C.O.S. (3M ESPE, www.3mespe.com).[10]

## Advancements in Jaw Relation Aids

Historically, a number of techniques have been suggested for registering interarch relationships during complete denture therapy. A graphic recording method dating to the turn of the 20th century, but recently updated, involves use of a central bearing device. This device can aid the practitioner in the clinical achievement and registration of both horizontal and vertical jaw relationships and is particularly useful when muscle deprogramming of habitual mandibular closure is indicated.[11] Use of this central bearing device has been shown to be very precise. The concept has recently enjoyed a resurgence of interest due in part to newly developed instrumentation (Massad Jaw Recorder System, Global Dental Impression Trays, Inc., www.gdit.us). Advantages of this new central-bearing device include: ease of attachment to record bases using conventional light-activated laboratory resin and a unique pivoting central bearing pin for adjustment in all dimensions during the recording process.

This new central-bearing device comes complete with all of the elements necessary to assist in the registration of centric relation in various clinical situations, including dentulism, partial edentulism, full edentulism, small-arch diameter, and large-arch diameter.

*Kavo arcus facebow:* A fully functional 3-dimensional computerized pantographic registration system to capture both, static and dynamic occlusal records for articulator programming and diagnostic set-ups. Accuracy and repeatability are unsurpassed with all records permanently archived.

Virtual articulator is another new concept. The virtual articulator can simulate the specific masticatory movement of the patient. During mandibular animation, the program calculates the sites where the opposing teeth come into contact. The studies made to assess the reliability of the virtual articulator show good correspondence in visualization of the number and position of the dynamic contacts. The virtual articulator is a precise tool for the full analysis of occlusion in a real patient.[12]

Complete denture occlusion simulation system (CDOSS) in the field of dental restoration is another new aid that is a useful tool to deal with the functional aspects of occlusal morphology in a diagnostical and therapeutical sense. With the aid of this software, the visualization and diagnosis of mandibular movement can be easily realized.

*Centric relation – a new concept:* A new concept of Centric Relation is defined as "A clinically determined position of the mandible in which both condyles are in their anterior and uppermost position in their glenoid fossae. This definition differs from the old definition in that the centric relation is the relationship of the mandible to maxilla when the condyles are at the most posterior portion of the glenoid fossa. Because some authors believe that in Centric Relation all the load of the mandibular residual ridge are transferred to the joint cavity pushing the head of the condyle against the avascular disc and the cavity wall. Recently it has been found that there is evidence of nerve and blood vessels in this posterior aspect which can get compressed causing pain to the individuals. But such pains are not noted in the patient thereby suspecting the actual position of this condylar head in the joint cavity. So recently authors have suggested their position to be anterior uppermost position of joint cavity.

## Advancements in Esthetic Concepts

Denture esthetics has essentially involved a subjective approach, employing long-standing techniques and principles to help reach a satisfactory esthetic and functional outcome for the patient and dental team. Particularly, this is the case with the clinical arrangement of the teeth in the trial-denture base. There have been no significant advances in recent years as far as concepts are concerned, however such principles have been well-described by few authors.[13]

## Advancements in Fabrication Techniques

### *Use of CAD/CAM System for Fabrication of Complete Dentures*[14]

The development of computer aided system for designing and fabrication of Complete Denture is a relatively recent development. So far the use of CAD/CAM has primarily being focused on fixed restoration such as inlays crown because difficulty in recording soft tissue morphologies of edentulous areas, and interocclusal relationship. Methods of recording and measuring 3D morphology have been greatly improved with recent advancement of optoelectronic measuring unit CAD software.

### *Procedure*

Involves three major steps
1. Impression procedure
2. Denture designing
3. Denture fabrication.

#### Impression procedure

1. As the first step, an impression of the load bearing area of the residual ridge and denture borders was made for the maxillary and mandibular arches using a specially designed double impression trays with Conventional Rubber Base or Silicone Impression Material.
2. Maxillary and mandibular impressions are held at specific vertical height and horizontal relation in patient's mouth.
3. The double impression trays are transferred and mounted on a 3D laser scanner that has a rod around which both the impression can rotate to full 360°. Two-dimensional images are recorded by spread laser beam and Four Charged-Couple device camera while the impression is made to move mearly. Surface images are obtained at three different angles time required - 15 to 20 mins.

#### Denture Design, Arrangement of Artificial Teeth

Denture space data are transferred to an engineering work station. Artificial teeth and denture surface data from the database are overlapped and matched with those of the denture space.

Placement of artificial teeth is done to achieve proper stress distribution.

### Denture Fabrication

Either a numerically controlled milling machine or 3-D laser lithography machine can be used.

Laser lithography create 3D models of new products based on CAD design.

Therefore, only two outer shells (occlusal/polished part and tissue surface part) are photopolymerized.

Tooth shade acrylic resin composites are used to fill inside the occlusal portion and two surface are connected using reference point.

Tissue colored autopolymerizing resin composite is then placed into the space and excess removed, and shells are polished using conventional manner.

**Orofacial prosthesis design and fabrication using stereolithography:**[15] The use of stereolithography for the manufacture of implantable prosthesis is relatively new aspects in dentistry. Until now, its use with the regard to mandibular resection has been to produce preoperative models that allows more sophisticated planning of the contour and better preparation of the metallic framework to be implanted. The framework rejoins the mandible restoring its function. Data extracted from Computed Tomography (CT) scan can be used to produce computer models of three dimensional (3D) anatomical structures. Using stereolithography, a rapid prototyping technique these computer models can be made into solid physical models.

The surface and internal structure of the anatomical site can be reproduced by polymerization of UV light sensitive liquid resin using a laser beam. The laser rays progressively polymerise photomonomer on the surface of the vat solution. The model is built vertically step by step as the polymerized section submerged beneath the surface of the solution. These models are then used for diagnosis and treatment planning of various cases.

## Miscellaneous Concepts

Effect of low energy laser application in the treatment of denture-induced mucosal lesion[16] has recently gained considerable attention. They are primarily used to relieve pain, reduce inflammation and edema and accelerate healing. Studies on the biologic effects of low energy lasers have been concerned with the ability of such light to increase blood circulation within regenerated tissues to increase production of collagen by fibroblast and to promote a suppresive effect on the immune system. Furthermore, increased mitotic activity has been reported, which indicates the growth stimulation occurs.

Recently, the bactericidal effect of light from a low energy laser was introduced as an alternative approach to Antibiotics and Antiseptics in eliminating cariogenic and periodontopathogenic bacteria from lesion. The greatest benefit of using a low energy laser is that its effects can be achieved without damaging host tissues and with protection to the operator. The effect of therapeutic laser treatment on both soft tissues and bone with subsequent improvement of denture foundation after treatment of denture-induced mucosal lesions.

## Recent Advances in Materials

*Vinyl-polyether Hybrids:* The newest class of impression material is the vinyl-polyether hybrids that include SENN. This new class of impression material combines properties from addition silicone and polyether impression materials. SENN is supplied as a 2-paste automixing system and contains a polymer with polyether and siloxane (e.g., addition silicone) groups that will combine elements and benefits of both impression materials. With the polyether groups, a hydrophilic material is provided without the use of a surfactant. With the siloxane groups on the polymer chain, a material that is dimensionally stable and recovers from deformation is combined with polyether properties. The material has a platinum catalyst, and the setting reaction is contaminated when powdered gloves are used to mix the material.

EXA'lence is another new generation of Vinyl PolyEther Silicone (VPES) impression material. EXA'lence is said to combine the advantages of both polyether and vinyl-polysiloxane silicone impression materials, resulting in excellent hydrophilicity, flow, dimensional accuracy, and high tear strength.

Silginat is an addition-curing, elastomeric polyvinyl siloxane (PVS) impression material to be used as an alginate alternative in a variety of anatomic impressions. Silginat boasts many advantages over alginate impression materials for both the practitioner and the patient. It was designed with a low-tear resistance to avoid inadvertently dislodging restorations or orthodontic appliances while providing excellent palatal definition and detail. Silginat has an optimized medium flow viscosity (medium-body viscosity per ISO standards) with heavy body hardness when set. Silginat is also highly thixotropic and flows properly under pressure, giving it an ideal workability. The thixotropic nature of the material also helps prevent patient gagging.

*Artex Rotofix facebow:* This is a new addition in the arsenal for successful prosthodontist. The Artex Facebow comes complete with 3-D universal joint, nosebar/nasion, pair of standard earballs, set of 10 disposable biteforks with thermoplastic bite compound, tray handle, and metal bitefork. Single lever eliminates torque distortion often found in facebows that require screws. The Artex opens symmetrically, which means alignment without sideshift or alteration of the sagittal distance.

A simplified clinometer has been designed with the intention of reducing the cost of the commercially available Hanau clinometer.[17] This clinometer can be fixed to the conventional three point articulator and used by undergraduate dental students to learn teeth arrangement in esthetic manner.

Biofunctional prosthetic system, and Premium Swiss Precision Dentures are the recent additions to the existing systems of denture fabrication. They include utilization of high end dental products like layered teeth, high strength flowable resins, and gnathometers and intraoral tracing devices.

## REFERENCES

1. Murthy VJ, Singh S, Shastri M, Rajaram S. Evaluation of complete denture patients using graphoanalysis: A clinical study. Indian J Dent Res. 2012;23(2):149-51.
2. Sudheer A, Reddy GV, Reddy G. Behavior shaping of complete denture patient: a theoretical approach. J Contemp Dent Pract. 2012;13(2):246-50.
3. Davidowitz, Gary et al. The Use of CAD/CAM in Dentistry Dental Clinics , Volume 55 , Issue 3 , 559-70.
4. Knyaz VA, S Yu Zheltov. "Photogrammetric technique for teeth occlusion analysis in dentistry." International Archives of the Photogrammetry, Remote Sensing and Spatial Information Sciences 36.5 (2006): 5.
5. Kathuria N, Prasad R, Bhide SV. Flabby alveolar ridges: a modified technique to treat this clinical challenge. Eur J Prosthodont Restor Dent. 2011;19(1):21-4.

6. Lynch CD, Allen PF. Management of the flabby ridge: using contemporary materials to solve an old problem. Br Dent J. 2006; 200(5):258-61.
7. Onur Geckili Altug Cilingir,Tayfun Bilgin Impression procedures and construction of a sectional denture for a patient with microstomia: A clinical report. J Prosth Dent. 2006; 96(6):387-90.
8. Alexandre M, et al. Modified functional impression technique for complete dentures. Braz Dent J.2005;16(2):135-39.
9. Massad JJ. Complete denture prosthodontics: modern approaches to old concerns. Inside Dent. 2008;4(8):2–6.
10. Birnbaum NS, Aaronson HB, Stevens C, Cohen B. 3D digital scanners: a high-tech approach to more accurate dental impressions. Inside Dentistry. 2009;5(4):70-7.
11. Massad JJ, Connelly ME, Rudd KD, Cagna DR. Occlusal device for diagnostic evaluation of maxillomandibular relationships in edentulous patients: a clinical technique. J Prosthet Dent.2004;91(6):586-90.
12. Bisler A, Bockholt U, Kordass B, Suchan M, Voss G. The virtual articulator. Int J Cont Dent. 2002; 5:101-6.
13. Leopardi A. Complete dentures: achieving superior anterior esthetics and post-delivery maintenance .Inside Dentistry. 2009;6(7):70-80.
14. Kanazawa M, Inokoshi M, Minakuchi S, Ohbayashi N. Trial of a CAD/CAM system for fabricating complete dentures. Dent Mater J. 2011; 30(1):93-6.
15. Morris CL, Barber RF, Day R. Orofacial prosthesis design and fabrication using stereolithography. Aust Dent J. 2000 Dec; 45(4):250-3.
16. Marei MK, Abdel-Meguid SH, Mokhtar SA, Rizk SA. Effect of low-energy laser application in the treatment of denture-induced mucosal lesions. J Prosthet Dent. 1997 Mar;77(3):256-64.
17. Rao NV, Sudheer A, Rao CS, Reddy KS. A starter's guide to preclinical teeth arrangement: simplified clinometer. J Contemp Dent Pract. 2012 Mar 1;13(2):236-9.

# PAPER IV QUESTIONS ASKED IN RECENT ADVANCES IN PROSTHODONTICS (1999-2014)

1. Advances in laboratory technologies for producing a prosthesis.
2. Maxillofacial prosthesis.
3. Osseointegration.
4. Nano-dentistry in prosthodontics.
5. CAD – CAM.
6. Implant supported prosthesis.
7. Lasers in prosthodontics.
8. Advances in maxillofacial materials and techniques.
9. "Titanium – A mystery material" – Explain the statement.
10. Luting – cements in prosthodontics.
11. Recent techniques in resin-bonded fixed partial dentures.
12. Immediate functional and non-functional loading of implants.
13. Role of mini-implants in extraoral prosthesis.
14. Adjustable articulators.
15. Recent developments in dental ceramic.
16. Smile design.
17. Recent advances in facial esthetics.
18. Preventive prosthodontics and its future scope.
19. Discuss the relationship of surface topography of implant and osseointegration.
20. Adhesive bridges.
21. Dental implant biomaterials.
22. Newer dental base materials and its applications.
23. Recent advances in removable partial dentures designing.
24. Maxillofacial and cranio facial defects management
25. Esthetic rehabilitation in implant prosthodontics
26. Discuss the concept of full mouth rehabilitation.
27. CAD-CAM technology in maxillofacial prosthesis.
28. Management of mandibular single complete denture patients.
29. Discuss in detail about the fundamentals and concepts of occlusion.
30. Management of temporomandibular joints dysfunction and their prognosis.
31. Discuss the role of implants in extraoral and intraoral prosthesis.
32. Precision attachments in RPD.
33. Retention in MFP.
34. Geriatrics in Prosthodontics.
35. Implant failures.
36. Comprehensive Denture service.

# Index

Page numbers followed by *f* refer to figure.

## A



## B

## N



## O